# BREAST CANCER ANSWERS

Practical Tips and
Personal Advice
From a Survivor

## *Judy King*

NEW PAGE BOOKS
A division of The Career Press, Inc.
Franklin Lakes, NJ

BREAST CANCER ANSWERS
EDITED BY JODI BRANDON
TYPESET BY EILEEN DOW MUNSON
INTERIOR ILLUSTRATIONS BY FIONA PRESTON
Cover design by Dorothy Wachtenheim
Printed in the U.S.A. by Book-mart Press

To order this title, please call toll-free 1-800-CAREER-1 (NJ and Canada: 201-848-0310) to order using VISA or MasterCard, or for further information on books from Career Press.

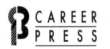 

The Career Press, Inc., 3 Tice Road, PO Box 687,
Franklin Lakes, NJ 07417
**www.careerpress.com**
**www.newpagebooks.com**

## Library of Congress Cataloging-in-Publication Data

King, Judith, 1945-
    Breast cancer answers : practical tips and personal advice from a survivor / by Judy King.
        p. cm.
    Includes bibliographical references and index.
    ISBN 1-56414-757-6 (pbk.)
        1. Breast—Cancer—Popular works. 2. Breast—Cancer—Miscellanea.  I. Title.

RC280.B8K53 2004
616.99′449—dc22
                                                                    2004048625

## Disclaimer

This book is not intended to replace medical advice or to be a substitute for a physician's recommendations. Always seek the advice of a physician before beginning any diet and/or exercise program or other treatment. Although prudent care has been taken for accuracy in the text, medical and complementary topics are constantly changing as new research is presented, so you are encouraged to check for the latest information available on the subject matter and consult a trained professional before making any decisions based on the material in this book. The author and publisher expressly disclaim responsibility for any adverse effects arising from following the suggestions in this book without appropriate medical supervision.

This book is dedicated to
Bonnie Burchard,
my head cheerleader who finished her own cancer journey
much too early,
and
the Rosebuds and Rosebuds II,
the ladies in my support group who give so generously of
their information, laughter, encouragement, and hope.

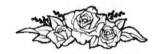

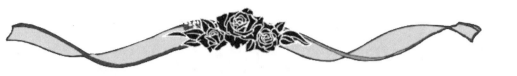

# Acknowledgments

I am grateful to every "cancer cousin" who shared her experience so that other women can benefit from her difficulties. In particular I thank these Rosebuds, ladies from my support group, who reviewed the manuscript and added gems from their experience and research: Suzanne Altenburg, Rosemary Barr, Florence Berger, Kathy Burrows, Annette Carr, Nancy Hannan, Pat Hanneman, Nancy Maranto, Leslie Munoz, Kelly Jo Myers-Madoian, and Linda Yarger.

Many thanks to my wonderful husband, Fred, who encouraged me to spend my limited energy in this pursuit, helped with research, took over even more household duties to free up my time, and generally cheered me on.

Also I profusely thank the following experts for reviewing the material in their fields (they are not responsible for the content because they did not see the final version, but their input was invaluable):

George Aaron, MHS, PT, OCS, MTC; Laura Baynham-Fletcher, MA, LPC, director, Place of Wellness, University of Texas M. D. Anderson Cancer Center; Sheila Kinberg Fisher, BS, University of California, San Diego; Sharona Hoffman, JD, LLM., associate professor of law at Case Western Reserve University School of Law; Mary K. Hughes, MS, RN, CNS, Clinical Nurse Specialist, Psychiatry Section, Neuro-Oncology Department, University of Texas M. D. Anderson Cancer Center; Dixie Melillo, MD, breast surgeon; Miguel Miro-Quesada, MD, oncologist; Cherie A. Perez, BS, RN, CCRP, RMT, Research Nurse Supervisor, Genitourinary Medical Oncology, University of Texas M.D. Anderson Cancer Center; Dena Reagan, RD, Clinical Dietician, University of Texas M.D. Anderson Cancer Center; Marilyn Robinson, Headwear Etc.; Nancy C. Russell, MPH (doctoral candidate), Integrative Medicine Program, Education, University of Texas M. D. Anderson Cancer Center; Andy Vorster, ND, CNC, Natural Health Associates; Maggie Williams, PT, CLT-LANA, MLD & PT Services LLC; and Garrett Wilson, City Wide Exterminating, Houston, TX.

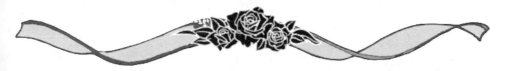

# Contents

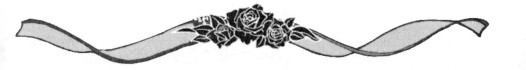

# *Introduction*

Terror. Fatigue. Nausea. Sadness. Anger. Limitations. Breast cancer brings a whirlwind of physical as well as emotional changes. A breast cancer survivor, I have been through chemotherapy, surgery, radiation, and metastasis, so I know what you are dealing with. Not only are breast cancer patients faced with dizzying choices about treatment, but then we are sent home to cope with uncertain futures and confusing day-to-day living, with little guidance from our physicians.

Although I much prefer that my oncologist be up to date on the latest treatment protocols than on how to choose a wig, I did cherish the friend who helped me select stylish headwear and gave her approval to my new shape after surgery. And daily I was thankful for the friend who told me I could qualify for a handicapped parking permit during chemo and the one who alerted me that depression was common after treatment was finished.

Yes, cancer alters our physical appearance, constitution, and capabilities, but it does not change who we are—it develops in us new dimensions, for sure, but we still face the same kind of daily issues as before diagnosis. I had the same pride in my appearance as before (although some days during chemotherapy no one would have known!). I ached in spots I never had before and wanted the pain to quit. I couldn't reach familiar places and angles and wanted to know how to regain that mobility so I could reach the dishes in the upper cabinets and hold the curling iron behind my head. I was SO TIRED and hated to complain and was frustrated that I couldn't perform all of my former duties (or pleasures).

You know the story. You try to be brave even as you hate some of the changes cancer forces upon you. You don't want to bother your busy physician with "little" things like how to get the radiation dye out of your favorite silk blouse or when you can comfortably wear a prosthesis and display a nicely curved profile.

You are not being silly to desire such answers. These concerns impact how we live our lives each day and how we feel about ourselves. Because stress affects us physically, it is unhealthy to stew about such things when solutions are available.

*Breast Cancer Answers* compiles the wisdom and solutions of hundreds of breast cancer survivors to help you get through each day—whether you are still in treatment or "free-floating" afterwards. The myriad treatment options is beyond the scope of this book. The many factors involved in choosing a medical course need to be considered by you and your team of doctors in planning how you will counter the cancer. Any treatment has potential side effects. This book is intended to help you cope with side effects you might experience as well as be prepared for the emotional and physical changes that are an inevitable part of breast cancer.

These practical tips have buoyed the spirits of thousands of women and made their lives easier and happier. I sincerely hope you will find in these pages ideas to repair your self-image, boost your energy, and fortify your optimism, knowing that many of the difficulties you are experiencing will eventually disappear and that those that linger can often be compensated for in acceptable ways. If these tips solve one challenge or answer one nagging question for you, then my mission has been accomplished.

I have presented information in a concise and easy-to-locate format so you can find what you need quickly and go on about your day. Together we can offset the impact of this disease—one day at a time.

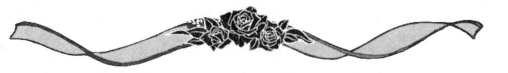

*Chapter 1*

# General Questions about Breast Cancer

You may want to jump right to the topic in this book that will improve the next hour of your day. At some point, however, you may be curious about some general cancer questions that are answered briefly here. (Refer to Resources on page 353 for places to research these topics further.)

## What Causes Cancer?

Unfortunately, the answer is still the subject of serious research at many leading institutions. There is not one single answer. Cancer has been described in medical literature since about 2500 B.C. Cancer cells are living cells whose growth and reproduction are out of control. Although the first cause of cancer may be merely a mutation of a gene or exposure to a certain chemical agent, researchers are identifying other factors that can stimulate the growth of cancer cells that, without those stimulators, might die. For breast cancer a few of the stimulating factors are now thought to be excess fat in the diet, a long period of estrogen exposure, obesity, alcohol consumption, and adult weight gain. The American Institute for Cancer Research (AICR) estimates that each of our more than 10 trillion cells takes 10,000 "hits" a day from agents that can cause mutations.[1] Our bodies have built-in systems for stopping the mutations or destroying mutated cells. What fuels these mechanisms is now the subject of much research.

The table on page 14 shows that three-quarters of cancers are the result of factors that are well within our control. Of course, some cancers may be the result of a combination of several factors, but the fact remains that we have much more impact on our cancer risk than we may have thought before.

| Risk Factors for All Cancers | | |
|---|---|---|
| **Factor** | **Percentage[2]** | **Total %** |
| **Genetic and Related Risk Factors** | | 14 |
| Family history of cancer | 5 | |
| Perinatal factors/growth | 5 | |
| Reproductive factors | 3 | |
| Prescription drugs/medical procedures | 1 | |
| **Environmental Risk Factors** | | 9 |
| Viruses/other biologic agents | 5 | |
| Pollution | 2 | |
| Ionizing/ultraviolet radiation | 2 | |
| **Lifestyle Risk Factors** | | 77 |
| Tobacco use* | 30 | |
| Adult diet/obesity** | 30 | |
| Sedentary lifestyle | 5 | |
| Occupational/job-related factors | 5 | |
| Alcohol | 3 | |
| Socioeconomic status | 3 | |
| Salt-food additives and other preservatives/ contaminants | 1 | |

\* *Secondhand smoke causes approximately 3,000 deaths a year.[3]*
\*\* *AICR estimates that 60 percent of all cancers in women and 40 percent in men are associated with diet.*

Three facts seem to support the theory that lifestyle is a major factor in breast cancer:

1. Thirty-three to 80 percent of women diagnosed each year with breast cancer have none of the typically recognized risk factors.[4]

2. Developing nations show similar rates of breast cancer as industrialized nations as their nutrition and lifestyle correspond more to Western ways.

3. Immigrants assume the breast cancer risks of their adopted country in the first generation.

## What Are the Risk Factors for Breast Cancer?

Some risk factors over which you have no control include:

- Gender. The disease is many times more common in women than in men.
- Age. Risk increases with age. About 77 percent of women are 50 and older at the time of diagnosis, 0.3 percent are younger than 30, and 3.5 percent are in their 30s. About 84 percent of breast cancer deaths occur in women older than 50.[5]
- Having an early start of menses (before 12) and/or having a late menopause (after 55). Your body is exposed to your own estrogen for a longer time.
- Having a mother or sister with breast cancer. Only 20 percent of breast cancer patients have a family history of the disease.[6] Dr. Valerie Beral of the Imperial Cancer Research Fund's Cancer Epidemiology Unit in Oxford, England, found that "four out of five women who have a mother and a sister with breast cancer will never develop breast cancer, and 12 out of 13 will not die from breast cancer." Based on a study (published in *Lancet*) of more than 150,000 women, Beral concluded that, for women with one close relative with breast cancer, the lifetime risk of being diagnosed with the disease was 8 percent. The risk was 13.3 percent for women with two first-degree relatives with breast cancer and 21.1 percent for those with three affected relatives. Women with affected relatives tend to develop the disease after age 50 if at all.
- Mutations in BRCA1 and BRCA2 genes. These mutations account for only 5 to 10 percent of total breast cancer. Of that number, BRCA1 accounts for only 20 to 40 percent of hereditary breast cancer; BRCA2 accounts for 10 to 30 percent of hereditary breast cancer. This leaves 30 to 70 percent of hereditary breast cancer caused by unidentified genes.[7]
- Having had cancer in one breast. There is a three- to fourfold increased risk of a new cancer (not a recurrence) in the other breast. A history of endometrial or ovarian cancer doubles the risk for breast cancer.[8]
- Race. White women have a slightly higher risk of developing breast cancer than women of other races.
- A previous breast biopsy of atypical hyperplasia increases the risk by four to five times. A diagnosis of proliferative breast disease without atypia or unusual hyperplasia gives a 1.5 to 2 times greater risk. Fibrocystic changes without proliferative breast disease do not increase risk.
- Radiation therapy of the chest at an early age.
- Having dense breasts.[9]
- Body fat around your waist.
- Being tall.

Factors over which you may have some control include:

- Living in North America or Europe.[10]
- No pregnancies of six months or longer.[11]
- Becoming pregnant for the first time after age 30.
- Exercising less than three times a week in the years before menopause.
- Postmenopausal obesity, excessive lifetime weight gain, or premenopausal thinness.[12]
- Alcohol consumption. For women not taking estrogen replacement, drinking two to five bottles of beer, 2.8 to 5.6 glasses of wine, or two to four shots of liquor per day increases the risk of breast cancer by 41 percent.[13] Women who drink one glass of alcohol a day have a 9-percent increase in risk.[14] Alcohol is believed to increase estrogen levels in the blood.
- Long-term use of hormone replacement therapy after menopause.
- Diet low in fruits, vegetables, or fiber, or high in fat.

So what does this mean to you? Researchers don't really know because overall health is such a complex issue. Although none of these factors is believed to cause cancer, they all describe the population that has contracted breast cancer. While we wait for more answers, all you can do is decide which risk factors you will eliminate from your lifestyle and what healthy measures you can continue or add—and hope for the best.

## What Are *Not* Risk Factors for Breast Cancer?

Claims about toxin accumulation from antiperspirants are not consistent with the science of cancer formation, although researchers in the UK believe parabens, a substance in antiperspirants, are worth more study. Studies have not proven that underwire bras cause breast cancer by obstructing lymph flow, that smoking causes breast cancer (although it does increase risk for other cancers), or that induced or spontaneous abortion (miscarriage) or silicone breast implants increase breast cancer risk. No studies show a correlation between breast cancer and coffee.[15]

## What Are Symptoms of Breast Cancer to Look For?

Symptoms, which also have benign explanations, may include a lump (usually hard and unmovable) or thickening in the breast, nipple discharge or inversion, change in the shape or size of your breast, enlargement of a node in the armpit, dimpling or puckering of the skin on the breast, or any other change not associated with a menstrual period.

## *Is Breast Cancer a Single Disease?*

No. Breast cancer is more than 100 different diseases in the breast with a common factor: genetic mutations.

## *Why Does Breast Cancer Risk Increase with Age?*

The process of cancer may be occurring several decades before the disease can be detected by current diagnostic procedures. Therefore, the longer you live, the more likely it is that a cancerous tumor could be developing. Also it is believed that the amount of time a woman is exposed to hormones, particularly estrogen, in her body (from the beginning of menstruation to menopause) may be a risk factor for breast cancer. The median age for breast cancer is 69. More than 80 percent of women with breast cancer are older than age 50.[16]

## *What Role Does Estrogen Play in Breast Cancer?*

With estrogen, there is good news and bad news. The good news is that in men and women estrogens (the three main estrogens are estradiol, estrone, and estriol) regulate the reproductive system and various metabolic processes and maintain the structure of blood vessels, bones, and the skin. However, prolonged exposure to estrogens and xenoestrogens (foreign estrogens not produced by the body) can have serious health consequences. Estrogens are broken down in the liver. There estradiol is converted into estrone, which further breaks down into 2-hydroxyestrone and 16-alpha-hydroxyestrone, the "bad" estrogen. The first form, 2-hydroxyestrone, forms into two other components: 2-methoxyestrone and 2-methoxyestradiol. These are "good" estrogens, which inhibit growth of malignant tumors. If production of the bad estrogens outpaces production of good estrogens, the body is susceptible to cancer-causing activity.[17] The compounds that estrone metabolizes into is affected by such factors as diet, lifestyle, genetics, and exposure to foreign estrogens in the environment. It is not known presently how to influence the production of the good estrogens. Approximately 70 percent of all breast cancers are estrogen receptor–positive, meaning that they feed off estrogen.[18] However, some common-sense precautions are available to reduce exposure to the foreign estrogens such as minimizing hormones intentionally given to pigs, chickens, and cows that we eat; minimizing effects from environmental factors such as pollution, agricultural chemicals, plastics, and even our water supply; and trying to prevent excess body fat, constipation, lack of fiber and exercise, poor diet, and stress. Obese women, particularly postmenopausal women, may produce a lot of estrogen in fat tissue. After menopause, women who are overweight, obese, or sedentary produce more estrogen than thin, active ones. A low-fat, high-fiber diet produces less estrogen whereas alcohol increases it.

## *How Is the Battle against Breast Cancer Progressing?*

The percentages are not encouraging at first glance. In the past 50 years, the lifetime risk of breast cancer has nearly tripled in the United States. In the 1940s, a woman's lifetime risk of breast cancer was one in 22. In the year 2003, the risk was one in eight.[19] Besides the more than 211,000 women who will develop invasive breast cancer this year, another 55,700 will be diagnosed with breast cancer in situ.

A ray of hope is that the range of drugs continues to expand. Although no new drugs were approved for breast cancer between 1976 and 1991, a dozen new ones were approved between 1991 and 2003. Currently, more than 400 pharmaceutical products are being tested for use against breast cancer.

## *Interesting Breast Cancer Statistics*

Breast cancer is the most commonly occurring cancer among Western women and the leading cause of cancer death among women ages 40 to 55 in most Western countries.[20] In the United States alone the frequency of breast cancer in women is exceeded only by skin cancer.[21]

## Frequency

A woman's chance of developing breast cancer increases with age, as you can see in the following table:

| Current age | Probability of developing breast cancer in next 10 years[22] | 1 in |
|:---:|:---:|:---:|
| 20 | 0.05% | 2,044 |
| 30 | 0.40% | 249 |
| 40 | 1.49% | 67 |
| 50 | 2.77% | 36 |
| 60 | 3.45% | 29 |
| 70 | 4.16% | 24 |

## Recurrence

Only 6 percent of breast cancers are diagnosed at an advanced or metastatic stage. The five-year survival rate for women diagnosed at this stage is 23 percent.[23]

More than 75 percent of recurrences occur in the first five years, and more than 90 percent have occurred within 10 years.[24]

## Survival/Death

Unfortunately, approximately 39,800 women are predicted to die of breast cancer this year.[25] More women have died of breast cancer over the last 20 years than the number of Americans killed in World Wars I and II and the Korean and Vietnam conflicts combined.[26] However, approximately three million American women are living with breast cancer.[27]

Fortunately, mortality trends have been improving since the 1990s. Breast cancer deaths in the United States were 46,000 in 1992. In 2002 they were 39,600.[28] Higher declines were seen for white women and for women younger than age 50.

Musa Mayer, author and breast cancer survivor, puts the raw numbers in a more helpful perspective in *After Breast Cancer: Answers to Questions You're Afraid to Ask.* She says that, adjusted for other causes of death, survival rates for women with invasive breast cancer are 86 percent at 5 years, 76 percent at 10 years, 58 percent at 15 years, 53 percent at 20 years, and 50 percent after 25 years. Now that sounds better.

Even those figures are always changing as treatments are refined. Someone treated 15 years ago would not have had the options we have now. Generally the longer you have gone since diagnosis without a recurrence, the longer you can expect to survive. But always keep in mind that statistics are averages or medians, meaning that half the people are on one side of the number and half are on the other side. You have as much chance of surviving disease-free for years as the next person. Plan wisely and enjoy every day.

Breast cancer is the second leading cause of cancer death in women, exceeded only by lung cancer.[29]

A study reported in the *Journal of the National Cancer Institute* (1993) reported that "the evidence that cancer patients die of non-cancer causes at a higher rate than persons in the general population is overwhelming."[30] More than half of the deaths are due to cardiovascular disease. This means you should adopt a heart-healthy lifestyle in addition to observing whatever breast cancer survival techniques you can.

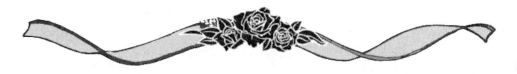

## Chapter 2

# Maximizing Treatment

After the shock of your breast cancer diagnosis, you face a maze of decisions—medical as well as personal. While reeling from the diagnosis, you have to consider financial and workplace matters and don't know where to begin. This chapter guides you through the confusing new landscape of medical decisions you don't feel prepared to make and experiences you don't want to have. Later chapters will deal with emotional and financial issues.

Begin by taking a deep breath. Realize that you have time, time to figure out the questions you need answered and time to find the answers. The topics presented here will help you start at the beginning. You don't have to decide everything today. Although you will probably want to discuss your decisions with your family or a close friend, you should be the ultimate decision-maker. You are not only the star of this show, you are also the director. You will depend heavily, of course, on your medical team, but you need to have the final say. The topics that follow will help you navigate the maze with some sense of control and competence.

## Finding a Doctor

If you do not have a doctor, there are many avenues to finding one qualified to assess your concerns. However you locate a doctor, try to find one who has had experience with breast cancer—the more, the better.

When selecting a surgeon, ask the office staff or the hospital administration how many operations similar to yours the surgeon performs a year and the success rate. They must tell you—but only if you ask.

Places to find a doctor to coordinate your cancer care include:

- Friends and family. If any have had breast cancer, ask about their physician(s).
- Support groups.
- Medical schools.

- Cancer centers.
- Local and national medical societies.
- American Cancer Society.
- Cancer Information Service of the National Cancer Institute.
- Your family practice doctor or PCP.
- Your insurance company.
- Your human resources department at work.

## Selecting Your Doctors

The most important characteristic of a doctor for your cancer treatment is someone whom you feel comfortable with and trust. You will deal with him or her for years, and you will rely on your doctor to guide you to the best treatment plan for you. Some women attach great weight to a doctor's surgical skill whereas others put compassion at the top of their list of traits they must have in a cancer doctor.

Other important characteristics of doctors for your cancer care are that he or she:

- Has experience with breast cancer (a specialist rather than a general oncologist if possible).
- Treats you with respect, dignity, patience, and compassion (like a person, not a case number or a disease specimen).
- Is easy to talk to; takes time for your questions.
- Explains medical terminology so you can understand it.
- Encourages you to participate in your treatment decisions rather than dictating a treatment plan.
- Is reasonably accessible in and after office hours.
- Has a nursing staff with knowledge and caring personalities.
- Has offices and gives treatment at a location convenient for you.
- Is in your insurance plan.
- Is willing to work and consult with your other doctors (surgeon, radiation oncologist, plastic surgeon, physical therapist, and so on).
- Has privileges at a hospital in your insurance plan or in which you have confidence.

## Doctor Visits

Because cancer treatment is a time of emotional as well as physical upheaval, you will find that you are not as mentally alert as you normally are.

This is especially true during doctors' visits when you may be hearing (or fearing you will hear) disturbing news or unfamiliar terms. Here are several ways to cope:

- Take your written questions or concerns. Keep a section in your Treatment Notebook (page 26) for questions. Hand a copy to the doctor at the beginning of the appointment to allow him to reserve enough time to answer them. Have a copy for yourself so you can be sure all were covered.

- Take someone else along. At many appointments you will feel stressed, anxious, and perhaps fearful. These emotions can interfere with your memory. When you get home, you may not be clear what was said about an important issue. If you take along a friend or family member, there is a better chance that one of you will remember what was said. Don't be shocked, however, if sometimes both of you fail to hear something. It's a stressful time for everyone, and forgetfulness is a normal reaction.

- Take notes. If you can take good notes quickly, jot down key points the doctor says. These will help jog your memory when you get home. If you are not adept at taking notes, however, this may produce more stress, make you miss what is being said while you are writing, and be counterproductive.

- Ask for any printed information on the cancer, treatment, medications, side effects, or other issues. Also ask for copies of test results.

- Take a tape recorder and ask your doctor if you can record the session. Doctors should not mind. They understand your emotional state and your desire to remember information accurately. A tape recording is handy to replay for family members who are interested in the details of your treatment. It also provides you a way to review the session to clarify anything you are confused about later.

## What to Expect during Each Office Visit

Even before you begin treatment, you may have several office visits to discuss test results and treatment options with your oncologist or physician. When each phase of treatment is completed, you will go back to discuss the effectiveness of the treatment, further treatment, and your follow-up schedule.

Although each physician's office procedure differs, it is not unusual to experience the following during routine office visits:

- Recording of weight, to track trends.
- Blood draw (a CBC [complete blood count]) to assess your red and white blood cell count and platelet levels, check for signs of infection, and assess such issues as liver and kidney function. Periodically an oncologist may test for tumor markers.

- Blood pressure and pulse reading. (If you had a mastectomy, be sure the reading is not taken on your affected arm.)
- Questions about your symptoms such as pain, side effects from medication, stamina, or new concerns. Be honest about these areas. Do not be concerned that you are complaining. Unless a physician knows about a symptom, he can't help you control it. This is not a time to grin and bear it. Most complaints can be treated, so speak up.
- Answering your questions and addressing your concerns.
- Discussion of when your next visit will be, what tests you need, what you can expect in your recovery, and so forth.

## Communicating with Your Doctor

Communication with your doctor is one of the most important factors in your treatment plan. You need to get the information you want. Some people find communicating with their doctors difficult because of their own biases. They feel a question is "dumb." They can't handle more information at the moment, so they don't ask. They are afraid of the answer, afraid the questions will make the doctor defensive, or are unwilling to reveal the real reason for a question or decision.

Doctors have probably heard anything you will say or ask. Your health is at stake. Doctors cannot read minds. Unless you tell, he won't know.

## Working with Medical Offices

Medical services these days can sometimes cause more stress than your medical condition. You may wait days or weeks for an appointment. You may have to wait in the waiting room a long time before being seen. Your calls may not be returned promptly. You may have to drive a long distance to receive care at a facility specified by your insurance company.

Although all of this is frustrating, try to remember that stress does not help your recovery. Stress can interfere with the immune system and can have myriad other effects on your body. So how do you avoid it in dealing with the medical community?

One way is to be proactive. That is, treat the personnel in the offices as you would want to be treated. Be pleasant. Learn their names and use them. Strike up casual conversations and remember details about their families or hobbies. Ask about these when you next talk to them. They will remember you and be glad to assist you.

Understand that you are not their only patient. When you call for information or have a request, be polite, not demanding. If you are not getting the service you need, be persistent, but try never to resort to anger or impatience. Express your frustration calmly and ask to speak to a supervisor if necessary.

If the information you are getting is vital, write down the name of the person you spoke to, the date, and the answer. Find out whom you should talk to about various aspects of your treatment: insurance payments, referrals, side effects, or general questions.

If the hassle gets too overwhelming, ask a spouse, family member, or friend to take over. You need to spend your energy getting well.

## *Records: They're Yours, and They're Private*

Your medical records belong to you, don't they? Yes and no. Although you may obtain a copy of your medical records, they actually belong to the provider who offered the service (doctor, lab, hospital, and so forth). Providers are allowed to charge for copies and to decide when to release them.

Be sure to request a copy of every test run, from the initial suspicious mammogram and biopsy to surgery, chemotherapy, and radiation. File them in your Treatment Notebook for handy reference.

Many facilities will not release a lab report for a week or so to give your doctor time to talk to you about the results. And that makes sense. Most of us need a physician's interpretation to know the meaning and significance of reports. If you have trouble getting a copy from the lab or hospital, ask your doctor for a copy instead. It's generally easier than hassling with a medical records department.

HIPAA, the federal Health Insurance Portability and Accountability Act of 1996, declares that healthcare facilities must take steps to keep your medical records confidential. The law spells out circumstances in which facilities may share your information, such as with another doctor treating you, for staff performance evaluations, for bill collection purposes, and to recruit research subjects. You must sign a form to allow a doctor to release your personal information to a spouse, parent, or child. You may request restrictions on who sees your information, although the facility does not have to agree. This law should protect you from disclosure of your medical records to an employer or prospective employer without your permission.

## *Organization*

You probably already know that when you feel bad, it's hard to concentrate and remember things. Add to that the fear of cancer, the confusion of being thrown into an unfamiliar language and circumstances and asked to make far-reaching decisions quickly, the toll of powerful emotions, and possible side effects from medications or treatment—and you realize you need help keeping up with everything.

## Treatment Notebook

Finding information efficiently is a time-saver and de-stressor. Devote a three-ring binder to your treatment information. Place dividers inside for:

- Patient Information. Include your name exactly as it appears on your medical insurance card, address, phone numbers where you can most easily be reached (if you don't keep your cell phone on, don't list it), Social Security number, driver's license number, birth date, emergency contacts, babysitters' contact information, dates of previous hospitalizations and surgeries, and so forth. All of these are commonly asked on new patient forms.

- Doctor Information (include information for your primary care physician, oncologist, radiation oncologist, surgeon, and other specialists you see). List the name, office phone and fax, emergency phone if different, address, and nurse and office staff names. To save time, tape business cards to this page.

- Diagnosis. Include a copy of the pathology and lab reports that determined you had cancer. Most doctors will want to see these.

- Appointments. Place a calendar here for your medical appointments. Also keep a separate piece of paper where, as you get further into treatment and your appointments are farther apart, you can record when you need to make your next appointment with each doctor.

- Medications. Keep a chart of each medication (whether cancer related or not), who prescribed it, for what condition, when you started taking it, the dose you take and how often, and what side effects you've had from it. When you stop a medication, record the date and reason. Also record herbs, supplements, and over-the-counter drugs, such as aspirin, that you take.

- Side Effects Charts. As you begin new medications, keep a chart of side effects. It does not have to be complicated. Just record, "Monday 6 a.m., woke up nauseated. Before 10 a.m. dose, ate oatmeal and nausea was better." Also keep records of any pain you experience.

- Questions. Label each doctor's name on a separate sheet of paper. Record the date of your next visit. Then each time you think of a question you want to ask, write it on this paper.

- Test Results. Obtain a copy of every test result: blood work, X-ray, bone scan, and so forth. File them by the type of test (get tabs to separate them) and file with the most recent first. Highlight dates and type of test for easier review.

- Reports, Letters. Obtain copies of letters between doctors such as second opinions. File here surgical and pathology reports.

- Insurance Information. Record company name, address, and phone number for customer service, and your ID number, plan number, and employer's name and address. File here bills, explanation of benefits (EOBs), referrals, receipts, and so on. Keep a chart of when a claim was filed and reimbursed and the amount reimbursed.
- Resources. Place here any handouts you'll need to refer to, such as do's and don'ts from your radiation oncologist.

Keep your binder in a tote bag so it's easy to grab and carry. Also carry in the bag a pen, notepaper, magazines or books, snacks, a bottle of water, and sweater.

## Basket Buddy

Pick a good-sized basket with a handle. Pack in it all the things you might need throughout the day such as pens, pencils, tape, phone list, cell phone, scissors, stamps, paper, tissue, water bottle, and reading material. On those days you are very tired, tote it along to your bed or couch. It will save you many steps in finding what you need.

Some patients devote a basket, tote bag, or box to cancer pamphlets, booklets, and so forth that they gather throughout treatment. They find that not having reminders of cancer scattered everywhere around the house helps tremendously with attitude.

### *Tests: What to Expect*

Tests may be the hardest part of breast cancer, not because they are painful but because they are stressful. You know that the person administering the test knows the results as she looks at the film or monitor screen—and she's not allowed to tell you. Most facilities will not give test results to a patient until her doctor has discussed the results with her. Even then most facilities will tell you to get copies from your doctor, not from them.

Know from the start that you will wait for test results. Several days may go by before the results are sent to your doctor. Ask your doctor's staff what the procedure is for informing you of results.

Some of my doctors' nurses would say, "We'll call you if something is wrong. Otherwise assume everything is fine." Don't settle for that. It is too easy for a test result to be sent to the wrong doctor, be misfiled, and so on. I always ask what day I can call to learn the results, and afterwards I ask for a copy to be faxed or mailed to me.

You may be tempted to postpone hearing test results. You may rationalize, "If it's good news, then nothing needs to be done. If it's bad news, I don't want to know." That is perfectly normal and understandable.

But think of it this way: If the news is good, you could be out celebrating instead of using energy trying to ignore the fact that you have a test result you should call about. If the news is bad, then you want time to consider your options. As with the initial diagnosis, a few days or probably even weeks won't make much difference as far as treatment is concerned, but you may as well get on with whatever therapy is recommended or have time to get other opinions.

## Initial Tests for Evaluation

There is no standard set of tests to determine whether you have breast cancer or, after you are diagnosed, to determine how the disease is progressing or regressing. Following are some tests often performed for diagnosis and monitoring your progress.

**Blood tests.** A complete blood work-up (blood chemistry and blood counts) will usually be done. In addition, two tests (CEA and CA 27.29) are used by some physicians to diagnose and then to predict recurrence. Some cancer cells produce substances that can be measured, known as tumor markers. The presence of these markers may indicate the presence of cancer, but the markers are not totally reliable. Doctors look more for a pattern of elevation in the marker numbers than for certain raw values. Certain conditions such as a virus, abdominal distress, or smoking can also raise the marker levels, so the markers are used more to indicate further tests than to identify recurrence absolutely.

**Mammogram.** An X-ray of the breast can sometimes detect tiny tumors that cannot yet be felt by an examiner's fingers. Some women worry about the radiation exposure in mammograms, but there is no need to. A mammogram exposes you to less radiation than when you fly across the country and back in a commercial airplane and less than a series of routine dental X-rays.[1] Mammograms may give false positives (25 to 30 percent) and false negatives (10 to 25 percent), so their use is somewhat controversial (especially in younger women), although they seem to be the best screening test we currently have for this purpose.[2]

New screening possibilities on the horizon are optical mammography, which uses a laser beam to detect physical and chemical changes in breast tissue; PET scans; and magnetic resonance spectroscopy (MRS), which measures the biochemical composition and metabolic state of breast tissue. MRIs are extremely sensitive, so much so that they sometimes mistake benign growths for tumors. Their expense also keeps insurance companies from paying for them for routine breast cancer screening. Digital mammography or digitized X-ray imaging sends pictures of the breast to a computer instead of X-ray film. This allows a radiologist to darken, lighten, or enlarge small areas and flag suspicious areas for future monitoring. The ImageCheckerM1000 works in conjunction with standard mammograms to find "regions of interest" (ROIs) that exhibit characteristics of cancer. The radiologist can then magnify these areas and reexamine them. Another technique to watch is Sestamibi imaging, also called scintimammography. A radioactive agent is injected into a vein and accumulates in areas of rapid cell division, which may indicate cancer. Although this imaging does a good job on dense breasts, it can miss small tumors.

Another exciting diagnostic tool that is just being finalized is the Breast Cancer Profile Chip (BCPC). It uses microarray technology to analyze the expression of more than 900 genes and suggests individualized treatment based on the genetic composition of the tumor.

**Thermography.** Some naturopathic physicians and doctors of integrated medicine are urging women to use thermography as an alternative to mammography. Thermography, or infrared imaging, measures changes of heat in the breast that could point to cancerous cells. The technique does not involve radiation exposure or compression of the breasts. It lacks precision, however, and has a high rate of false negatives and positives.

**Ultrasound.** Working on the principle that tissues of varying densities reflect sound waves differently, this technique is most reliable for detecting fluid-filled cysts. It cannot distinguish between cancerous and benign solid tumors. It is often used for young women whose breasts are too dense for mammography and is very safe. Because of its limitations, it should never be the only reason for proceeding to surgery unless there are corroborating tests.

To obtain sonograms, the patient lies on a table, gel is spread on the area to be tested, and a small sensor that is connected to a computer is slowly pushed around the area. The technician will periodically take pictures. The process is painless unless the area is sore to the touch.

A new technique, harmonic imaging, is being studied as a more precise alternative to sonograms.

**Chest X-ray.** As with any other X-ray, you stand in front of X-ray film while a few images are taken. Chest X-rays may be taken to check for spread of the cancer to the lungs or to check for conditions such as infection during chemotherapy or scarring from radiation.

**CAT scans.** Computerized axial tomography, or CT scans (computed tomography), synthesizes X-rays of cross-sections of the body into one comprehensive picture. CAT scans are taken of the abdomen, brain, liver, or other area to check for metastasis or to evaluate response to treatment.

**MRI scans.** Magnetic resonance imaging visualizes soft tissue and anatomic structure similar to a CAT scan, but without the radiation.

**PET scans.** Positron emission tomography is a new technique in which radioactive material, which is taken up by metabolically active cells such as cancer cells, is injected. Once an active area has been identified, other tests may be run for further evaluation.

**Bone scans.** These are run to check for the spread of cancer to the bones. Approximately three hours before the scan, radioactive material, which is absorbed by cells that make bone, is injected into the bloodstream. Areas of intense activity show up dark on the film. Drink lots of fluid to help the dye diffuse through your body thoroughly. Be sure to empty your bladder before you begin the scan! For about 20 to 45 minutes you will lie on a table that slowly moves through an opening while multiple images are taken. This is an open machine. There is no pain. After the scan, drink soda pop containing phosphoric acid to flush the radioactive agent out of your system as quickly as possible.

**Biopsies.** Suspicious lumps will probably be biopsied. There are several ways to obtain a sample of the suspected tissue or fluid: fine needle aspiration (taking a very small sample from a lump), core needle biopsy (removal of tissue in the suspicious area with a hollow needle), or surgical (excisional) biopsy (removal of the total lump and some surrounding tissue). Ductal lavage is a new technique available in major medical centers to detect ductal cancers. Tiny tubes are inserted into the nipple, a liquid injected, and a sample removed. Cells recovered by any of these techniques are then sent to a lab for further study.

**Ductograms.** This X-ray is done to examine nipple discharge. A fine plastic tube is inserted into the opening of the duct into the nipple and a contrast medium injected to show any mass inside the duct.

**Transillumination.** In a dark room the physician will hold a powerful light near the lump to determine if it is solid or filled with fluid.

**Diffusion MRI.** This is a new development to watch. It tracks movement of water in and out of cells. This tells researchers whether a cell is dying or, in other words, whether treatment is working. It can read more subtle indications than conventional scans. Also, results may be available with this information weeks earlier than the current "wait and see" method. More studies are needed, but it is an encouraging area.

## Blood Draw

No one likes to have blood drawn, but, unfortunately, you'll have to get used to it. Many oncologists take a blood sample every office visit (sometimes just a finger prick). That's because a blood test can provide a wealth of information, such as blood counts, presence of infection, and function of organs.

## In advance

- Ask the nurse about using a butterfly needle, which is smaller than the normal needle.
- Ask the technician to wipe off the alcohol with a dry cotton ball before inserting the needle to avoid alcohol sting.
- Eat foods high in bioflavonoids to strengthen the tissue of the blood vessels. Plant foods that are blue, yellow, red, orange, and purple qualify.
- Ask a trained herbalist and your oncologist about taking hawthorn berries, blueberries, turmeric, or gingko biloba.
- Drink nettle tea to strengthen your veins.

## Calm down

- Chit-chat with the technician about something pleasant or about him or her to take your mind off yourself.
- Don't look at the needle.
- Ask if you can use a portable CD or tape player with soothing music or relaxation instructions.
- If one nurse or technician finds your veins easier than another, ask for her each time.

## Positive pressure

To facilitate a blood draw from a vein, try any or all of the following to increase blood flow and keep your veins plump:

- Hydrate. Drink generous amounts of fluid the day before and morning of your blood draw.
- Move. Take a walk just prior to your blood test.
- Exercise. Regular arm and hand exercises will help with frequent blood draws.
- Warm up. While waiting for your blood draw, stay warm with a sweater or towel. If your veins are really difficult to find, take a heating pad to the doctor's office and warm your arm and hand for 15 minutes before the blood draw. Place a warm rice bag (page 160) on your arm during the drive to the office.
- Hang out. Let your arms dangle down to increase blood pressure in the veins.
- Medicate. If nurses often have trouble finding a vein, ask your oncologist to prescribe an EMLA cream to be applied to the site at least 60 minutes before an IV is started. It numbs the area for up to 20 minutes. Ethyl chloride spray can be used immediately before the stick.

## *Understanding Your Pathology Report*

Your pathology reports from biopsy and surgery are the roadmaps to your cancer journey. Most of the factors that will determine your doctor's treatment recommendations come from those few pieces of paper. There are many varieties of breast cancer, and each has a number of characteristics that respond to different treatments. As an informed patient, you will want to get to "know" your cancer so you can better evaluate information you read and determine what might apply to you.

Be sure to file copies of the reports in your Treatment Notebook so every healthcare professional involved in your treatment can review them.

What will the report tell your doctor?

- Size of tumor. A small tumor (less than 2 centimeters) gives a better prognosis than a large one (more than 5 centimeters).
- Type of cancer. Breast cancer may be found in the ducts (ductal carcinoma), in the lobules (lobular carcinoma), in the chest wall margins, or elsewhere. A cancer is called *in situ* if it is confined to one anatomic area and has not spread to the fatty tissue around it or to other organs. If it has spread, it is called *invasive* (*infiltrating*).
- Lymph node involvement. If cancer is found in the lymph nodes under the arm (axillary), recurrence is more likely. If no malignant lymph nodes are found, the report is "negative"—and that's good! However, many breast cancers have metastasized on such a microscopic level they are not detectable by current tests.
- Histologic grade (sometimes called a Bloom-Richardson grade, Scarff-Bloom-Richardson grade, or Elson-Ellis grade). Used for invasive carcinomas, this number describes how unlike a normal cell the cancer cells are. *Differentiated* means the extent to which the cancer cells look and act like normal cells. Pathologists grade breast cancer cells 1 to 4, with 1 being well differentiated and less aggressive.
- Nuclear grade. This number gives a description of the size and shape of the nucleus of the tumor and the number of cells that are dividing. Nuclear grades are 1 to 3, with 1 being closest to normal.
- Van Nuys Prognostic Index. This indicates the likelihood of a DCIS (ductal carcinoma in situ) cancer returning after a lumpectomy.
- Hormone receptor status. Estrogen and progesterone are two hormones necessary for normal breast tissue. Hormone receptors are chemicals in the cell membranes that bind to hormones and allow them into the cell. If your tumor was hormone receptor-positive, it contained these chemicals and you are sensitive to estrogen and progesterone and compounds that mimic them. The presence or absence of estrogen receptors (ERs) or

progesterone receptors (PRs) has been called the most important biomarker in breast cancer. Assessment of these biomarkers is essential to determining the best intervention to use. About two-thirds of breast cancers are ER positive; about 40 to 50 percent are PR positive.

- HER-2/neu status. This measures a growth factor protein. A positive status means a more aggressive tumor and sometimes a poorer prognosis. About 20 percent of breast cancers are HER-2/neu positive.

- S-phase fraction. This is the percentage of cancer cells that are dividing. A higher "proliferative capacity" means a faster-growing and more aggressive tumor.

- DNA content. The ploidy of cancer cells means the amount of DNA they contain. If the amount is normal, they are called diploid. If the amount is abnormal, they are called aneuploid and tend to be faster growing.

- p53 gene. This gene normally inhibits the growth of tumor cells and is altered by some types of cancer so it cannot perform its task.

- Margins. The lesion or breast tissue removed during surgery is inked on the surface. Then when it is sliced and examined, the pathologist determines how close to the inked margins the cancer cells appear. If they touch the surface (dirty or involved margins), they may exist outside the tumor in other parts of the body. If they don't touch the inked margins, they are referred to as clean.

- Stage. This is determined by the size of the tumor and degree of spread and is an important factor in deciding treatment. The Staging System of the American Joint Committee on Cancer is called the TNM system. The letter "T" is followed by a number from 1 to 4. A higher number indicates a larger tumor and/or more extensive spread to tissues near the breast. The letter "N" is followed by a number from 0 to 3 to indicate whether the cancer has spread to lymph nodes under the arms and whether they are fixed to other structures under the arm. The letter "M" followed by a 0 or 1 indicates metastasis to distant organs. The TNM numbers determine the stage grouping.

| Stage 0 | Carcinoma in situ |
|---------|-------------------|
| Stage I | Tumor 2 cm or less with no regional or distant metastasis |
| Stage II | Tumor up to 5 cm with lymph node involvement and no distant spread, or more than 5 cm without lymph node involvement |
| Stage III | Tumor of any size with lymph node involvement and no metastasis but possible skin or chest wall involvement |
| Stage IV | Tumor of any size with or without regional involvement and with metastasis |

In general you can evaluate your pathology report with the following table:

| Characteristic | A Better Report | A Worse Report |
|---|---|---|
| Tumor size | Less than 1.5 cm | More than 1.5 cm |
| Type | DCIS, LCIS | Invasive, infiltrating |
| Axillary lymph node status | Negative nodes | Positive nodes, more is worse |
| Estrogen/ progesterone receptors | Positive | Negative |
| HER-2/neu oncogene | Negative (absent) | Positive (present) |
| p53 | Negative (absent) | Positive (present) |
| Histologic grade (1–4) | Well differentiated, low grade | Poorly differentiated, high grade |
| Nuclear grade (1–3) | 1 | 3 |
| DNA content | Diploid | Aneuploid |
| Histologic tumor type | Tubular, papillary, medullary, colloid (or mucinous); ductal is most common and is neither good nor bad | Inflammatory |
| S-phase | Less than 5 percent | More than 5 percent |
| Margins | Clean | Dirty, involved |
| Stage (0–4) | 0–2 | 3–4 |

## *Deciding on Treatment*

Although a cancer diagnosis is certainly a catastrophe, it is not usually an emergency. An exception is inflammatory breast cancer, which needs immediate treatment. Fortunately it is rare.

You don't necessarily have to begin treatment the day you hear the frightening news, or the next day, or even the next week. Different kinds of cancer cells divide at different rates: some within 30 days; others not for as long as 200 days. Most tumors stay localized until they are 1 cm (approximately 0.4 inch) in diameter, and they usually take years to reach that size. You have time to learn about your particular diagnosis and treatment options.

Before you shake your head and declare, "I don't know anything about cancer. I'll just do what my doctor recommends and get on with fighting this disease," consider that cancer treatment protocols are constantly evolving and, in some cases, two treatments are equally effective. Each treatment has different side effects, some of which you may be willing to endure and others of which you may not. Also, what was standard treatment even a year ago for one type of breast cancer may be different today because of information gleaned from a clinical trial. If your doctor is a general oncologist or maybe not even an oncologist, it is possible that he or she is not up to date on the latest treatments for breast cancer.

Because treatment decisions affect your health and your physical condition and your life, you have the greatest motivation to choose what suits your preferences best. Some women whose cancer has a high probability of recurring in the other breast will choose a prophylactic bilateral mastectomy whereas others say, "I'll take my chances. Keeping one breast is very important to me." Research has shown that in some cases of ductal carcinoma in situ, a lumpectomy and radiation are just as effective as a mastectomy. Again, some women choose to have the entire breast removed, hoping to reduce the chance of recurrence. Other women prefer to conserve as much of the breast as possible.

Many factors contribute to your treatment decision. These include your physician's recommendation, your age, other health concerns, self-image, stage and characteristics of the cancer, personal preferences, and risk factors. Only you know what inconveniences, difficulties, and risks you are willing to put up with. Discuss your preferences with a trusted friend or relative or a counselor. Ask that they not try to talk you into or out of a particular treatment option, but that they listen to your reasoning and give their candid feedback. Ask that they verbalize their fears so that you can consider their comments in light of their emotions and perspective.

Another important factor in choosing your treatment is benefit versus risk. All breast cancer treatment options have benefits for a percentage of patients; all have risks of varying scope. Ask about all the risks, even the rare ones, before you decide. Weigh the information carefully, remembering that there is no perfect treatment that will cure you with no possible side effects.

There is no one right answer for breast cancer treatment, so you should be the one to decide what sounds right for you. If your doctor does not offer alternative treatments, ask questions and do your own research. Help with research is often an excellent way to involve your husband or other family members or friends who feel helpless in the face of your diagnosis. They can read books and search the Web for information. Be sure anyone helping in this way knows the particulars of your diagnosis. Also request that they limit their search to reliable sources.

## Evaluating Online Information

As the number of Web sites soars, so does the risk of obtaining tainted or misleading information from the Internet. How do you know what to believe? The best you can do is to evaluate a Website by asking the following questions:

- Who runs the site? Is it a government agency (address will end in ".gov"), a university (address will end in ".edu"), a nonprofit (address will end in ".org"), or a manufacturer (address will end in ".com" or ".net")?

- Who pays for the site? Advertisers? A drug or supplement company? Funding sources can influence content. If ads proliferate, be concerned about the site's objectivity.

- What is the source of the information? Claims and statements should be referenced.

- How is information selected for posting? Is there an editorial board? What are the qualifications of its members?

- How current is the information? Medical information needs to be up to date. If listings are old, be wary of the validity of the information.

- Does the site require you to "become a member" and share personal information? Many commercial sites sell your information to other vendors. Understand the use of your information before giving it.

- Does the site have a seal of credibility? Just because the site may not have one does not mean it is not credible. Health on the Net monitors health Web sites for security, confidentiality, and qualified sources. Check *www.hon.ch/HONcode* to be sure a seal is legitimate. To verify a seal from the Utilization Review Accreditation Council (URAC), visit *www.urac.org.* This group reviews sites for 14 principles and 53 Web standards.

- Are studies the site mentions published on PubMed? The National Library of Medicine (NLM) and the National Center for Biotechnology Information allow public access to their Medline database (*www.pubmed.com*) that archives articles from more than 4,500 journals as far back as 1966. Studies not found there may not have been published in a peer-reviewed journal, a standard for credibility.

- Is there another study on the topic? A sole study may mean the results did not generate enough interest for further investigation or that the results are so new that they are not adopted into mainstream protocol yet. If there are other studies, read them, because studies with different criteria can yield very different results.

# Talking to Your Doctor about Information from the Internet

Some doctors encourage their patients to research their condition and ask questions. Others want to be the final authority—no questions asked. If you have found information on treatment or symptoms or other aspects of your cancer, you have a right to have your questions answered. To help your doctor give a valid opinion, do the following:

- Bring him a copy of the article with your areas of interest or concern highlighted and a written list of questions.
- Tell him the source. That alone may give him good information about the claims being made.
- Inquire; don't confront. Say you have found information on XYZ Website that you want to ask about. Summarize the article in two or three sentences and say you'd be interested in his opinion.
- Give him time. Offer to let him read the article at his leisure and get back to you at the next visit or fax it a few days before your appointment and say you'd like to discuss it then.

# Understanding Risk

Statistics can say almost anything you want them to, and getting survival statistics for various cancer treatments can certainly be a time your mind plays tricks on you—for better or worse.

When your doctor mentions survival statistics, remember foremost that the numbers are only that: numbers. They are not your agenda or a blueprint for your life. Someone has to make up the long-term survival group. Why not you? I wanted to know how my disease might progress, and I did fall briefly into the "death by statistics" trap. You probably will too at some point. Just hop right out once you realize you have done so.

The most confusing part of statistics is comparing relative risk and absolute risk. For instance, women with a particular breast cancer profile might have a 15-percent chance of dying in 10 years. A certain chemotherapy drug might provide a *relative risk reduction* of 15 percent. Does that mean all women on that drug will be cancer free in 10 years (15 percent – 15 percent)? Unfortunately, no. The reduction is off the initial percentage (15 percent of 15 percent, or 2.25 percent). So women who choose this particular drug increase their survival rate by 2.25 percent (15 percent – 2.25 percent) to 12.75 (or 13) percent.

**Absolute risk reduction** would mean that the drug would reduce the risk of dying in the next 10 years from 15 to 13 percent.

**Absolute survival benefit** of the drug would mean that the rate of survival for the next 10 years is 87 percent (100 percent – 13 percent) instead of 85 percent (100 percent – 15 percent).

All of these numbers say the same thing, but they sound different. Patients desperate for hope are inclined to add risk reduction numbers (15 percent + 15 percent = 30 percent) instead of multiply them (15 percent × 15 percent = 2.25 percent). When you hear statistics, be sure to restate them to your doctor and ask if you have understood them correctly. Your treatment decisions will often be based on such statistics and you want accurate information for making decisions. If a chemotherapy protocol will increase your chance of survival for another few months by 1 to 2 percent and the treatment will make you very sick, you may decide against it. If it will increase your chances of survival by 10 to 15 percent and still make you sick, perhaps you would decide to try it.

Keep an open mind when you hear statistics and make decisions based on accurate numbers. Only you can decide what treatments you are willing to put up with.

## Fact and Opinion

Many women have found that knowledge drastically reduces fear and helps clear their mind. I suggest you find pictures taken after the various surgeries you are contemplating. Although the sight is shocking at first, many patients find it helpful to begin getting used to their new look through the impersonal tool of a photograph. It is not unusual in a support group for a woman who has had a particular surgery to offer to "show and tell" someone in the decision-making stage. My daughter was horrified that I had "flashed" a new woman in my support group, and I had to laugh when I realized that, modest as I am, I never hesitated. The sisterhood that comes from breast cancer will amaze you—and encourage you.

One suggestion that survivors do stress repeatedly, however, is to get a second opinion before you commit to a treatment.

### *Second Opinions*

If your primary doctor is not a breast cancer specialist, do try to locate someone who is a specialist for another opinion on treatment. Many women are afraid this step will insult the doctor they have consulted. To the contrary, most physicians understand the reason for second opinions and consider them routine. In fact, be wary of a doctor who balks at the idea.

Where do you find a helpful second opinion? It is best to see someone who is not in the same practice as the first doctor. You want a totally new approach to your diagnosis, and doctors who practice together may tend to view cases similarly. If someone totally divorced from your first doctor agrees with the treatment plan, you will probably feel more comfortable pursuing it.

Also try to find a breast cancer specialist. Unfortunately, there is no board certification for breast or cancer surgeons. You will have to ferret out someone with extensive or exclusive experience in breast cancer surgery.

Call the National Cancer Institute (NCI) (1–800–4–CANCER) for the location of the nearest Comprehensive Cancer Center and go there if at all possible. NCI recognizes 48 such centers, which are at the forefront of research and treatment of cancer.

You can also call a local medical association or regional chapter of the American Cancer Society for doctors' names. Your gynecologist, your family physician, university hospitals, academic health centers or teaching hospitals, or a large hospital in your area may be willing to provide names of breast cancer specialists. Just be aware that anyone can name a practice "Cancer Center." Check them out just as you would any other doctor.

In smaller or rural locations a general surgeon may perform breast cancer surgery as well as surgery for other cancers. Do ask about his or her experience with breast cancer surgery.

When you go for your second opinion visit, take reports from all your tests or have them faxed before your appointment. Ask whether you are to bring the film (from mammograms or scans) or just the reports. Ask if there is anything else you need to bring or send.

Also check with your insurance company to see how second opinions are paid for. They may require you to go to specific doctors for the company to cover the cost. Evaluate the credentials and experience of their doctor as thoroughly as you would one you plan to see at your own cost. If the insurance company does not offer to send you to a breast cancer specialist, consider paying for a consultation out of your own pocket. A specialist will be more likely to know the latest findings and treatment protocols. The general surgeon my insurance company limited me to recommended an immediate mastectomy. After consulting three breast cancer specialists on my own, I found that for my particular circumstances, chemotherapy was the first step to take and a bilateral mastectomy was something for consideration. I am so thankful I got the best information before making my decision.

Once your treatment is determined, it may be perfectly adequate to be under the care of a general surgeon or family doctor, but the selection of treatment is as much an art as a science and you want the best input you can find.

## Clinical Trials

Although new treatments often are born in a laboratory, they eventually must be tried on humans to determine their safety and effectiveness. There are various kinds and stages of experiments that a treatment goes through before it is approved for routine human use.

But before a treatment gets to the testing phase, it may have had its beginning in a more amorphous and yet equally important kind of study called an **epidemiological study**. These studies look at large populations of people for trends that point to further investigation.

**Population studies** compare, for example, rates of various forms of cancer to the total population of a country or region. Then researchers compare rates for different populations and try to determine factors that might account for differences. For example, in 1999 the death rate for breast cancer in the United States was 21.2 deaths for every 100,000 persons; it was 4.51 per 100,000 in China.[3] From looking at the differences in diet between the two countries (and other countries with similar diets), among other factors, researchers are now exploring the possible role of soy in reducing breast cancer incidents. The low incidence of breast cancer in Japanese women and their better survival rate if they do develop breast cancer led to the realization that Japanese women eat fat as only 10 to 12 percent of their diet whereas American women consume 37 to 40 percent of their calories as fat. Japanese immigrants to America adopt our Western diet and their rates of cancer begin to increase to the U.S. rate. Such observations lead to carefully controlled studies to confirm or deny the possible role of soy and fat in breast cancer.

Another theory that has benefited from population studies is the role of early menstruation in breast cancer. Studies show that American girls, who are raised on a high-protein, high-fat diet, have their first period earlier than girls from less developed countries, where meat is scarce. As Americans rely more and more on animal products (compared to the early 20th century), the age of menarche decreases a little in each generation.[4] This allows for longer exposure of our bodies to estrogen, which may be a factor in breast cancer.

**Animal models** are health experiments conducted on animals before theories are tried on humans. Researchers experiment with animals to see how a mechanism works or what the condition responds to. Obviously, a rat's or mouse's body functions differently from a human's, so these studies cannot be considered conclusive. Some ideas involving breast cancer that were learned from animal studies are: (1) dietary fat is involved in producing breast cancer in animals, (2) once breast cancer is present in animals, excess dietary fat promotes spread of the disease, (3) reduction of fat hinders the growth of breast cancer tumors in animals, and (4) when breast cancer is induced in animals, those on low-fat diets live longer than those on high-fat diets.[5]

When results from animal models are positive and promising, new treatments may advance to laboratory studies, which look at cells and tissues and how they respond to the treatment, to pilot studies, or to clinical trials. **Laboratory studies** are necessary for the wealth of information and lack of risk they offer, but they are not the final step. What happens in a test tube is not always what happens in a complex human body. These studies do help define other areas to be studied.

**Pilot studies** are studies conducted at non–National Cancer Institute facilities such as universities or pharmaceutical companies. Studies are usually not randomized, meaning participants take the new treatment and are not compared with a similar group taking the standard treatment. Participants in pilot studies are usually women with advanced cancer who have limited options for cure and are willing to risk unknown side effects for the possibility of benefit.

**Clinical trials** are rigidly controlled research studies using humans to determine more about causes or treatment of medical conditions. Groups such as the National Cancer Institute, National Surgical Adjuvant Breast Project (NSABP), Southwest Oncology Group (SWOG), or Cancer and Leukemia-Group B (CALGB) select a group of participants with certain characteristics and divide them randomly into at least two groups. One group receives the most up-to-date treatment. The other group receives the protocol being tested.

A further refinement of a randomized trial is double-blind studies, in which neither participants nor doctors nor researchers know who is in which group. This eliminates most bias that may creep into results. One bias that is almost impossible to eliminate, however, is the placebo effect, by which people not taking the "real" medicine think they will get better and so they do. This is a proven effect, which just shows the power of the mind over the body.

## Myths about clinical trials

Currently, only 3 to 5 percent of adult cancer patients participate in clinical trials. A recent survey found that most were unaware they could participate.[6] Others are afraid because of misinformation.

*Myth: I may be given a placebo instead of treatment.* If a standard treatment exists for a condition, participants will receive either the standard protocol or the protocol being tested. It would be unethical to withhold care from a patient when an effective therapy exists. Placebos are used only when there is no known therapy, so they are rarely used in cancer trials.

*Myth: I'll be a guinea pig.* Clinical trials are approved by institutional review boards (IRBs). These consist of members of the community such as clergy, attorneys, ethicists, and scientists as well as physicians, nurses, social workers, and other healthcare professionals. Their responsibility is to protect the safety and the rights of the study volunteers.

## Phases of clinical trials for humans

Before a drug or therapy has reached the clinical trial stage, it has undergone testing in the laboratory and/or in animals and/or has been researched in people groups or cultural groups. In other words, there is strong evidence to indicate that it may work. Clinical trials have three stages:

- Phase I trials test for tolerance and optimum dose. These are reserved for those with metastatic disease and usually involve only a dozen or so participants because the risks are unknown.
- Phase II trials measure the amount of reduction in particular diseases. These are also reserved for those with metastatic disease and rarely involve more than 100 participants. If at least 20 percent in the trial respond favorably to the new protocol, further testing follows.
- Phase III trials compare standard treatment with the promising new protocol. Usually participants are newly diagnosed and hundreds or thousands of participants are involved. This is the last step before approval by the U.S. Food and Drug Administration.

## Possible benefits of clinical trials

- You receive high-quality cancer care and attentive monitoring.
- You may experience a better outcome than if you had a standard treatment.
- A new treatment may have fewer side effects than the standard treatment.
- You have a chance to help others and yourself.
- Some costs are usually covered by the organization sponsoring the trial.

## Possible drawbacks of clinical trials

- New treatments are not always better than, or even as effective as, standard treatments.
- Health insurance does not always cover costs associated with clinical trials because the treatment is considered "experimental," and you may incur additional costs. For instance, you may have to pay to park for all the trial appointments or hire a baby-sitter more often. Most trials, however, cover tests and medications required.
- Clinical trials involve more of your time and more organization (scheduling and so forth).
- Your participating in a clinical trial costs your oncologist extra time and money to fill out required paperwork.

Discuss with your doctor whether he knows of any clinical trials (see Resources) and whether he recommends that you participate.

## Questions to Ask about a Clinical Trial

The first question to ask is "Am I eligible?" Participants are selected according to strict criteria so that results can be measured with some assurance. Interested patients will be screened according to age, stage of disease, previous treatments, or other factors such as ethnicity, place of residence, or lifestyle. If you seem to meet the criteria for a trial, then begin asking questions, such as those that follow. Continue asking them until you are totally comfortable with your decision. It helps to take along a trusted friend when you discuss the trial with your doctor or the researchers. She can help you understand what you are hearing and may think of other questions to ask.

- What are the goals of the study? What is the expected outcome?
- How long will the study last? Will there be follow-ups after the study is completed?
- What phase study is this? Has this treatment been tested before? What were the results? Why do researchers feel the treatment may be better than the standard? Were there any fatalities in the previous phases?
- Who is the study sponsor? Who has reviewed and approved the study? Who will monitor patient safety?
- What are long- and short-term risks of the new treatment? What side effects can be expected? What percentage of participants developed various side effects? How might the study affect my daily life?
- How might the study benefit me? Is there a standard treatment for this condition? How do the study risks and benefits compare with the standard treatment?
- Will I have to pay for tests, medications, parking, or anything else? Will someone help me determine if my health insurance covers any of the costs? Medicare now reimburses enrollees for office visits and tests associated with trials.
- Does the sponsoring group accept financial responsibility if I should develop a long-term condition or die as a result of the trial?
- What kind of treatment, medical tests, and procedures are involved? Where will they take place? How long will each procedure take? How often will I receive treatment? Will the study involve hospitalization? Where and for how long?
- How will I know if the treatment is working?
- Who will be in charge of my care? Will I continue seeing my own doctor? Will I have to change any of my current treatment?

## Your Rights as a Participant in a Clinical Trial

You have the final say about participating in a clinical trial.

**Informed consent.** Before you agree to participate in a clinical trial, you will be asked to sign a release or consent form. Read every paragraph carefully and ask questions about any part you do not understand. If it is not included in the consent form, ask to see the protocol, or action plan, for the study. This explains the treatment plan, medical tests involved, possible risks and benefits, and any responsibilities you may have. For example, you may be asked to modify your diet, keep a journal of side effects, meet monthly appointments, or agree to follow-up phone calls for years after the study is completed.

**Ongoing information.** As a trial progresses, the investigators may learn that parts of the treatment being studied are more dangerous than they knew or that the new treatment is so much more effective than the standard that it is unethical to keep some participants on the standard. Ask what will happen if such conditions arise. Investigators, however, rarely release results of a study until all data have been collected and analyzed.

**Freedom to withdraw.** You are free to leave a clinical trial at any time for any reason. If you do withdraw, be sure to remain in contact with your doctor about other treatments.

## Evaluating Study Results

The newspaper headline reads: "Fruit Cures Stomach Cancer!" Can you believe it? Does it mean anything for you?

Answering those questions is not straightforward. Reading results of clinical trials and other studies in the popular press is one of the best examples I know of your need to educate yourself about breast cancer and your disease in particular.

Perhaps a trial did show that a particular food or substance produced a positive response in the study participants. Before you rush out and buy that substance, ask yourself a few questions:

- Who conducted the study? If the manufacturer of the drug or substance conducted the study, the possibility of bias may exist.
- What kind of study was it? Was it randomized and double-blind, the gold standard, or some other kind? Was the kind of study appropriate for what was being studied?
- How many participants were there? A dozen or even a few hundred patients may not be enough to offer clinically significant results.
- Over what time was it conducted? Was the length appropriate for what was being studied? Testing survival over one year is not as convincing as over 10 years.

- What type of cancer did the participants have? A therapy that brings response in lung cancer may or may not have the same result in brain or breast cancer.
- What were other characteristics of the cancer: stage, size, estrogen/progesterone-receptor–positive or -negative, HER-2/neu status? What were other characteristics of the participants: late- or early-stage detection, age, gender, previous treatment, life stage (such as pre- or postmenopausal)?
- What exactly did the results show? Longer survival? If so, how long? What tradeoffs were there (side effects, quality-of-life issues)?
- What is the reputation/mission of the publication/medium? Is it a reliable source of news or is it selling the very commodity in the report?

Although it is tempting to pin our hopes on what we read, be an astute consumer. If the answers to these questions line up with your situation, ask your doctor about the usefulness of the information for you. To clarify the results of a study, call the American Institute for Cancer Research Nutrition Hotline (1–800–843–8114).

## Hospital Visits

Being in the hospital is stressful, and situations that might not bother you on a regular day may seem overwhelming while you are sore or scared or sick. Also, most hospitals are short-staffed and, although the majority of nurses truly want to help you, their patient load may mean that you wait for the care you need. Whenever possible, have a close friend or family member with you to run interference when necessary.

## Patient Advocates/Liaisons

If you have a problem that is not getting solved after repeated requests, find the facility's patient liaison. Almost all hospitals have an employee whose job it is to resolve problems between patients and the staff. When I called one hospital's switchboard and asked for a patient advocate, I was connected to the executive offices. Surprised, I politely repeated my request.

"Do you mean a patient *liaison*?" the crisp voice inquired.

"I guess," I answered. "I just need someone who can coordinate with the kitchen to follow my special diet. I'm not having any success on my own."

"Our patient *advocates* deal with legal issues," the voice explained.

"Well, I don't need an advocate...yet," I replied.

Do be reasonable about your requests. Try first to get satisfaction from your nurse, the nursing supervisor, your doctor, and/or her office. If none of these produces the result you need and the situation is serious enough, don't hesitate to seek out this line of help.

## *Medications*

Almost any breast cancer treatment will include a variety of medications—either as primary treatment or to manage side effects. You can facilitate this part of your treatment by keeping two lists (on the computer is most helpful so you can print out a list for every doctor's appointment).

One list is current medications: name, dose, how often taken, prescribing doctor, when you started it, and any side effects (positive and negative). Make a second section of over-the-counter medications or supplements you take on a regular basis.

The other list is the same information on medications you have taken in the past. Include in that list when and why you stopped taking them and any adverse reactions.

# Questions to Ask about New Prescription Medication

When your doctor prescribes a new medication, ask the following:
- How much should I take and how often?
- Under what circumstances could I take more? How much more?
- Should I call you before increasing the dose?
- What if I forget to take it on time?
- Should I take it with food?
- How much liquid should I drink with each dose?
- How long does it take to start working? How will I know if it's working?
- Should I avoid any food, beverage, or activity while on it?
- What drug interactions should I be aware of? What over-the-counter medications should I avoid?
- What side effects may occur and what can I do to prevent them? What do I do if they should develop?
- What are long-term side effects?

Every medication has side effects, some more common and some more serious than others. For example, tamoxifen, the gold standard in hormone therapy for years, can cause endometrial and uterine cancer, increase the risk of stomach and colon cancer, and cause depression and bone loss.[7] Each of these represents a tiny risk. The benefits are numerous, but you have a right to know such things before you agree to a treatment. For information on common cancer medications, see the American Cancer Society's guide to cancer drugs at *www.cancer.org/docroot/CDG/cdg_0.asp?pagKey=E* or MedLine's drug information at *www.nlm.nih.gov/medlineplus/druginformation.html.*

## Common Breast Cancer Medication Side Effects

Every chemotherapy drug will have its own set of side effects. Some of the most common are nausea, bone pain, weight gain, headache, hot flashes, diarrhea, constipation, or lowered white or red blood cell count. Some have serious, but rare, side effects such as infertility, enlargement of the heart, and increased risk of other cancers.

Ask your doctor for a list of possible side effects, particularly the long-range ones, for your medications. Always keep in mind that serious side effects are more rare than benefits from taking the drug, but you need the information to make an informed decision.

## Tips on Taking Medications

- If you have more than one medication to take at specified times, buy a couple of alarm clocks and set each one for a different time.
- If your pills are taken around meal times, buy a pill case labeled "Morning," "Noon," and "Evening." Some even have four compartments, including "Bedtime." Divide your medication into these compartments for several days at a time.
- Swallow medications with tap water. Ice water constricts your throat muscles and makes swallowing harder.
- Separate drugs and herbs by about two hours to reduce interactions.
- Do not skip doses. Know whether it is safe to take two doses at once if you do miss one. Usually it is not recommended.
- If you experience side effects, tell your doctor.
- Inform each doctor of all the medications you are taking to avoid interactions.
- Never take any one else's medications or share yours.

## Be Aware of Dangerous Interactions

Be sure that your doctor as well as your pharmacy has a list of all medications and supplements you are taking, even something you consider harmless. Drugs, herbs, and even vitamins may interact with each other in dangerous or counterproductive ways. Some vitamins may interfere with the effectiveness of your chemotherapy. Some herbs should be stopped two weeks before surgery; others may mimic the effect of medications you are taking and intensify them. Opposites may cancel out the effectiveness of each other.

Also be aware that most MDs have not been trained in nutrition or herbs. Many will roll their eyes if you mention an interest in such things. Do not let this deter you from informing him or pursuing an interest in such complementary possibilities. MDs with extensive training in nutrition may now earn the Certified Nutrition Specialist (CNS) designation from the American College of Nutrition. Naturopaths are trained in both herbs and drugs and may be a specialist to consult with.

Herbs are not the only substances that may produce adverse individual reactions. Prescription medications may also cause problems. This is why you must inform your health team about everything you are taking. Following are just a few examples of interactions to watch for:

- Coumadin (a blood thinner) may interact with foods such as broccoli and spinach and with such substances as feverfew, garlic, ginger, ginkgo biloba, vitamin E, or aspirin.[8]
- Grapefruit and grapefruit juice react with many prescription drugs.
- St. John's wort can compromise the effectiveness of Coumadin or other prescription blood thinners. Do not take it with antidepressants.
- Do not take passionflower or valerian root with tranquilizers such as Valium or Xanax.[9]
- Aspirin and other NSAIDs (nonsteroidal anti-inflammatory drugs) can reduce absorption and speed up the breakdown of vitamins, making them less effective. There is no optimal spacing for taking these substances, but wait two to three hours between them if possible.
- Fish oil, ginkgo biloba, garlic, and vitamin E can increase aspirin's ability to inhibit blood clotting, leading to a risk of abnormal bleeding.[10]
- Avoid garlic supplements if you take blood thinners.
- Kava-kava is a depressant. Don't take it if you are being treated for depression. Also, do not mix it with sedatives, sleeping pills, alcohol, or other medications that might exhibit liver toxicity. It has the potential to interfere with some medications and anesthesia.
- Do not take ginseng with Coumadin or estrogens. It can cause swollen breasts and vaginal bleeding, so some researchers do not recommend it for women with breast cancer.
- Chamomile may interact with blood thinners. It should not be taken with alcohol or other sedatives.
- Published studies disagree whether ginger may interfere with blood clotting. Be safe and ask your doctor before using it to control nausea.
- Ginkgo biloba may interfere with blood clotting, anesthesia, and some medications.

## What to Do with Leftover Medication

You usually take a full prescription of most medications. However, occasionally you will encounter one that does not work for you or one that you do not need to complete. Don't throw away your leftovers!

Some hospitals, university religious groups (especially Baptist Student Ministries), and medical schools sponsor mission programs that can use your leftovers. These programs send medical personnel to poor areas of the world to help as they can. Your medication may be useful.

When you donate, leave the medicine in its original bottle. With black marker, obliterate your name, prescription number, and other personal information. Leave visible the medication name and strength.

If you cannot locate such a group, keep excess medication that you might need until the expiration date, then flush any left down the toilet.

## Chemotherapy

Chemotherapy is probably the most dreaded treatment for breast cancer because of stories you have heard about the experiences of others. Although there is no guarantee that you will sail through chemo as if nothing is happening, there is also no guarantee that you will be deathly sick and unable to function—or that you will lose your hair.

Different drugs have different side effects, and each woman reacts differently to the same drug. In other words, there is no way to predict how you will react to chemotherapy. Many patients are able to continue working. Some feel bad for a few days, then are able to function normally until the next treatment. Even if it were guaranteed that they would be sick, most women would choose the treatment anyway because it can lengthen their life.

Until you know how you will react, have someone with you for the first treatment to drive you home. If you feel fine, celebrate with a light meal on the way home! Also have someone available to keep your children during the first week in case you are sick or too tired to take care of them.

If you work outside the home, ask your doctor before the treatment when side effects typically occur and ask your supervisor for flexibility the first time until you know how you will react. Then you can plan your treatments so you are home on the days you expect to feel poorly. Some employers may be required by federal or state law to arrange your work schedule to fit your treatment needs.

Chemotherapy drugs are given in different ways and over different periods of time. Some are given every three weeks. Some are given once a week. The choice of drugs and the regimen will depend on many factors about your disease such as stage, characteristics, and kind of breast cancer.

Some patients have chemotherapy at the doctor's office or clinic. Others go to the outpatient department of a hospital or even have it administered at home. Occasionally, someone will take treatments as an inpatient of a hospital.

It is very important that you keep all your treatment appointments. Your schedule reflects the timing that has been determined to give the optimum benefits from the drugs. If you delay or miss a dose, you may compromise the effectiveness of the chemo. Adjustments can be made for holidays or other special situations. If timing of appointments is a big issue with you (because of job or childcare requirements), discuss these with your doctor when he is deciding on your treatment. Sometimes there will be an equally effective drug that will accommodate your schedule.

The doctor may decide to postpone a treatment based on the results of certain blood tests. If your blood count is low, for instance, she may decide to wait until it reaches a certain level before continuing treatment.

Be sure to inform your doctor about all medications, over-the-counter remedies, herbs, supplements, vitamins, laxatives, and pain relievers you are taking; the dose; the frequency; and the reason you take it. Some medications and supplements can interfere with your chemotherapy, magnify a side effect, or have dangerous interactions. For instance, there is controversy whether antioxidant supplements can interfere with chemotherapy or radiation, and we know that some herbs should not be taken with antidepressants. During treatment, ask your doctor before you begin a new medication or stop one.

Before starting chemotherapy, ask your doctor to explain what side effects to expect and when they might occur. He may ask you to sign a consent form that details possible side effects. Take your time reading the form. However, remember that such forms include rare side effects as well as more common ones, just as do forms you are asked to sign before a surgery. Ask about any concerns you have, but don't panic over some effects you see listed.

## Purpose of Chemotherapy

Most commonly, chemotherapy is used in combination with other treatments rather than as the only treatment. Neo-adjuvant chemotherapy is that used to shrink a tumor before surgery or radiation. This may allow breast-conserving surgery. It does enable a patient to begin combating the cancer systemically without having to wait for surgery and healing.

Adjuvant chemotherapy helps destroy cancerous cells that may remain after surgery or radiation. Radiation and biological therapies may work better in conjunction with chemotherapy than alone.

Chemotherapy can help destroy cancer that has spread from the site of the original tumor or that has recurred in the original location. Some drugs are used to relieve symptoms caused by the cancer.

Drugs work in different ways to kill cancer cells or interfere with their growth or reproduction. Although chemotherapy can damage healthy cells as well as malignant cells, most healthy cells can repair themselves once treatment has stopped.

Chemotherapy drugs continue working sometimes for months after they enter the body because they interact with cells at various stages of the cell cycle. They may kill cells immediately or they may interfere with cell division that will happen weeks from the time of treatment. Because chemo drugs are so potent, they need to be flushed out of the body quickly after each treatment. Your doctor will advise you to drink lots of fluids if this is the case.

# Questions to Ask Your Doctor about Chemotherapy
## About chemotherapy
- What chemotherapy medications will I be taking? Why do you recommend these medications over others?
- Are there alternatives to chemotherapy?
- Are there any clinical trials I might want to consider in lieu of these medications?
- What percentage of patients responds to this medication?
- How will we know if the medication is successful?
- What are the risks and benefits of this chemotherapy?

## About your treatment
- From what you know now, will you recommend other treatment before or after the chemotherapy?
- What is the goal of this treatment: remission, easing discomfort, other?
- Where will I receive treatments?
- How many treatments will I have? At what intervals?
- How long will each treatment take?
- How will the medications be administered? Orally? Intravenously?
- Should I eat before I come for treatment? After treatment?
- Should I take my regular medications (if applicable)?
- Are there any medications I should avoid (such as Tylenol, aspirin, or ibuprofen)?

## About side effects
- What side effects might I experience during treatment?
- When are side effects likely to occur?
- What treatments are available to deal with or avoid side effects?

- Will the side effects get better or worse as treatment progresses?
- Will side effects interfere with the effectiveness of the chemotherapy?
- Will my treatment plan affect my daily activities?
- What long-term side effects have been identified for this medication?
- Will I lose my hair?
- What side effects should I notify you about? Whom should I call if I have a problem? Daytime number? Nighttime number?

## How Chemotherapy Drugs Are Administered

Different drugs are administered in different ways:

- By mouth (pills or capsules). Most hormonal therapies are pills.
- Intravenously, through an IV in the arm or hand. Tell your nurse if you feel any burning, coolness, or other unusual sensation where the needle enters the vein. Also mention any swelling, redness, pain, burning, or discomfort at the site during or after each treatment.
- Through an injection.
- Through a CVC (central venous catheter), a thin, flexible tube that is placed in a large vein in the chest and remains for the duration of treatment. If you have an external catheter, you cannot shower during chemo because you should not get the catheter wet. It will cause a small bulge under your blouse that will hardly be noticeable to anyone else. The incision will leave a slight scar.
- Through a portacatheter or mediport, a plastic or metal container about the size of a quarter that has been surgically implanted, usually under general anesthetic, just under your collarbone and is noticeable as a bump on the skin. With it you can swim, shower, and lie on your stomach but not on a hard surface. Although the chemotherapy drugs are injected into the port, you still feel a needle stick each time. Ask about EMLA numbing cream that can be applied an hour before your treatment is scheduled or ethyl chloride spray that can be used immediately before. Notify your doctor if you see signs of infection around the port. The port does not require the same level of care that a catheter does. At the end of treatment, the port is removed, usually in the surgeon's office under local anesthetic. You will have a scar from this implant. A portacatheter may be recommended because some chemotherapy drugs can irritate small veins and burn surrounding skin or because of lymph node removal, you can receive chemo in only one arm and the veins in that arm might become overused and unable to tolerate more chemo.

- Through a PICC line, tiny tubing usually inserted into a vein near the elbow. Patients must be careful not to break the fragile tubing. Cases have been reported of lymphedema developing as a result of numerous chemotherapy treatments into the same vein, so varying the vein used is something to ask your physician about. (See also "Lymphedema," page 137.)
- Through a pump. Pumps are either external (outside the body) or internal (implanted during surgery). Pumps control the flow of medication into the vein so patients can continue their daily activities. External pumps are usually carried in a pouch over the shoulder, the way you would carry a purse.

If properly placed and cared for, catheters, ports, and pumps cause no pain, although you will be aware of their presence. The external devices require disciplined cleaning. Both internal and external devices carry the risk of infection and formation of blood clots along the line. Your doctor may place you on a blood thinner to help prohibit clotting.

Discuss any fears or concerns with your oncologist or oncology nurse. Also inform them of any side effects you may experience. There are solutions and medications for most side effects, but unless you tell them what is happening, they can't help you.

## What Does a Chemotherapy Treatment Feel Like?

In general, the initial discomfort from chemotherapy comes from the needle stick in the arm if an IV is used or in the skin covering the port. This is usually instantaneous and feels like a quick bee sting. Usually the patient does not feel anything while the drugs are flowing into the vein. You may be given medication before the chemo to try to minimize any nausea.

Some drugs may make you sleepy right away or toward the end of the injection. Swelling or stinging or redness at the site of the injection is not normal and should be brought to the attention of the nurse.

Many times nausea or vomiting, if they come at all, or other side effects are delayed and do not occur until 24 to 48 hours after administration of the drugs.

## Things You Can Do to Prepare for Chemotherapy
### Before beginning chemotherapy

- Go to the dentist, especially if you know you need dental work. Chemotherapy can put you at risk for infection, so dental work should be avoided during this time. Any undetected oral disease or source of infection could complicate your overall health. Also, your dentist may be able to suggest ways to manage mouth problems that might arise, such as mouth sores or dry mouth.

- Get a pap smear. Chemotherapy can affect the cells on the cervix for up to a year after it is finished and give false abnormal results.
- Get a wig if you will need one.
- Arrange to be off work at least a few days after your first treatment. Many patients are able to arrange treatment late in the week so they'll have the weekend to recuperate. Warn your boss before your first treatment that you have no idea how you will react to therapy and what your schedule will be. Plan what you hope will work, but if you feel sick or tired, don't force yourself to go to work.
- Ask about having a MUGA scan to check heart function if you are to use Adriamycin or Herceptin, which can affect the heart.

### Before each treatment
- Arrange transportation. Have someone go with you for your first treatment and drive you home. Some antinausea medications can make you drowsy. Until you know how you will react right away to chemo, don't depend on driving. Many women are able to drive themselves to and from therapy, but don't count on it until you've been through the cycle once.
- Arrange for childcare during and after your treatments. You will not be able to take your children to chemotherapy and you may not feel up to caring for them when you get home. The first round will let you know how to prepare for the next times. Often you will feel reasonably well for 24 to 48 hours before side effects begin. Their duration varies considerably from person to person.
- Prepare meals for at least a few days and freeze them. Accept meals from friends if they are offered. Stock up on foods that need little or no preparation such as puddings, peanut butter, tuna, cheese, crackers, pretzels, or Popsicles.

### Within 24 hours
- Plan something relaxing or pleasurable the night before a treatment. Go to a movie, have friends over for dessert, or take a long relaxing bath in lavender water.
- Drink at least 8 to 10 cups of water a day for several days before a treatment and eat well-balanced meals to give your body the nutrients it needs to keep you healthy.

### Before you leave the house
- Have your bed ready for when you return from the clinic. Keep a list of emergency phone numbers beside the phone.
- Arrange for someone to stay with you the first 24 hours or longer, depending on how you react to your drugs.

## Tips for Going to a Chemotherapy Treatment

- Fatigue may mean a low white blood cell count, so be sure to mention your fatigue to your doctor before treatment begins.

- Take a pillow, blanket, and barf bag in the car, just in case. You'll feel better being prepared.

- Take a portable CD, DVD, or cassette player with earphones so you can listen to soothing music or a relaxation tape during your treatment.

- Breathe out deeply, rather than hold your breath, while the IV is being placed.

## Dressing for Chemotherapy

- Wear comfortable clothing. Ask where you will receive the chemo (near the wrist, bend of your arm, and so on). Wear clothing that will accommodate access to that area—something that opens in front, preferably two pieces, to accommodate an IV line in your upper chest area, for instance.

- Lounging pajamas or pants with an elastic waistband are good choices. It is difficult to maneuver tight pants if you have to use the bathroom with an IV in one hand.

- Choose socks or knee-highs so you don't have to undress totally when you get home and want to rest. Wear shoes you can just kick off.

- Often doctors' offices are chilly, so take a wrap with you.

## Eating during Chemotherapy

If chemotherapy makes you nauseated and takes away your appetite, try some of these suggestions. You need to fortify your body with nutrients as much as possible.

- Have something light in your stomach when you go for a treatment.

- Drink as much liquid as you can during the first 24 to 48 hours after treatment. This helps wash the chemicals out of your body (and, no, they are not more effective if they stay in your body longer).

- Avoid alcohol because it may interfere with how some chemotherapy drugs work. If you feel a glass of wine might relax you, check with your physician about your particular drug.

- Nibble on "comfort foods"—whatever that is for you, whether mashed potatoes, canned peas, rice, bread, applesauce, or chicken soup. Starches and carbohydrates are more easily digested than greasy, heavy, or spicy foods.

- Eat by the clock instead of when you feel hungry. Your body may not signal hunger the way it usually does and you need to keep your strength up.

- If your treatment lasts more than an hour or you have to drive a long way to the treatment site, take healthy snacks or a light meal in an insulated sack or small cooler.

- Breakfast foods are usually tolerated well during chemo. Try egg dishes, muffins, pancakes, and hot cereals.

Cancer treatment weakens your immune system by causing blood cells to be less effective in fighting infection, foreign substances, and disease. Therefore, it is important while recovering from chemotherapy to limit/avoid foods that are likely to contain high levels of bacteria such as:

- Raw and undercooked meat (including game), poultry, fish and shellfish, eggs, hot dogs, sausage, bacon, and tofu.
- Cold smoked fish (salmon), lox, and pickled fish.
- Unwashed raw vegetables and fruits and those with visible mold; all raw vegetable sprouts.
- Unpasteurized milk and milk products including yogurt and cheese; aged cheese such as blue, brie, camembert, sharp cheddar, Roquefort, and Stilton.
- Refrigerated cheese-based salad dressings and cheese requiring refrigeration.
- Unpasteurized honey, commercial fruit and vegetable juices, and beer.
- Moldy and outdated food products.
- All miso products, tempeh, and maté tea.
- Raw, uncooked brewer's yeast.
- Well water that is not tested and found safe annually.
- Herbal preparations and high-dose supplements.

## Common Side Effects

A prevalent myth about chemotherapy is that all patients get violently ill and nauseated—and if you don't, the therapy is not working. Neither of those statements is true.

The extent of your illness or side effects has nothing to do with how the treatment is affecting the cancer cells. Remember also that every instance of chemotherapy may trigger a different reaction as your body becomes used to the drug or as the effects of the drug accumulate in your body. Be sure to inform your doctor or nurse of bothersome side effects so they can assist you in overcoming them. They may be able to adjust the dose of your drugs to prevent or minimize them.

In general, chemotherapy is drying and leaves your immune system weakened so you want to keep your body and skin hydrated and take precautions against infection and germs. The simplest and most helpful things you can do are to drink 8 to 10 cups of fluid a day and practice every form of hygiene you know. (See Chapter 3, page 97, for coping with common side effects.)

## Less-Common Side Effects

- Accelerated tooth decay, gum disease.
- Acne.
- Darkening or loss of nails.
- Excessive sensitivity to sun.
- Vein darkening. Sometimes the veins that receive the chemotherapy infusions turn very dark. They usually return to their normal color within a few months after therapy ends. Some women wear long-sleeved shirts to hide the veins. Others apply makeup to make them less obvious.

## Long-Term Side Effects

Chemotherapy is a trade-off. The drugs can interrupt the cancer cell cycle, and they also can sometimes raise your risk for other health concerns in the near or far future. Although you may want to ask about the long-term effects of the drugs you are taking, do remember to weigh the benefits of the drug against the possibility of side effects.

## Types of Chemotherapy Drugs

Because cancer cells are in differing stages of growth at any given time, often a combination of drugs will be given at the same time for maximum effect. Different types of drugs affect cells in different ways.

Antibiotics such as Adriamycin (doxorubicin), Epirubicin, or Novantrone (mitoxantrone) interfere with copying the DNA, the blueprint of the cell.

Vinca alkaloids such as vinblastine, Oncovin (vincristine), and Navelbine (vinorelbine) interfere with some parts necessary for cell division as well as damaging cell structural elements. These drugs are obtained from the vinca or periwinkle plant.

Antimicrotubule agents such as the taxanes (Taxol [paclitaxel] and Taxotere [docetaxel], made from the Pacific yew tree) are deadly to cancer cells by inhibiting cell division.

Akylating agents such as Cytoxan (cyclophosphamide) interfere with several phases of cell division so that cells cannot reproduce their genetic material.

Antimetabolites such as methotrexate and 5-flourouracil hamper the manufacture of DNA, RNA, and proteins so the cell can no longer grow and divide.

A heavy metal such as Platinol (cisplatin) prohibits cell division.

Aromatase inhibitors such as Aromasin, Arimidex, and Femara block the production of aromatase, an enzyme that produces estrogen in many body tissues.

Bisphosphonates such as Aredia (pamidronate) and Zometa (zoledronate) are used with bone metastasis to help reduce bone pain and slow damage to the bone from the cancer.

Monoclonal antibodies are proteins produced by the immune system that attach to foreign cells. They can be mass-produced in laboratories. Herceptin is the first drug of this type to be approved for preventing HER-2/neu protein from promoting excessive growth of breast cancer cells.

Antiangiogenesis drugs reduce cancer growth by preventing new blood vessels, which feed the cells, from growing. Cancer cells seem not to develop a resistance to these drugs.

New cancer drugs are building on new information about tumor suppressor genes, which restrain cell growth; oncogenes, which promote cell growth; proofreader genes, which repair defective DNA; and growth factors and their receptors, hormonelike secretions and receptors that usher them into the cells. Researchers hope to find drugs to assist when these genes stop performing their intended tasks.

## How Will I Know if the Chemotherapy Is Working?

Your doctor may order a test for a tumor marker at some point during treatment. Because tumor markers are not reliable for everyone, she may skip this test. Other tests that may be ordered are a bone scan, X-ray, or CT scan. Sometimes the doctor can feel the tumor with her hands and estimate the effect of the chemo.

The presence or absence or intensity of side effects has no connection to the effectiveness of the chemo.

## Radiation

If radiation is part of your breast cancer treatment, it will probably start about four to six weeks after any surgery. This gives the surgical incision time to begin healing. The purpose of radiation is to disable cancer cells in a specific area of your body whereas chemotherapy can affect cancer cells wherever they are in the body.

Radiation therapy is the treatment of cancer with penetrating, high-energy waves or streams of particles called radiation. Radiation is many times more powerful than the waves used for X-rays. The beams are created in special machines called linear accelerators. Radiation treatment is carefully planned by your doctor; the radiation oncologist, a doctor trained in using radiation in treating cancer; the dosimetrist, who calculates the amount of radiation to be used; the radiation physicist, who maintains the equipment; and the radiation therapist and nurse, who position you for treatment and run the equipment. The beams may kill cancer cells on the spot or may disable cells so they die when they try to reproduce, so, in effect, radiation keeps working for weeks as different cells in different stages of the cell cycle mature.

Radiation therapy for breast cancer usually lasts up to six or six and a half weeks. Patients go every weekday for a treatment. The first appointment can last for an hour or more. Each subsequent appointment lasts about 15 to 30 minutes, with only about 10 minutes of actual treatment. Skipping a treatment may reduce the effectiveness of the radiation therapy.

For various reasons, some patients require additional radiation, called a boost, to the tumor site. This typically involves five to 10 extra treatments with the linear accelerator or another type of machine. Less frequently, a doctor will implant small seeds of iridium, a radioactive material, into the surgical area and leave it for 48 to 72 hours.

Radiation is sometimes used to alleviate bone pain in breast cancer metastasis.

## Common Concerns about Radiation Treatment

- Will I become radioactive? No. The dose has been carefully determined for safety and effectiveness. Only the irradiated part of the body is affected. You may kiss, hug, and have sexual relations as normal.
- How does radiation work? The radiation given for breast cancer causes a biochemical change in the cancer cells that inhibits their growth and reproduction.
- May I take vitamins or herbs or food supplements during treatment? Little research has targeted this question, so answers are incomplete. There is some concern that high doses of antioxidants such as vitamin C or A may interfere with what the radiation is trying to accomplish. Many doctors feel that standard amounts (Dietary Reference Intakes) are safe. The American Institute for Cancer Research recommends that people undergoing chemotherapy or radiation "stop taking dietary supplements with antioxidant properties for several weeks before and during treatment unless advised by their radiation therapist or oncologist."[11]
- Do the effects stop once radiation treatment is over? No. The biological changes in the body can still be active for weeks and months after treatment stops.
- What is the risk of radiation? About 1 percent of younger women who have radiation develop a second cancer. This is extremely rare for older women. However, the benefits far outweigh this slight risk. The usual dose of radiation is 4,500 to 5,000 rads (radiation absorbed dose) delivered at a rate of 160 to 180 rads per day for about six weeks with a booster dose being 1,000 to 2,000 rads to the site of the tumor. For comparison, a mammogram issues approximately 0.3 rads.

## First Visit

The first time you see the radiation oncologist is usually a consultation to review the treatment and answer your questions. The end of that visit or the next one will involve a simulation. You will lie on the treatment table while the staff enters into a computer just how much radiation the oncologist has ordered and exactly where the radiation is to be directed. Then the technician marks your chest with either tiny, permanent tattoos or indelible ink so that the doses are aimed at the same spot each day. The purpose of the permanent tattoos is to inform any doctor who gives later treatment exactly where this radiation was administered because there are lifetime limits of radiation to specific areas of the body. The tattoos are placed with needles just as any other tattoo is.

Some facilities use ink or dye instead for semipermanent markings. The ink or dye used for markings will stain your clothing, so be sure to take an old T-shirt to wear under your outer garment as you leave the office and for the remainder of your treatment time.

Your radiation oncologist may fit you with a board to lie on during each treatment. The board holds your arm on the affected side over your head. The material is molded to fit your body. When you lay on the form for each treatment, the radiation penetrates the same spot each day. Others position you using a grid on the table or special plates that are placed over the "eye" of the machine that line up with the markings on your chest.

## What Is a Radiation Treatment Like?

Radiation treatments themselves do not hurt. In fact, you will not feel, see, or smell anything emitting from the linear accelerator. Your arm that is raised over your head may ache from the uncomfortable position and your skin may become dry or irritated during the course of treatment, but you will not feel any sensation from the treatment itself.

You will first be asked to remove your top garment and put on a surgical gown. Then you will be taken to the treatment room. You will lie on the table, on the form if your doctor uses one. The nurse will expose your chest so the machine can be aimed at the markings. You will be asked to raise your arm above your head to expose the area under your arm that is to be radiated. If you have limited range of motion or tenderness in the surgical area, inform the nurse and she will make the necessary accommodations.

Once the nurse has lined up your body with the machine, she may cover your abdomen area with a shield to protect it from radiation. Then she will leave the room and turn on the machine, which is very large. You may hear thumping or humming while the machine is working. All you do is lie still, breathing normally. A therapist often watches you through a television screen or window in the control room, so you are not really alone.

This is a good time to pray, sing to yourself, or think of fun activities you want to participate in. Some people use this time to meditate or practice visualization.

The actual radiation emission will last only four to five minutes. The nurse will return and reposition the machine to radiate other areas if needed. You may have two or three areas to be radiated.

In most practices you will see the radiation oncologist about weekly.

## Dressing for Radiation Treatments

Wear something that is easy to remove, preferably pants and a top. Wear loose, soft clothing during the weeks of treatment. Natural cotton feels very good, especially if your skin becomes tender. Avoid heavily starched tops.

All during your treatment you will need to protect your clothing from the dye or ink on your chest. Purchase some men's T-shirts you can discard after treatment. Wear one all the time under your clothes. Wearing sleeveless garments will be difficult because you may have ink marks under your arm, so you will need at least a small portion of the T-shirt over that area.

If the dye does stain your clothing, it may be hard to remove. Bleach white cottons. Pretreat synthetic or colored material with Amway's LOC or another presoak for at least 30 minutes, then wash separately so the dye does not bleed onto other clothing.

## Other Tips for Radiation Treatment

- Buy inexpensive towels and washcloths or use old ones you can throw away. The dye may stain these when you pat dry.
- Inquire about the advisability of a baseline mammogram before radiation (although you probably have had one already in the diagnosis process).
- Tell your doctor if you develop any unusual symptoms such as pain, fever, coughing, or excessive perspiring.
- If you are nervous, ask the nurse to talk to you during treatment. All medical personnel will leave the room while the machine is on, but they can hear you. Ask if they will say something to you every minute or so—even to tell you how much longer a treatment will last.
- Plan a special outing after some of your treatments so you have something to look forward to—lunch with a friend, an afternoon movie, an hour in an armchair on the porch—anything that brings you pleasure.
- Eat a nutritional, high-calorie diet during treatment. Increase protein and fluid intake to help repair tissue damage.

## Most Common Side Effects of Radiation

- Raw, red skin that looks (and unfortunately sometimes feels) sunburned. It may crack, peel, or blister. If this happens, ask your doctor whether you can use any kind of cream. Some doctors allow unscented Lubriderm, 100-percent pure aloe gel (clear), RadiaCare (available at medical supply stores), Nivea skin cream, or goat milk soap. Ask if you can apply the fresh gel from an aloe vera leaf. The reaction may increase for a week or so after your final treatment before it begins to subside.

- A mild rash, particularly in the underarm area.

- Itching when the skin is peeling. Cornstarch may relieve the itch. Do not use talcum powder unless your radiation oncologist approves it. Do not scratch the area, because you are trying to avoid infection. If you find that you scratch it while you sleep, cover your hand with a sock or cotton glove.

- Tender skin. The treated areas may remain tender to the touch (even if not burned) for months after treatment. You may not be able to tolerate wearing a bra. Don't scrub when bathing. Soap is not necessary unless the area is dirty. Avoid extremes in temperature (ice packs or heating pads) on the treated area or the skin opposite the area on your back.

- Fatigue. This side effect is cumulative and often does not show up until the third or fourth week of treatment. If this happens to you, by all means give in to it. Nap. Cut back your working hours. Delegate home responsibilities. Your body is using all the red blood cells it can produce to repair healthy tissue, and the fatigue tells you it can't keep up with the demand. Your body heals itself while you sleep, so rest is what you need during this time. This is not the time to play superwoman. That role will only slow your healing. The fatigue may last several weeks, months, or even years after treatment is over while your body plays catch-up. A rule of thumb is one month of fatigue for every week of treatment you received. Although that seems like a long time (and it is), at least you know that it will eventually end. If you are still fatigued after that time, check with your doctor for other possible causes such as depression, improper diet, lack of exercise, and so on.

- Difficulty swallowing. Occasionally, if the lymph nodes behind the breast bone are radiated, the lining of the esophagus may become irritated. Avoid extreme temperatures in your food and liquids and try liquid antacid to prevent acid reflux and coat the lining of the esophagus.

- Pain, soreness, or tenderness of the remaining breast or nipple. Generally this is only a mild discomfort and will disappear about two weeks after treatment is over. Apply compresses of warm water on the sore breast.

- Stiffness of the shoulder.

- Added fibrous (scar) tissue in the area of radiation.
- Hot sensation in area being radiated.
- Decreased perspiration.
- Diarrhea.
- Moist, weepy areas on the skin.
- Slight swelling of the nipple or treated area.
- Shrinkage of the irradiated breast. Women who gain weight after radiation find that the irradiated breast normally does not change in size whereas the nonaffected breast enlarges.
- The irradiated breast may not produce enough milk for breastfeeding later on, but the nonaffected breast should function normally.
- Reduced elasticity and sensitivity of the skin in the irradiated area. This poses a risk for lymphedema. Gently stretch your arms and chest several times a day to keep the skin in those areas supple.
- Tenderness of ribs. This may last up to several years. Your ribs may also be more brittle than normal so a mild trauma, even coughing, could fracture them. Unfortunately, there is nothing you can do other than be aware of the possibility.
- Decrease in red or white cell blood counts or platelets.
- Although it's very rare, radiation can weaken the heart muscle. It may take up to five years for this effect to show up.

## Lumpectomy and Radiation

Many women are able to choose breast-sparing treatment for breast cancer: a lumpectomy and radiation rather than a modified radical mastectomy. Radiation may cause additional changes to the treated breast. These may appear after the radiation therapy is completed and may last for a year or longer. Occasionally, telangiectasias, small red areas of dilated blood vessels, may appear months after therapy. If you notice these or any other change in breast size, texture, shape, or appearance after about a year, mention them to your doctor.

Common changes that may occur the first year after radiation treatment include:

- Red areas may fade to tan, leaving some skin darker than before.
- Enlarged pores in the skin.
- Change in sensitivity in the skin on the breast, either increased or decreased.
- Thicker and firmer skin and tissue on breast.
- Change in size of breast: larger due to fluid buildup or smaller due to scar tissue.

Some women have implants of radioactive material temporarily placed near the site of the lumpectomy a week or two after the external radiation therapy is completed. This is done with an anesthetic. The implants may make your breast feel tight or tender. After they are removed, you may experience any of the changes just mentioned. Keep your doctor informed.

The implantation of radioactive material into a malignancy is known as brachytherapy. It has been used as a booster treatment following standard radiation treatment as well as the sole treatment for small, localized tumors. The advantages are a much shorter course of treatment than the standard six weeks and improved cosmetic results because only a portion of the breast is treated.

Brachytherapy, still considered experimental by some, is administered several ways. One is inserting several hollow nylon tubes into the affected part of the breast under local anesthetic and administering high-dose iridium 192 isotope for five minutes twice a day for five days. This method delivers a homogeneous dose to the affected area. A second method called MammoSite inserts a catheter with a balloon and one dose of iridium in the center of the biopsy cavity. The disadvantage is that the dose cannot be modified for the portion or size of breast being treated and some normal tissue may be affected.

Some physicians will use this technique only if the patient has a tumor less than 5 centimeters in diameter and has no more than four positive lymph nodes. Some doctors will not treat anyone with this technique if she has any positive lymph nodes. A benefit of this method is that it can be performed shortly after a lumpectomy and before chemotherapy. It is also a consideration for patients who live a distance from a radiation site. A five-day stay is much more tolerable than six weeks of long drives or lodging away from home.

## Symptoms to Tell Your Doctor About

Not all changes in the treatment area carry any serious meaning. However, your doctor is the one to decide. Tell her about any of the following or any other side effects that bother you:

• Signs of infection (redness, heat, rash, and so on).
• Changes in skin color.
• Itching, flaking.
• Tenderness.

Very rarely are other organs impacted by radiation for breast cancer. Ask your radiation oncologist about any side effects to watch for, such as swelling of the arm or difficulty swallowing.

## Skin Care during Radiation

The most important thing to remember during radiation is not to wash the marks off your skin. These are critical for lining up the area for treatment each day. The marks will fade with time, and the doctor or technician may reapply them. Bathe that area with a soft washcloth and clear, warm water. Do not use soap or creams that may leave a layer on the skin that could interfere with treatment. Pat the area dry gently.

Other precautions include:

- Do not rub, scratch, or irritate the skin in the irradiated area. Do not use soap on the markings on your chest. Just let water run lightly over marked areas so you don't wash them away. They can be re-marked, however, if they fade.

- Avoid sun exposure in the treatment area. Do not use sunscreens on the area during treatment and until skin has healed completely.

- Do not use cosmetics, perfumes, medications, soaps, lotions, talcum powder, deodorant, or home remedies in the treatment area during treatment. Especially avoid aluminum in products because it (and other metals) can deflect the radiation and diminish the treatment. Ask about water-based moisturizers you can use. Amoena makes a product called response powder that contains cornstarch and silica, absorbs moisture and perspiration without caking, and is a dry lubricant. Other options are dusting under your arms with cornstarch or using an all-natural deodorant.

- Do not apply skin lotions within two hours of a treatment. Aquaphor, a lotion, or Natures Sunshine Healing AC, a cream, can soothe dry, itching skin.

- Avoid temperature extremes in the area such as heating pads or ice packs, saunas, hot tubs, whirlpools, or sunlamps. Use lukewarm water for bathing.

- Avoid shaving in the treatment area until the skin has completely recovered. If you must, use an electric razor. Do not use preshave lotion or hair removal products on the treated area.

- Minimize rubbing and irritation by wearing loose-fitting clothing made of natural fibers such as cotton or silk. If you are large-breasted and need the support of a bra, wear a cotton sports bra with wide straps and support around the collarbone. You can usually resume wearing a bra three or four weeks after treatment if your skin has healed. If you will be wearing a prosthesis, you should wait about six weeks after treatment because it is heavier than your breast was.

- Expose the irradiated area to air as much as possible.

- Avoid contact with adhesives, tapes, Band-Aids, and medication patches in the treated area.

- Avoid necklaces or jewelry that could rub the area being treated.
- If you dye your hair, be careful that the chemicals don't drip onto your skin and irritate it.

Even after treatment is completed, it is important to take special care of the irradiated area. Continue to avoid sun exposure and heat extremes and protect against scrapes and infections. Use a moisturizer until the skin is no longer dry.

## Common Emotional Reactions to Radiation

Although radiation does not hurt in the sense a wasp sting or a broken arm hurts, it can be uncomfortable for some women. Many problems are emotionally based. For instance, Hester Hill Schnipper, chief oncology social worker at Beth Israel Deaconess Medical Center in Boston, has identified two groups of women who have difficulties during radiation treatment: women with a history of sexual abuse (lying still while a powerful object hovers over them releases past fears) and women whose main coping strategy is to avoid a problem (the daily treatments are reminders of their diagnosis, which they may have been able to ignore until now).

Other women are afraid because of the terrible effects they have seen from radiation in industrial accidents or wartime actions. The dose of radiation cancer patients receive is carefully measured and directed at a specific area of the body. The dose is adjusted for how deep the radiation is to go into the body so that tissue and organs near the target site are not affected.

## After Treatment Ends

You'll want to throw a party when your everyday appointments come to an end. Do so! And follow these recommendations:

- Continue gentle washing of the treated area for at least a month. Rinse well to keep soap from staying on the skin.
- Use moisturizers or the special cream your doctor gives you.
- Avoid sun exposure to the treated areas—for life. If you must be in the sun, use a sunscreen with SPF of 15 or higher or sunblock.
- Follow-up visits are important. The period between them will lengthen as time goes on.
- Follow a heart-healthy diet. Radiation leaves you at higher risk for heart disease.[12]

Although most side effects disappear within a few weeks, some may linger or be permanent. For instance, your treated skin may remain slightly darker than the rest and may continue to be sensitive to the sun. Skin elasticity may be diminished forever. Your fatigue could last many months. Check this book for tips on dealing with side effects or consult your doctor about any that bother you.

## Surgery

Often the only information your doctor thinks to tell you about your surgery is the medical name (biopsy, lumpectomy, modified radical mastectomy, and so on) and when to report to the hospital. For most women, fear of the unknown is almost as strong as their fear of cancer.

## Questions to Ask Your Surgeon about Surgery

Here are some questions to ask your doctor or nurse. Knowledge is a powerful sedative.

- How long will the surgery take? How long will I be in the hospital?
- Is there any preparation at the hospital such as taking blood?
- How long can someone stay with me? Can my husband, daughter, or friend stay with me in the holding area?
- What will you do if you find something you are not expecting?
- Where will the incision be?
- How long will it take the incision to heal?
- If you are considering reconstruction: Is it possible to do reconstruction or prepare for reconstruction at the same time as this surgery? What are the advantages and disadvantages of doing both procedures at the same time?
- How will I feel when I wake up? Will I be nauseated? If so, for how long?
- How much pain might I expect? What can be done about it?
- What side effects might occur? How long might they last? Might any be permanent?
- Will I have to do anything special to care for the wound/site? For how long?
- Will I have any restrictions in my activities? For how long?
- When will I know the pathology report? How will I receive it?
- How do I take care of the drains?
- When should I begin moving/using the arm? What exercises should I do? Will you set up an appointment with a Reach to Recovery volunteer (an American Cancer Society program)?
- When can I wear a bra again?
- When can I wear a prosthesis and what kind?
- What should I eat and not eat?
- When should I make a follow-up appointment?

Also ask your doctor about two options that will make your postoperative experience more tolerable. Ask if she can use dissolving stitches so you can avoid staple removal (although that is not painful, just uncomfortable). Also inquire about a special plastic dressing on the wound that would allow you to shower immediately after surgery. Feeling fresh again is powerful in your emotional recovery.

## Sentinel Node Biopsy

It is becoming more common for a surgeon to perform a sentinel node biopsy before or at the beginning of surgery for breast cancer. This is a procedure in which a radioactive tracer is injected into the tumor or the adjacent tissue before surgery or a blue dye, isosulfan blue, is injected during surgery and the path of that substance is examined. The first lymph node the dye travels to, sometimes called the gatekeeper node, is identified and carefully examined during surgery. If it is free of cancer, then it is assumed that no cancer cells have spread elsewhere in the body and usually no further lymph nodes are removed. Without this procedure, a surgeon has to remove a section of tissue, hoping to retrieve 10 or more nodes for later examination. Of course, once those lymph nodes are removed, your lymph system is permanently impaired.

Ask your surgeon about this procedure and check with your insurance company about coverage. Ask also about false negatives. In about 10 percent of cases further examination of the sentinel node will reveal cancer after all.[13] You may want to know how your doctor would handle that news should it occur and what his experience has been with false negatives.

There are some situations in which sentinel node biopsy may not be appropriate, including very large tumors, preoperative chemotherapy (unless sentinel node biopsy is done first), pregnancy, or prior axillary surgery. With this procedure your urine will be blue afterwards.

## Preparing for Surgery

Prior to surgery, your surgeon may order additional tests such as blood work, a chest X-ray, and an electrocardiogram. These are routine for many surgeries, not just breast cancer, to be sure you are fit enough for surgery.

Prepare your body by consuming high-protein and calorie-dense foods to compensate for the time you will not be allowed to eat or may not feel like eating. Concentrate on nutritious foods to give your body tools for rebuilding after surgery. Other helpful tips are:

- Drink at least eight glasses of water before midnight on the night before your surgery because some pain medications you might require can cause constipation.

- Ask your doctor if you can take vitamin C for two weeks prior to surgery to support your immune system.
- Avoid drugs that thin the blood such as vitamin E and nonsteroidal anti-inflammatories such as aspirin, Motrin, Advil, and Naprosyn for five to seven days before surgery.
- Inform your doctor of all other substances you take on a regular basis, including herbs and over-the-counter medications, in case any might interfere with surgery. For instance, garlic, ginkgo, ginseng, and green tea can cause bleeding; kava and valerian can make anesthetics more potent; St. John's wort can interfere with some drugs; echinacea can alter immune function; ginseng can lower blood sugar levels; and ephedra can elevate heart rate and blood pressure.[14]
- Discuss "ghost surgery" with your doctor. This is a situation in which a doctor or resident other than the one you have met with performs the actual surgery. Although credentials may not be an issue, a doctor who just shows up in the operating room does not know you and may not have been informed about your concerns and preferences. Though this is an accepted medical practice, discuss it with your surgeon if it concerns you. Some women draft a written agreement that they ask their surgeon to sign saying that only he or she will perform the surgery.
- Ask your surgeon or anesthesiologist to talk to you during surgery with positive affirmations or to play soothing music. Evidence shows that our subconscious is aware during surgery and that hearing positive messages can help healing.

## Special Breast Cancer Preparations

Before a complete axillary dissection (not a sentinel node biopsy):
- Measure both arms in several places (wrist, 3 inches below your elbow, 3 inches below your armpit, around the palm of your hand, and a couple of fingers especially on your dominant side) as a baseline for measurements for lymphedema, a possible complication of surgery that involves swelling of the arm, hand, fingers, or chest wall.
- Ask the hospital for a pink "Lymphedema Alert" band for your arm on the side of your surgery.
- Post a sign over your bed that reads, "No blood pressure or injections to be given in right/left arm."
- Before you are medicated, tell the anesthesiologist that you do not want to use the surgery side for blood pressure or IVs. Ask her to be very careful with that arm during the surgery and while moving you to and from the operating table. Write on your arm in marker: "No BP, no stix."

## Home Preparation

- Leave your home prepared for your return from the hospital. Clear a path to the bathroom (no cords, rugs, and so forth) so you can get there safely if you are groggy.

- Arrange for someone to stay the first night with you because anesthesia can leave you woozy, sleepy, or nauseous.

- Place a small bell next to your bed to alert your caregiver when you need something or use a baby monitor with a plug-in unit and a portable receiver. Your caregiver can then move about the house and yard and still hear when you call.

- Stock up with bendable straws and plenty of soft foods and liquids. (See "Clear liquid diet" and "Soft diet," page 93.)

- Have a comfortable bed ready with lots of pillows to prop up your arm and support your back.

- Have beside the phone a list of phone numbers for doctors, the hospital and pharmacy, and family and friends.

## What to Take with You

Although we think of hospitals as self-contained communities, sometimes it is comforting to have a few personal items along. Consider taking the following:

- Another person! It will be especially helpful if you can have your husband, mother, daughter, or close friend stay in your hospital room the night after surgery. You might be groggy or not feeling well and might not understand or remember much of what the doctor tells you when he visits after surgery. That person can be your advocate for getting a meal that was forgotten, medication you need, or an appointment with a social worker, dietician, or other hospital specialist. Also she can encourage you and assist in getting any information you need.

- An ID, a referral, an insurance card, or any other paperwork, if needed. Will you need to make a payment before you are admitted? Before you check out?

- Comfortable clothing to go home in. Take a top that buttons in front, not one that slips over your head or buttons in back. You'll need a roomy top, not a body-hugger. If you want a bra, take a loose-fitting, soft one that fastens in the front. Tight, back-fastening bras (or underwires) are not appropriate. Ask your surgeon if you can even wear a bra.

- A tape recorder with earphones and some favorite tapes; light reading material.

- A toothbrush and toothpaste.
- A comb or brush.
- A headpiece for sleeping if you have lost your hair from chemotherapy. (It's generally cold in hospitals.) Or bring a headband to keep hair under control if you can't wash it for several days.
- Makeup. Some women like to apply foundation or blush; others could care less.
- A robe and socks in case you get cold.
- An eye mask if you are sensitive to lights.
- A teddy bear. Even if you're 60, those little critters are wonderful companions and comforters. Be bold and ask if you can have it in the recovery room.

Leave all your jewelry (including wedding ring and watch) at home. Do not take a purse or wallet if you have another family member to handle any payments for you.

# What Happens during Surgery and Right After?

If you have reconstruction at the same time as your surgery, these guidelines will not apply to you and your hospital stay will be longer.

### Sentinel node biopsy

This procedure identifies the first lymph node into which the tumor might drain. Sometimes this surgery is done a few days before a surgery to remove the tumor and sometimes it is done at the beginning of the surgery.

### Axillary dissection

This surgery removes axillary lymph nodes, which are located in the underarm area. These are then reviewed by a pathologist. The amount of tissue removed is determined by an assessment of the likelihood of affected nodes. The exact number of lymph nodes taken is not known until the pathologist examines the tissue.

When you wake up, you will probably have a drain under your arm to prevent fluid buildup. You can carry it in a fanny pack or a pocket. (See "Drains," page 73.) One study reported that 72 percent of women with this procedure reported pain, weakness, numbness, or loss of range of motion over their lifetime.

### Lumpectomy/breast conservation surgery

This procedure involves removal of the tumor, some surrounding breast tissue, and sometimes a few lymph nodes. Often a lumpectomy is day surgery. Expect some numbness and tenderness at the surgical site. Numbness may last six months or forever. Tenderness generally fades in a few months. Wearing a supportive sports bra to bed for several nights may help stabilize the breast and speed healing. If your incision was near the nipple, the numbness may interfere with your sexual pleasure. Your skin may feel leathery or thick, and sutures (thread) may emerge through the incision site. As long as they are not accompanied by pus, ignore them and they will disappear. Some women experience shooting pain in the chest wall and breast for up to several months. A cold pack may help relieve pain.

If the lumpectomy was for invasive breast cancer and lymph nodes were removed, you may experience side effects similar to those after a modified radical mastectomy.

## Simple mastectomy

During this surgery, the entire breast and nipple are removed but not the underlying pectoral (chest) muscle. A sampling of lymph nodes may be taken. This is the surgery used for prophylactic mastectomies, elective surgeries for women with high risk for developing breast cancer or those with early-stage breast cancer (DCIS) who choose a very conservative treatment.

When you wake, you will have gauze and tape or an elastic bandage wound tightly over the incision site, and the incision will be stapled or sutured closed. Many women feel no real pain with this procedure because generally nerves are not cut. If nerves are cut, you may experience numbness or tenderness at the incision site and in the adjacent area. Skin will feel tighter when you reach or stretch; with gentle exercise, this usually corrects itself.

Some women develop a hypersensitivity to touch or have odd sensations in the area that may last many months or even years. This may make it hard to wear a prosthesis; sometimes even clothing is painful. One woman reports that a physical therapist had her gently pull a common, dry washcloth across that area three times a day. She worked up to three minutes. The washcloth felt like sandpaper to her chest, but eventually the sensitivity went away.

Some women have the experience of "something tight plastered to my chest." Sometimes, as the nerves grow back, these sensations disappear.

## Modified radical mastectomy

This surgery is similar to the simple mastectomy. The entire breast and most axillary lymph nodes are removed. This procedure is sometimes called a total mastectomy.

Many women are pleasantly surprised to experience little or no pain after this surgery. The incision may pull and feel uncomfortable, but some feel no sharp pain because no muscles have been cut as in other types of surgery. Other women are quite sore and have difficulty lifting their arm. The axillary node dissection can leave your shoulder sore and the muscles there tight. Tenderness under the arm and in the chest area from fluid buildup or swelling usually goes away in six months, although it may last much longer. Numbness under the arm and in the chest area is another common result of this surgery. Feeling may return or you may be numb forever. One woman described her numbness "like having a brick inside me there."[15] While numb, use an electric razor or Magic Shaving Powder depilatory to avoid cuts while removing underarm hair.

You may be stiff and have limited range of motion. (See "Frozen Shoulder," page 120, for tips on assessing this condition.) Swelling under the arm and in the surgical area is common and usually short-lived.

If you experience pain, tell your doctor and have it assessed. Sometimes nerve damage happens in surgery. The acute pain can become chronic if not treated immediately. In one study, 12 to 55 percent of mastectomy patients experienced phantom breast pain; 35 to 39 percent experienced pain of the chest, axilla, or arm; 61 percent reported chronic pain; and 100 percent reported decreased sensation.

The two things you will notice when you wake up in the recovery room after surgery are that the top half of your chest is wrapped snugly in gauze or an elastic bandage and that you have a plastic bulb dangling from your rib cage on each side where a breast was removed.

Generally you will stay in the hospital overnight after this procedure.

### Radical mastectomy

This used to be the standard treatment for breast cancer, but it is not common today. In this surgery, the entire breast, the pectoral muscle (behind the breast), and the axillary lymph nodes are removed. Lymphedema and shoulder weakness were real concerns.

### Mastectomy with reconstruction

Postsurgical effects will depend on the type of reconstruction you had. If you had a tissue transfer, the area the tissue was taken from will be sore for several days or weeks in addition to the breast area. If you had an expander, the skin at the breast will be tense and the pain can be intense. Generally by a month out, the discomfort can be controlled by over-the-counter pain relievers. Scars from the surgeries will fade in a year or two but will always be visible.

## Drains

The Jackson-Pratt drain is to drain any fluid buildup from the surgical area outside the body. Sometimes a patient will have one drain below the armpit and another below the chest area. Although you may notice the drains, they normally do not cause much discomfort, though sometimes they can be painful. Talk to your doctor about the cause if pain develops.

The drains, which are 12 to 18 inches long and snaked through your tissue, usually stay in for the first one to two weeks, although sometimes a patient will drain for several weeks. If the drain is removed too early, fluid can collect under the skin to form a seroma, which feels like a golf ball in the armpit and can be very uncomfortable. Seromas must be aspirated in one or several visits to the doctor's office.

The doctor will ask you to empty the fluid into a container, record the amount and color of fluid collected, and bring the record to the next office visit. Ensure that the drain is not tugging unduly on your skin. Wearing a cloth belt to which you can fasten the drains helps relieve the pressure as the fluid builds up. Inform your doctor if the fluid is bright red (which might indicate bleeding) or if the skin around the drain is red (which might indicate an infection).

When the drainage fluid has diminished to almost nothing, the surgeon will remove the drains during an office visit. Some women report no pain with this procedure whereas others find it very painful. Ask your surgeon what can be done to prevent pain.

## After-Surgery Concerns
### Postoperative pain

Although 10 to 30 percent of patients experience postoperative pain after breast cancer surgery, many physicians do not discuss this before surgery or treat it adequately if it does occur. In the first four to six weeks after surgery, many patients will experience a range of normal discomfort or pain in their arms or chest wall. It is not unusual for the surgical area to tingle the first few weeks and then be numb.

However, after 30 to 90 day,s some women may begin to have sharp, stabbing pain, burning, tingling, itching, or numbness. Some women describe it as a spasm or charley horse of the armpit or breast or as the pain and sensation of a phantom breast. Others report sleep disturbances. This pain is thought to be the result of cutting of the intercostobrachial nerves during axillary node dissection. This cutting is necessary because the nerves are located in the middle of the lymph nodes that have to be removed. However, sometimes the pain begins after chemotherapy or radiation. It is more common after a mastectomy than after a lumpectomy.

This type of pain is sometimes called postmastectomy/postaxillary dissection pain syndrome (PM/PADPS), post-breast surgery pain syndrome

(PBSPS), postmastectomy pain syndrome (PMPS), postaxillary pain syndrome (PAPS), or post-breast therapy pain syndrome (PBTPS). It is not a formally recognized medical condition (in insurance code books). The pain can be chronic or involve serious sensory disturbances such as pain with movement, touching, or change of temperature. Sometimes wearing a prosthesis or even clothing of any kind can be unbearable. It can develop in your arm, shoulder, chest, or even back. A more debilitating condition can occur when nerve endings grow back abnormally. This is called reflex sympathetic dystrophy (RSD). The increasing use of sentinel node biopsy seems to be reducing the incidents of postsurgical pain because fewer women are having extensive axillary dissection.

If you develop postmastectomy pain, tell your doctor. Remedies may include antidepressants (not because it's in your head, but to reprogram nerve pathways in the brain that send pain signals), anticonvulsants such as Neurontin, anti-inflammatories, pain medications, biofeedback, or surgery. If you keep hearing, "It'll go away," ask to consult with a pain specialist. If movement causes the pain, you may inadvertently restrict arm activity, which could lead to frozen shoulder.

## Eating
- Immediately following surgery you will probably be on a clear liquid diet until your bowel and digestive functions return to normal. Then you may be allowed a soft diet for a short time before you resume your normal diet.
- If you have limited networks for support after surgery, freeze some meals in individual portion sizes before surgery and stock up on your favorite snacks. You will need to keep up your strength and should reserve your energy for healing rather than household chores.
- This is not the time for restrictive dieting! Eat healthy foods and enough to rebuild your strength. There will be plenty of time for diets later. Now is the time to give your body the nourishment it needs to heal.

## Healing
- Slight postsurgical swelling in the upper arm and chest is common and does not mean you have lymphedema.
- You may experience numbness or tingling in the upper inner arm and armpit. Numbness usually diminishes, although not always. Because of this, be careful shaving under your arms.
- Do not use deodorant until your stitches are removed under your arm. Do not rub hard when drying off after a bath.

- Sleep with a small pillow under your affected arm for at least 24 hours after surgery. This may prevent swelling. Use the arm as needed, but don't overdo and avoid as much stretching and pulling as you can while the drains are still attached.
- Graciously accept all offers of help for at least a few days. Your body has undergone a major trauma, and you need to rest to promote healing.
- After the surgeon gives permission, apply vitamin E cream or aloe vera gel (or liquid straight from the leaves of the plant) to the scars to help them fade more quickly.
- Some European surgeons order compression sleeves to be worn as a preventative measure, although American doctors have not adopted this practice.

## Posture

- Resist the tendency to droop your shoulders forward. This is natural either to protect your tender area or as a subconscious attempt to hide your "new" look. Holding your shoulders back and your head high will help not only your physical healing (the muscles will be stretched) but also your emotional health. You eventually will realize that discomfort with your profile is something the other person has to resolve for herself and is not your problem.

## Dressing

- Reach to Recovery volunteers can bring you a light mastectomy bra and fluff filler that is soft and comfortable to wear after surgery—after your surgeon gives permission.
- Neither you nor your doctor will probably want a regular prosthesis rubbing against your incision site for up to six weeks. Even after the doctor gives you permission to wear a bra, the weight of the prosthesis may be irritating.
- For several days or even months after surgery, you may prefer a soft camisole or undershirt to a bra. Some catalogs and stores carry camisoles with pockets for prostheses; some versions even come with lightweight cotton fillers. Ladies First, Inc., makes the Softee postmastectomy camisole. One style has a discrete pocket for the drainage bulb. The camisole can be stepped into if raising your arms is painful. Stretch straps and lightweight breast forms provide shape and practicality.
- If you are self-conscious about your flat profile, wear vests or jackets, loose tops, or scarves that hang over your shoulder. Pockets in top garments can be stuffed with tissue for a fuller effect.
- For sleeping or lounging, pick loose nightgowns or pajamas that fasten in the front. You will have limited use of your arm for a while and may not be able to raise it over your head to slip on clothing.

## Exercises

Because you will not be moving your shoulder and arm very much while you are healing from a mastectomy, you are at risk of developing adhesive capsulitis, commonly known as frozen shoulder. This is a painful limitation of your range of motion. It occurs somewhat more frequently if your nondominant side is the side of the surgery. As soon as the surgeon gives you permission (usually after the drains are removed), you should begin prescribed exercises to encourage the return of motion, stretch the shoulder joint, and keep the affected muscles toned.

Use your shoulder for any task that does not produce pain, and stop if pain occurs. This is not a situation when you want to work through the pain. The healing period will be characterized by periods of progress and plateau. At first you may find it easier to do exercises under a warm shower. The warmth loosens the muscles. Gentle moving in a warm pool is also easy on your muscles.

The first week after surgery, with your doctor's permission, raise your affected arm above your heart level and open and close your hand 15 to 25 times. Then bend and straighten your elbow. Repeat three or four times a day to reduce swelling by pumping lymph fluid out of your arm. Avoid sleeping on your affected side.

Following are some exercises to include in your stretching/strengthening routine after your surgeon says you can begin exercising. Do them slowly and smoothly. Never bounce or jerk when you exercise. When you begin to hurt, hold that position for two seconds and release the hold. Never force painful range of motion.

- **The Shrug.** While sitting or standing, gently lift your shoulders towards your ears. Hold for three seconds and slowly lower them. Build up to 10 repetitions. Next roll your shoulders forward in a complete circle, then backward. Build up to 10 repetitions.

- **The Bird.** Sitting or standing, stretch your arms to each side and raise them to shoulder height. You may not be able to do this initially. Raise them together as far as you comfortably can, then raise one all the way if the other hurts to do so. Flap them gently a few times like a bird. Slowly lower them to your sides. Repeat 10 times. Then raise your arms again to shoulder height and slowly rotate them in a circle while fully outstretched.

- **Don't Bow.** While standing, hold a rod (a piece of PVC pipe or dowel from a hardware store or part of a broomstick) horizontally behind you. Keep both arms at the same height. Keeping your back and arms straight, slowly lift your arms behind you as high as you can, then lower the rod to your buttocks. At first you may lift the rod only an inch or so. That's okay. Progress is gradual.

- **Lifting the Veil.** Lie on your back with your legs straight in front of you. Hold a rod with both hands, resting it on your thighs. Keeping your arms straight, slowly raise the rod in an arc, over your head until your arms are beside your ears. Again, it will take time for you to be able to do this. Don't rush it.

- **The Prize.** Have someone place a small reward (such as a piece of candy or a gift certificate to your favorite store) on a high shelf or tape it to the wall at arms' length above your head. Crawl your fingers up the cabinet or wall until you reach the prize. At first you may not be able to climb very high, so place some treats at increasing distances for encouragement.

- **The Chicken Walk.** Place your hands on your shoulders. Gently raise your elbows until they are level with your shoulders. Repeat 10 times. Once you can do this, rotate your elbows in a slow circle before lowering them.

- **The Nap.** Standing or lying down, cross your fingers behind your head. Now gently stretch out your elbows until they are perpendicular to your shoulders.

- **Samson Stretch.** Standing in the center of a doorway with your feet slightly apart and your toes 6 inches back from the threshold, place your hands at shoulder height on both sides of the door frame. Gently lean forward, keeping your back straight. Stop when you feel pain in your shoulder or chest. Hold for the count of 10 and release. Repeat 10 times. As your muscles stretch, move your hands further up the door frame and/or step back further from the threshold.

- **Scissors.** Lift your arms to shoulder height, with arms straight in front of you and palms down. Slowly cross one hand over the other, then switch the top hand. Repeat with the palms facing up to use different muscles. Repeat 10 times.

Ask your doctor to refer you to the American Cancer Society's Reach to Recovery Program for additional exercises.

## Recuperated?

As with any surgery, expect several weeks to months before you regain total use of the affected areas. Depending on the restrictions your surgeon gives, you should be able to do the following without pain four to six weeks after a lumpectomy, axillary node dissection, or modified radical mastectomy and about three months after reconstruction surgery. If you cannot, ask for a referral to a physical therapist to evaluate your progress.

- Move your arm in all directions.
- Fasten your bra in back.

- Easily reach into an overhead cabinet without pain.
- Carry bags of groceries or the laundry basket without pain. (Don't carry more than 10 pounds until your doctor gives permission.)
- Have energy to do your normal housework.
- Stretch your arms to each side at shoulder height and above your head.

Once your surgeon gives permission, consider water aerobics as an exercise option. The buoyancy of the water lessens the impact of exercise on your muscles and joints, and the water itself has a calming effect in addition to increasing resistance for a better workout. I can exercise about twice as long in a pool as I can on land because my muscles don't tire out as easily.

## Reconstruction

Breast reconstruction means surgically re-creating the shape of a breast complete with nipple and areola (dark circle around the nipple). Although reconstruction sounds like a perfect solution for the removal of a breast, some women find that is not the case. A reconstructed breast, whether from your own flesh (transflap) or an implant, will not have the sensations your breast had. The feel of the skin may be different also. Some women are very pleased with their new look; others are disappointed in the additional surgeries and medical care needed and the "permanent lump" now attached to their bodies. Although there is no way to know how you will feel afterward, take this possibility into consideration when making your decision.

By all means, ask to see pictures of actual breasts reconstructed by the surgeon you are considering and using the type of procedure you are considering. Even the saline and silicon implants have a different look and feel. You need to know exactly what you are choosing.

Probably the most important aspects of your decision regarding reconstruction are these:

- What are the dangers? Although most plastic surgeons will paint a rosy picture of reconstruction, there is another side of the story for some women: complications, some of which last for years; hardness around the area that requires additional surgery; leaking or rupturing of the implant; and so forth. Talk with several plastic surgeons and ask specifically about the percentage of their patients who have problems, what kind of problems, what was required to solve them, and so on. Talk to other women who have had reconstruction and learn about their experience. This may give you additional questions to ask.
- Do you smoke? Women who smoke have more complications, regardless of the type of reconstruction. One study showed that stopping smoking at least three weeks before surgery reduced the rate of complications.

- How much of your self-esteem is wrapped up in your breast? Can you be a "whole" person without a breast? Your answer to this is important. If you feel you absolutely must have two breasts to have value, then you may have issues that not even a perfectly shaped breast can resolve. Although breasts are fun, pleasing, and a significant part of our sexuality, we are more than our breasts. No one wants to forfeit a breast, but there is life after a mastectomy, even a bilateral mastectomy. If you depend upon your breasts for your self-image, then there is a high probability you will not be pleased with your new look because it will be different from your previous standard.
- Is it best to have reconstruction at the same time as a mastectomy or later? There is no right answer for everyone. The decision depends upon your treatment plan, your insurance benefits, and other factors.

## Immediate Reconstruction

A woman can choose to have a breast reconstructed at the same time as a mastectomy or later. If you choose immediate reconstruction:

- You may eliminate one surgery.
- You may adapt to the reconstructed breast faster if you have it when you wake up from the mastectomy and never see yourself without a breast.
- Sometimes your cosmetic results are better because the cancer surgeon and plastic surgeon consult during surgery to ensure adequate tissue for reconstruction and an incision that lends the optimal medical and cosmetic results.
- Radiation sometimes hardens breast tissue and can make reconstruction more difficult or, in some cases, impractical. Discuss this possibility with your oncologist before you begin any treatment.

## Delayed Reconstruction

If you may want reconstruction later, consult with a plastic surgeon before the mastectomy so he can discuss options with the surgeon that may give you better cosmetic results.

If you are scheduled for chemotherapy after a mastectomy, you probably should delay reconstruction. Any infection or delay in healing of the reconstructed breast could delay the chemotherapy.

Anticipate restrictions for several weeks after reconstruction surgery. Your doctor will tell you what activities to avoid.

## Types of Reconstruction

There are several types of reconstruction. Your type of breast cancer surgery, further treatment, general body composition, and other factors will determine which one(s) you are eligible for.

## Implant

A pouch filled with silicone gel or a saline solution in a silicone envelope is placed under the skin and chest muscle. The surgery takes one to two hours. The saline feels more like water than a real breast but apparently is harmless if the solution leaks into the body. Studies are being done to determine the safety of silicone breast implants although they are still available for women having reconstruction after breast cancer.

## Tissue expander

An inflatable device is inserted behind or on top of the pectoral muscle and will be filled with saline over several weeks or months so that the skin stretches slowly. Once or twice a week for six to 10 weeks you will go to your surgeon's office to have more fluid injected until the expander is about the size of your other breast. Then the expander is removed and either a silicone or saline implant is inserted in the doctor's office under local anesthetic or in the hospital. The expander can be inserted at the time of a mastectomy or later. The surgery takes about one to two hours. You might stay in the hospital about three days.

The safety of silicone in breast implants continues to be debated. Women still choose this option because of the realistic appearance. However, all women who use the silicone have to enroll in a study of its safety. After the implant is positioned, your body makes scar tissue around it. In about 5 percent of cases, this scar tissue is so hard it is painful and distorts the shape of the breast. Special exercises and massage may reduce the likelihood of this complication. If it does develop, you must replace the implant. Another possible complication is leakage. After 10 to 15 years, leakage is almost inevitable although it may not be significant. Again, do your homework about the danger of silicone in your body. A leaking implant should be replaced.

## Transfer of tissue

Tissue is transferred from another part of your body along with the underlying layer of fat, muscle, and blood supply to the breast area. Usually this tissue is taken from the lower abdomen (TRAM flap, transfer of rectus abdominal muscle), the upper back or side (latissimus dorsi flap), or the buttocks (gluteal flap). In the first two surgeries, the original blood vessels are not cut.

In the latissimus dorsi flap, an incision is made under the scapula. Part of the muscle from the upper back and the fat and skin covering it are pulled through a tunnel to the breast area. Although these surgeries eliminate any concern about a foreign substance in the body, such as saline, they are much more extensive surgeries, require a large incision (and leave a long scar), and involve healing in two areas of your body at the same time. Recuperation is longer and discomfort is more pronounced. The latissimus dorsi scar is covered by a bra or swimsuit. The TRAM incision is covered by a one-piece bathing suit or relatively high two-piece swimsuit. Women who smoke have a higher rate of complication from these surgeries because of vessel damage. Women with little fat or with previous scars in the affected areas are not generally good candidates for this surgery. A more complicated procedure than an implant, the tissue transfer operation lasts three to six hours and requires a hospital stay of up to seven days. Taking tissue from the back usually has the least number of complications, although the texture and color of the skin differ from those of the breast area.

The TRAM operation gives you the extra benefit of a tummy tuck. You will have a scar from hipbone to hipbone about midway between the top of your pubic hair and your navel—and you may have a new navel if it was displaced or distorted in the surgery. Although the cosmetic results may be very nice, be aware that the sensations of your real breast will not exist. You also may be numb in the abdominal area where the tissue was removed.

If tissue is taken from the buttocks, the scar is usually hidden in the buttocks crease. This is a more complicated surgery because blood vessels must be disconnected, then reconnected. The surgery can last up to 12 hours. If any of the blood vessels do not regenerate, then additional surgery may be necessary.

### Free flap transfer

This is similar to transfer of tissue, but the substitute tissue and blood vessels are severed from their original area and reconnected to the new blood supply in the chest instead of being tunneled through the body as in the regular transfer operation. Less muscle needs to be removed for this surgery, so healing may be faster. This surgery is very delicate and may take longer than a regular TRAM surgery. It should be done only by a plastic surgeon with experience in microsurgery.

### Skin-sparing mastectomy

This technique removes the breast tissue but does not compromise the blood supply to the outer skin around the breast. This skin is used to cover an implant or a tissue transfer and gives very natural results. There is some risk of recurrence in the skin flap, but it can easily be detected by manual examination.

If only one breast is removed, a woman generally wants the reconstructed breast to match her natural one in shape and fullness. To accomplish this, it may be necessary to operate on the natural breast to make it larger (augmentation) or smaller (reduction) or to lift it (mastopexy).

The most common postsurgical complication of reconstruction is formation of scar tissue (capsular contracture), and this usually occurs only with implants. If this occurs, the reconstructed breast feels hard and is often painful and may require additional surgery to correct the problem. To help prevent scar tissue, ask your surgeon when you can begin gentle massage in the operated area. With the pads of your fingers, gently stroke the area up and down, side to side, and in a circle several times a day to assist healing.

The implant is the simplest surgery, although there is controversy about safety. The flap procedures are much more complicated surgeries, requiring longer time under an anesthetic, with more possibilities for complications and a longer recovery time. Although reconstruction at the time of mastectomy is becoming more popular, some doctors do not recommend that amount of surgery at once. Know your options and discuss them thoroughly with the plastic surgeon as well as your cancer surgeon.

## Limitations of Reconstruction

Although the immediate results of reconstruction may be just the emotional lift you need, be aware of issues that may arise later:

- Your reconstructed breast can remain swollen for several months so symmetry won't be immediate.
- Complications are always a possibility in surgery. In breast reconstruction, scar tissue may form and become hard (about 20 percent of cases).[16] Implants can leak. Transferred tissue can refuse to grow or get infected. You can experience pain or bleeding. Ask your plastic surgeon about the frequency of such complications and ask to see photographs of the good and the bad results of her work.
- A natural breast can be altered surgically to match the reconstructed breast in shape and sag. However, over time a natural breast will begin to droop again, whereas the reconstructed breast retains its original shape. A bra solves this problem, but it will be noticeable in the buff.
- Your scars will always be noticeable.
- You may have weakness in your abdominal area from a TRAM flap or your arm and upper back from a latissimus dorsi flap.

## How Safe Are Implants?

In 1992 silicone implants were banned for breast enlargements, but they remain an option for postmastectomy patients. In June 1999 the Institute of Medicine concluded a review of all past and ongoing research on silicone breast implants. The report said:

First, reoperations and local and perioperative [right after surgery] complications are frequent enough to be a cause for concern and to justify the conclusion that they are the primary safety issue with silicone breast implants. Complications may have risks themselves, such as pain, disfigurement, and serious infection and they may lead to medical and surgical interventions, such as reoperations, that have risks. Second, risks accumulate over the lifetime of the implant, but quantitative data on this point are lacking for modern implants and deficient historically. Third, information concerning the nature and the relative high frequency of local complications and reoperations is an essential element of adequate informed consent for women undergoing breast implantation.

Go to *www.fda.gov/cdrh/breastimplants/birisk.html* for the FDA update from 2000.

## Insurance Issues

In 1998 the Women's Health and Cancer Rights Act was passed to compel group health plans to provide coverage for "all stages of reconstruction of the breast on which the mastectomy has been performed; surgery and reconstruction of the other breast to produce a symmetrical appearance; and prosthesis and physical complications of mastectomy including lymphedema." If the plan covers mastectomy, then it must cover the other stages mentioned. Of course, deductibles, co-pays, and other limitations or caps may apply.

## The Choice Not to Reconstruct

In our breast-obsessed society, some women may feel confused about breast reconstruction. They wonder if they are normal if they don't want to do it. Yes, they are. There are many reasons women opt out of reconstruction. Some are:

• They fear complications.
• They've had enough surgery and doctors, thank you very much.
• They feel comfortable with their self-image without breasts.
• The surgery is very expensive and not all insurance plans cover all costs.
• They are ready to put cancer behind them and don't want to delay even a few more weeks to heal from reconstruction.
• They realize that even beautiful reconstructed breasts will not bring back sexual stimulation in that area, so they decide not to bother.

A study done in 2000 at Park Nicollet Clinic in Minneapolis, Minnesota, showed that women who had postmastectomy reconstruction reported more mood disturbances and a poorer sense of well-being than those who had mastectomy alone. The researchers suggested that this might be due to a longer recuperative period that kept them from normal activities and greater postoperative pain.

Try to separate your personal feelings from those of your spouse or others. Talk to women who have had reconstruction about their expectations, experiences, and eventual outcomes. Then decide what you want for you. You can usually choose reconstruction later, so if you are at all ambivalent, don't rush into it. Do get information up front because some situations may preclude later reconstruction (such as radiation).

## Concerns about Lymphedema

Reconstruction carries risks for developing lymphedema just as any breast cancer surgery does. Discuss your concerns thoroughly with your plastic surgeon and don't take a "that's not going to happen" answer. Lymphedema complications are not common, but they happen enough that you should educate yourself about the risks and feel confident that your plastic surgeon understands your concerns. Unfortunately no one can predict who will develop lymphedema.

The risk with a tissue expander is the pressure in the axilla. The TRAM flap procedure weakens the abdominal wall and reduces the options for re-routing lymph fluid. Scar tissue is the concern with the latissimus dorsi flap because scars can block lymphatic flow and limit options for drainage.

Consider intensive manual lymph drainage before surgery to optimize your lymph system and take the same precautions after surgery that are recommended for breast surgery.

## Other Potential Problems

Besides the cosmetic results of reconstruction, consider other possible scenarios:

- Recovery can take a few weeks or a few months.
- Your range of motion may be limited permanently.
- With implants capsular contracture is a possibility. This is when the implants or the tissue around them hardens. This can be painful and look abnormal. If this happens, the implants will have to be replaced in another surgery.
- Implants can wander from their initial location.
- Implants can rupture.

- If both stomach muscles were involved in the TRAM flap procedure, a graft or mesh underlining may be necessary to prevent hernias, although the risk of hernia is still higher than normal.

- Mammograms are harder to read through an implant because they are not transparent on the X-ray. This is especially true if the implant was placed in front of, instead of behind, the chest muscle; if scar tissue has formed; or if the silicone has leaked into nearby breast tissue. Additional X-rays called implant displacement views can be taken for a more complete exam.

## Nipple Reconstruction

Nipples may be reconstructed—in a separate surgical procedure. Usually tattooing is used—and you have a choice of colors! The look is nice, although the nerve endings will not bring sexual pleasure as they once did. Tissue for nipple reconstruction can be taken from the vulva at the entrance to the vagina or from the inside of the thigh. If you take tissue from your other nipple, you might lose sensation in both. Nipple surgery is usually delayed for two months after reconstruction to allow time for the breast swelling to dissipate. Some women use removable polyurethane nipples, available at stores that sell prostheses.

## Hormone Therapy

Unlike cytotoxic drugs that kill cancer cells, hormone therapies are sometimes given as treatment for breast cancer to prevent cancer cells from getting the hormones they need to grow or to change the way hormones work in the body. Hormone therapy can affect normal cells in the body just as chemotherapy does. The presence of estrogen or progesterone receptors predicts a good response to hormonal therapies.

Any hormone therapy can cause a "flair" reaction, a painful protest of the cancer cells being starved. The pain is usually short-lived. Most hormone therapies are pills.

Nolvadex (tamoxifen) is the most common antiestrogen drug used. Evista (raloxifene) and Fareston (toremifene) are other antiestrogens, substances that bind to hormone receptors in cells so "bad" estrogen cannot. They are often referred to as SERMs (selective estrogen receptor modulators).

Aromatase inhibitors are another kind of hormone therapy. Arimidex (anastrozole) has been shown to be as effective, and maybe a bit more effective for postmenopausal women, than tamoxifen. These drugs slow breast cancer growth by blocking the enzyme cells needed to produce estrogen. Femara (letrozole) and Aromasin (exemestane) are two others in this class.

Gonadotropin-releasing hormone (GnRH) agonists, such as Zoladex (goserelin), block the release of some hormones, which causes the ovaries to stop ovulating and producing estrogen.

Estrogen receptor downregulators (SERDs) block estrogen in all tissues and are being investigated for use against metastatic breast cancer. Faslodex (fulvestrant) is one such medication.

Megace and Halotestin are progestins (hormones produced in the ovaries) that decrease available estrogen, the number of estrogen receptors, and the estrogen's effect on the cancer's growth. Progestins can cause fluid retention.

Other hormone therapies include androgens (male hormones), which can cause masculine characteristics such as more body hair or deeper voice. Oophorectomy, removal of the ovaries, used to be common treatment, but it is rarely used now except in premenopausal women.

Some side effects reported by women on these hormones are hot flashes, weight gain, blood clots, and cramps and numbness in the legs and hands. Some women have found relief from the leg cramps by taking quinine sulfate (by prescription). Tell your doctor if you experience spotting or vaginal bleeding.

## Eating during Treatment

Cancer can interfere with the body's system for regulating appetite, so appetite changes are often a side effect of the disease. In breast cancer treatment more women gain weight than lose it. Unfortunately, some women also lose their appetites during chemotherapy and, less often, during radiation— just when their bodies need all the nutrients they can get to rebuild normal tissue that has been damaged by treatments and to counteract the emotional and physical stress a cancer diagnosis brings.

One of your primary goals during all of treatment should be to eat as healthy as you can. Vitamins and minerals, especially zinc, strengthen your immune system to fight the cancer. A healthy diet can prevent the breakdown of body tissue, rebuild tissue, and bolster your stamina and strength. However, there are times—for instance, if you are nauseated—that eating anything, be it a Popsicle or a bowl of ice cream, is better than waiting until you can handle broccoli.

Treatment is also not a time to worry about dieting if you are battling side effects. If your appetite is unaffected by treatment, then you can begin shifting your food choices in a healthy direction, but if your appetite diminishes, eat enough calories from healthier foods to fuel your body.

Many women find that they "graze" during the day, nibbling and eating five or six small meals, instead of holding out for three big meals. To get enough calories, eat when you are hungry and ask your caregivers not to force you to eat something that does not sound appetizing. If you are not able to handle much regular food, try a liquid nutritional supplement. Women who gain weight during treatment are not necessarily eating more calories. Their body is just metabolizing food differently than before.

Some sources report that a large number of cancer patients do not tolerate animal protein as well as vegetable protein. If this is true for you, remember that you can get more than enough protein from beans and legumes, peas, corn, and soy products (see page 309). Fish and poultry seem to be tolerated better than beef. (See also "Eating during Chemotherapy," page 55.)

## Quick Snacks

Keep a supply of snacks on hand that need no preparation so you can have a few bites whenever you feel the urge. Some healthy and easy snacks include:

- Applesauce.
- Whole-grain crackers.
- Unsalted pretzels; air-popped popcorn (spray with olive oil).
- Whole-grain bread with jam or peanut butter.
- Dry cereal (mix equal portions of bran flakes, oat circles and squares, and miniature shredded wheat).
- Cheese.
- Soup in a cup.
- Fruit (canned, fresh, or dried).
- Hard-boiled eggs.
- Frozen or regular yogurt.
- Liquid meal replacements (such as Ensure or Boost).
- Nuts/nut butters. Nuts lowest in fats are almonds, hazelnuts, pistachios, walnuts, peanuts, and pecans. Cashews and macadamia are highest in saturated fats.
- Puddings/custards.
- Raw vegetables.
- Water, 100-percent vegetable or fruit juice, or club soda with lemon or lime.

## How to Add Protein to Your Diet

Protein is a building block of healthy cells and helps your body maximize strength, immune function, energy, and skin integrity, so be sure you get enough during treatment. High-protein foods include eggs; lean beef, pork, fish, chicken, and turkey; beans; low-fat milk, yogurt, cheese, and cottage cheese; nuts; peanut butter; and soy foods.

To add protein to your diet:

- Add low-fat hard or semisoft cheese to scrambled eggs, meat and starch dishes, sandwiches, or vegetables. Melt on tortillas, meats, pies, hamburgers, or eggs.
- Top fruits or vegetables with cottage cheese or ricotta cheese or add a dollop to casseroles, pancake or muffin batter, gelatin salads, or pasta dishes.
- Substitute milk for water when possible with canned soups, casseroles, hot cereals, and hot beverages.
- Add small amounts of powdered milk to casseroles, mixes, milk shakes or fruit smoothies, meatloaf, baked goods, mashed potatoes, and milk-based desserts.
- Drink complete nutrition drinks such as Ensure or Boost as snacks.
- Indulge in low-fat ice cream, yogurt, or frozen yogurt. Mix in blender with complete nutrition drinks, carbonated beverages, fruit, or desserts. Make "sandwiches" with graham crackers and low-fat ice cream or frozen yogurt.
- Add extra eggs/egg whites to casseroles, stuffing, rice dishes, or potatoes.
- Add nuts, seeds, or wheat germ to cereals, casseroles, desserts, baked goods, salads, fruit, and vegetables.
- Use nut butters on fruit slices for snacks. Spread on pancakes or use as a vegetable dip.
- Add beans or legumes to salads, pastas, rice and grain dishes, and soups.
- Add lean meat or fish to casseroles and pasta or rice dishes.
- Add low-fat cottage cheese to casseroles, spaghetti sauce, omelets, pancake batter, or pudding desserts or use to stuff pasta shells.

## How to Add Calories to Your Diet

If you weigh less than a healthy level, you obviously need to increase your calories. Try to get them from healthy sources, but limiting the weight loss is the highest priority. Once you have stemmed the loss, then you can switch to healthier sources of calories. High-calorie foods include such things as sauces, gravies, salad dressing, sour cream, butter/margarine, jams, sugar, syrup, whole-milk products, nuts, dried fruits, or cream cheese.

To increase calories:

- Use honey or jam as glaze for chicken, meat, or fish.
- Add powdered milk or egg white protein to baked goods, casseroles, or cooked cereals.

- Add granola to baked goods and eat as a snack; sprinkle on fruit, desserts, vegetables, ice cream, or pudding and custard.
- Sprinkle nuts on hot or cold cereal or combine with dried fruit for a trail mix.
- Add dried fruit or nuts to baked goods, cereals, or stuffings. Eat as a snack.
- Add extra eggs to baked goods, batter for pancakes or quiches, mashed potatoes, or sauces. Add hard-boiled eggs to salads, vegetables, or casseroles.
- Add avocado to sandwiches or salads.
- Bread meats and vegetables. Pan fry or sauté food instead of baking or broiling. Add gravies or sauces.
- Make a smoothie from a can of VitalCal or similar product, a banana, low-fat ice cream, and fruit. Add protein powder or nonfat dry milk powder for an added boost.
- Stir chocolate or strawberry syrup into milk.
- Add olive or canola oil to soups, sauces, casseroles, hot cereals, grains, potato dishes, and cooked vegetables. Mix with herbs to flavor meats, burgers, and fish.
- Top fruit, pudding, desserts, hot drinks, and waffles with whipped cream. Fold a little into mashed potatoes or vegetable purees.
- Substitute cream or sour cream for milk in recipes, hot cereal, canned soup, and egg dishes.
- Roll cream cheese into balls and roll in wheat germ, granola, nuts, or coconut. Spread cream cheese on crackers, breads, fruit, or pancakes.
- Add sour cream to baked potatoes and potato dishes, sauces, or soups. Use as topping for cakes, fruit, gelatin, or breads or a dip for fresh fruits or vegetables.
- Add cheese to vegetables, casseroles, potatoes, omelets, or sandwiches.

## Grocery Shopping Tips

Take a little extra time in selecting your groceries and protect yourself from hidden bacteria by following these tips:

- Choose only the freshest products. These are often in the back of the row. Do not buy products, including meat, poultry, and seafood, whose "sell by" or "use by" date has passed.
- Pick the prettiest fruit and vegetables. Do not buy blemished or bruised pieces.
- Do not buy dented, rusted, swollen, or otherwise damaged cans of food. Be sure packaged and boxed foods are sealed.

- Check the eggs in a carton and choose another if any eggs are cracked. Do not buy unrefrigerated eggs.
- Resist free food samples that have been sitting out and have had many hands and mouths near them.
- Do not buy food from self-serve, bulk containers.
- Avoid delicatessen and bakery foods such as unrefrigerated cream and custard products. Avoid ice cream and yogurt from soft-serve machines.

Make the frozen and refrigerated sections of the store your last stop. Don't leave groceries in a hot car; take a cooler to put them in if you have a long commute home. Store cold and frozen items promptly upon arriving home.

## Food Handling Tips

Now is the time to be fastidious about cleanliness in your food preparation. Begin by washing your hands thoroughly with warm water and soap before and after preparing food and before eating.

Also observe these basic food preparation precautions:

- Wash your hands before and after handling produce and raw meat.
- Wash tops of canned foods with soap and water before opening. Routinely clean your can opener.
- Wash fruits and vegetables under running water before peeling or cutting. Vegetable washes that claim to remove more pesticides than water have not been proven independently[17] to be more effective than water, especially on nonwaxed foods such as broccoli, strawberries, or spinach.
- Do not sample foods that smell or look strange. Toss them!
- Thaw food in the microwave or refrigerator in a dish to catch drips rather than at room temperature.
- Use defrosted food immediately; do not refreeze.
- Do not use the same utensil for stirring as for tasting.
- Cook meat to well done, with no pink in the center.
- Return perishable food (including cut produce) to the refrigerator within two hours of serving or dispose of it. Dishes with eggs, cream, and mayonnaise should not be out of the refrigerator more than an hour.
- Cook eggs until the yolks have begun to thicken.
- Boil tofu in half-inch cubes for five to 10 minutes before using.
- If your microwave has no turntable, rotate dishes a quarter turn several times during cooking to prevent "cold spots" where bacteria could survive. Use a lid and stir during reheating.

## Tips for Dining Out

Observe these safety tips, especially during chemotherapy treatment:

- Avoid food sources that are high risk for bacteria: sidewalk vendors, delicatessens, buffets, potlucks, salad bars, self-serve machines, and bulk supplies.
- Eat early to avoid crowds.
- In fast food establishments, ask that your food be prepared while you wait.
- Request condiments in individual packages rather than use those from the self-serve containers.

## Kitchen Hygiene Tips

To sanitize surfaces, use a solution of one part household bleach to 10 parts of water or a disinfectant cleaner.

### Sink area

- Have soap available for washing hands.
- Use paper towels instead of cloth. If you use cloth, change them daily.
- Change dishcloths daily.
- Sanitize sponges daily and replace weekly.
- Do not store food near cleaning supplies and chemicals.

### Refrigerator/freezer

- Keep the refrigerator clean: wipe up spills immediately, and sanitize shelves and doors weekly.
- Keep the refrigerator at 34 to 40°F and the freezer less than 5°F.
- Cool hot food uncovered in the refrigerator. When it is cool, cover it tightly.
- Freeze what you will not eat in the next three days. Throw away food that has been in the refrigerator more than three days (not, of course, condiments, jellies, cornmeal, and so forth).
- Throw away cracked eggs, food with expired "use by" dates, food with freezer burn, and/or entire packages that contain mold.

### Work surfaces and equipment

- Keep counters and cutting boards sanitized and free of food spills.
- Disassemble blenders and mixers to wash the container. Wipe down and sanitize toaster oven, microwave, can openers, and blender and mixer blades.
- Use separate cutting boards for raw and cooked foods or wash with soap and hot water, dishwasher, or 3-percent hydrogen peroxide after cutting raw foods and before cutting anything else, even in the same recipe. Sanitize once a week.

## Pantry

- Throw away any cans that have bulges, leaks, cracks, or indentations in the seam area.
- Take precautions against rodents or insects in food storage areas.
- Use home-canned foods within one year of canning. Check jars for signs of spoilage and sealed lids. If a lid bulges or does not snap when opened or if the food inside has any unusual characteristics, toss it.
- Abide by "use by" dates on packaged foods.
- Store new food in back of the food already in your pantry.

## Special Diets

Your doctor may recommend a special diet for parts of your treatment. They may include:

### Clear liquid diet

*Used after surgery until digestion returns to normal or during periods of diarrhea or vomiting.*

Liquids you can see through—such as water, apple juice, grape juice, cranberry juice, ginger ale, fruit-flavored drinks or punch, clear soup (such as bouillon or consommé) or fat-free broth, flat carbonated beverage (clear), sports drinks, fruit ice without fruit pieces or milk, plain gelatin, Popsicles, coffee, weak tea. If these make you nauseated, try diluting them with water. A clear liquid diet does not provide sufficient nutrients, so don't stay on one more than three to five days.

### Full liquid diet

*A step up from clear liquids or for patients with mouth sores.*

Milk and milk shakes, fruit juices/nectars, pureed fruits, carbonated drinks, fruit drinks or punch, coffee, tea, bouillon or broth, yogurt without fruit, ice milk, sherbet, smooth ice cream, pudding, custard, hot cereal, cream or cheese soups, butter/margarine/cream/oil, liquid meal replacements, pasteurized eggnog, plain gelatin, potatoes or tomatoes pureed in soup, tomato or vegetable juice, water.

### Soft diet

*For patients with mouth sores.*

Avoid all raw fruits and vegetables, foods with skins, nuts, seeds, and dry, crisp foods. Well-tolerated foods include:

- Apricots, pears, beans, squash, and peas.
- Dairy products: ice cream, yogurt, frozen yogurt, cottage cheese, chocolate milk, Popsicles, ices, sherbets.

- Scrambled or soft-boiled eggs.
- Milk shakes or smoothies.
- Mashed potatoes, macaroni and cheese, baked potatoes without the skin, noodles.
- Applesauce, bananas, watermelon, soft canned fruits, fruit nectars and juices.
- Flavored gelatin, puddings, custards.
- Cooked oatmeal, cream of wheat, buckwheat, other cooked cereal.
- Cooked vegetables or soups at room temperature; cold soups.
- Baby food, pureed meats or vegetables (mix them with broth into a soup).
- Liquid meal replacements such as Carnation Instant Breakfast, Boost, or Ensure.

## Water

Drinking plenty of fluid is essential during chemo (and during health also!). Although conventional wisdom dictates eight 8 -ounce glasses of water, the source of that figure is illusive. As with other nutritional goals, it makes sense that a 110-pound woman in her 30s would have different fluid needs than a 200-pound man in his 60s.

Work with a dietician or doctor to determine your daily fluid goal, then find a jug or thermos that holds that much water. Fill it up each morning and drink from it all day so you can have an accurate account of your intake. Another way to keep track of how much you drink is to place on the counter a fork or spoon for each glass you want to drink. As you drink a glass, return that utensil to the drawer. Or do the same with toothpicks or paper clips or rubber bands. As you drink a glass, place the item into a container. When you see no more, you have accomplished your goal.

Herbal teas and vegetable and fruit juices may count towards your total fluid intake. Coffee and alcohol are mildly dehydrating but do contribute some fluid value.

If you don't want to bother with counting, just check out the color of your urine. If it's pale, straw-colored yellow, you're in good shape for the moment. If it's brighter or darker, you have not had enough fluids in the last few hours, so drink up.

## How Much Treatment?

Sometimes patients feel that the benefits of treatment do not outweigh the poorer quality of life from that treatment and decide to stop treatment. This is a serious decision you will want to discuss first with family, clergy, and caregivers. Your choice will depend upon what you think about life and death.

Refusal of treatment does not mean an immediate or painful death. You can still receive medications for pain, and you can change your mind at any time.

The Patient Self-Determination Act (PSDA) is a federal law that requires all medical facilities that receive Medicaid or Medicare payments to inform patients about some choices they have about the extent and type of medical care they want to receive. Tools you can use to make your wishes known are called advanced directives. State laws differ on advanced directives. Contact your state health department for information. Three of these tools are:

- **Living will.** This is a notarized legal document that allows you to refuse any type of treatment you wish.

- **Durable power of attorney for healthcare.** Through this legal document, you appoint someone to make medical decisions for you, based on your wishes, if you are unable to do so for yourself.

- **Will to Live** (*www.nrlc.org*). This differs from a living will in its "general presumption for life." Some groups are concerned that some terms in a living will are so vague ("extraordinary measures," "terminal condition," "irreversible condition," and even "medical treatment") that your wishes may not be carried out. For instance, "medical treatment" now includes food and hydration. The vague terms can be interpreted by the healthcare facility or a court of law. Consult an attorney to discuss exact meanings and court rulings about terms used. Then compare the two documents to see which you are more comfortable with. Few healthcare facilities will tell you about the Will to Live.

## *End-of-Life Issues*

Death is a difficult subject for most of us. However, families whose members plan ahead are saved many hard decisions—and oftentimes considerable money. At least be sure you have a valid will so your property will go to the persons you want and won't be distributed according to state law. If you have children younger than 18, be sure you have designated a legal guardian. Social Security and other groups may require a legal guardian for your children to qualify for benefits. Money spent consulting an estate planner or lawyer may be well spent.

Decisions about treatment can be confusing. Ask all the questions you need to and discuss your preferences with your family so you can make a decision that feels right for you.

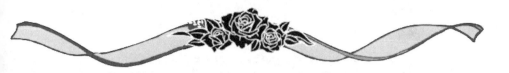

*Chapter 3*

# *Managing Side Effects*

How you will react to your treatment is as individual as your facial features. Don't assume that just because your friend got sick, you will also. Your medications, dosage, general health, stage of the disease, and other factors will determine how well you tolerate your treatment. All treatment options have some common side effects, *but you may not experience any of them.*

If you do, look here for tips from other breast cancer patients that will help you cope. Most side effects disappear after treatment is completed. Try to think of them as fellow warriors fighting alongside you to combat this disease.

## *Abdominal Cramping or Pain*

Some chemotherapy drugs can alter the bacterial flora in the intestines or the movement of the stool through the bowel. Either of these shifts can cause cramping or pain in the abdomen. A dull ache is not an uncommon side effect of chemotherapy. However, a sharp pain should be checked by a physician.

To relieve the cramping, try:

- Increasing your fluid intake to eight to 10 glasses a day, particularly between meals.
- Eating small amounts of bland foods every few hours.
- Lying still and breathing deeply, but avoid lying flat for two hours after eating.
- Gently massaging your abdomen in a circular motion or placing moderate heat on it for no more than 10 minutes.
- Avoiding cigarettes and alcohol, which may irritate the stomach.
- Avoiding NSAIDs (nonsteroidal anti-inflammatory drugs), narcotic pain medications, or aspirin unless your doctor has prescribed them.
- Avoiding very hot or very cold foods/fluids, lactose, or spicy or greasy foods.

## Anal Fissures

An unusual side effect of breast cancer treatment is the development of small ulcers around the rectum. Because the lining of this part of the body replaces itself every few days, it is sensitive to cancer-killing drugs. Your oncologist can prescribe a cream to apply should this occur. Keep the area clean with moistened wipes. Apply liquid vitamin E or tea tree oil to the area. If your stool is hard, increase your liquids and take a stool softener.

## Anemia

The bone marrow manufactures red blood cells, which carry oxygen to all parts of the body so the tissues can function properly. Chemotherapy, radiation, or excess blood loss during surgery can interfere with this process and cause a condition known as anemia, or decreased red blood cells. Red blood cells usually live about 120 days, but during cancer treatment they last about 90 days.

If your red blood count is low, your doctor may prescribe a medicine such as Epogen, Procrit, or Aranesp to increase the number of such cells. Side effects, although usually mild, may include dizziness, headaches, joint aches, nausea, or diarrhea. If your red blood count is severely low, your doctor may order a blood transfusion.

## Symptoms of Anemia

Approximately 60 percent of cancer patients develop anemia.[1] If you develop any of these symptoms during your treatment, notify your doctor immediately:

- Dizziness or feeling faint or unusually cold.
- Heart pounding or beating very fast.
- Shortness of breath.
- Fatigue.
- Pale, dull, or grayish face coloring; a washed-out appearance.

## Coping with Anemia

- Rise slowly from a sitting or lying position to prevent dizziness.
- Eat a well-balanced diet.
- Get most of your sleep at night, and nap during the day if you are tired.
- Ask for help with routine tasks to conserve your energy.
- Do only essential activities.

(See "Fatigue," page 111, for other tips for low-energy days.)

## *Anxiety*

Feeling anxious about a cancer diagnosis is perfectly normal, but if the anxiety interferes with your ability to make decisions, handle routine tasks, or think clearly, consult your doctor about possible remedies.

In addition to anti-anxiety medications, you might consider nonpharmaceutical approaches. Do not self-medicate. Consult your doctor or health professional with training in herbs and complementary medicine.

Mind/body work and regular exercise can help relieve anxiety. Also, writing out what you are anxious about can put things in perspective. Break the anxiety into small pieces and see what solutions you can find for each part. Also ask questions of people who will have reliable answers, such as your medical team. Perhaps something you are anxious about is not applicable to you. (See also "Depression," page 227, and "Fear," page 225.)

## *Appetite Loss*

You cannot predict whether your appetite will increase or decrease during treatment. However, know that whatever the effects, there are ways to counter them.

Loss of appetite or early satiety (feeling full after eating only a little food) can have consequences other than weight loss. Without proper nutrition, you can begin to feel weak and your body will not be as efficient in many of its processes.

Try some of the following tips to stimulate your appetite. If they don't work, your doctor can prescribe an appetite stimulant such as Megace or Marinol. Some of these suggestions conflict with the recommended anti–breast cancer diet or diets recommended for other conditions. Remember, however, that your body needs different attention at different times depending on its focus at the moment. Although broccoli is a healthy food, if you are losing weight and it gives you gas and prevents you from eating, it's *not* what you need to be eating *just now*. Approach your diet one day at a time and base your choices on what your goal is at the moment.

Eating involves other factors besides food and appetite. For instance, you can lose your appetite if you are fatigued, depressed, or sensitive to smells. Nausea or mouth problems may make eating difficult. Review specific side effects in this book for more coping techniques.

## Eating Tips

- Eat small amounts of high-calorie (see page 89) or high-protein (see page 88) snacks every few hours. Avoid low-calorie versions of foods such as diet soda.

- Bland foods such as rice, toast, pretzels, grits, or fruit juices are usually well tolerated.
- Concentrate on healthy, nutrient-filled foods and beverages so what you can get down does you some good. For instance, choose fruit juice or nectars, fruit smoothies with yogurt, or milk instead of coffee, sweetened tea, or soda.
- Avoid foods that can cause gas (see page 122) and further interrupt your appetite.
- Herbs and substances that may stimulate appetite are fennel seed, peppermint, ginger, ginseng, gotu kola, and papaya.[2] Check with your doctor before consuming the herbs.
- Try new recipes.
- Consume a complete nutrition supplement such as Ensure, Carnation Instant Breakfast, or Boost.

## Environmental Changes
- Make meals fun. Prepare foods with color. Set the table with cheery placemats or decorative napkins and paper plates. Add fresh flowers or candles.
- Change your surroundings for eating. Eat in a new room or on the patio. Watch a favorite TV show or eat with family or friends.
- Keep conversation pleasant and relaxed.
- Avoid unpleasant smells while you eat.

## Non-Food Tips
- Many people have a better appetite in the morning when they are rested. If this is true for you, eat your largest meal then.
- Use a small plate with small portions so the amount of food is not intimidating.
- Do some mild exercise each day or take a walk before meals. Fresh air and muscle movement can stimulate your appetite.
- Have someone else cook so you conserve your energy for eating.
- Use ready-to-eat or prepared foods. Take advantage of time-saving appliances such as microwaves and blenders.
- Ask your doctor about taking vitamin B supplements. Vitamin B helps release energy from food and may enhance appetite. Also ask about drinking a small glass of wine or beer, both appetite stimulators.

(See also "Fatigue," page 111; "Taste, Changes in," page 170; "Mouth Sores," page 147; and "Dry Mouth," page 110.)

## *Bladder/Kidney Effects*

Some drugs will change the color of your urine or emit a strong odor. Adriamycin, for instance, turns urine a bright red, and Epirubicin turns it pink for one or two days after treatment. Ask your doctor if your particular medications will have this effect so you are not unduly alarmed.

Cytoxan can cause bladder hemorrhage, so tell your doctor if you see blood in your urine. Other chemotherapy drugs can cause bladder spasms or infections. You are more prone to bladder infections when your white blood count is low.

## Call Your Doctor if You Have Any of These Symptoms

- Inability to urinate even though your bladder feels full.
- More frequent urination than normal for you.
- Pain or burning when you urinate.
- An urgency to urinate.
- Red or bloody urine, unless your medication causes this.
- Chills, especially with shaking.
- Fever.

Void as soon as you feel the urge. Drink at least two quarts of liquid (not carbonated) beverages a day. Cranberry juice is particularly good for urinary tract infections.

## *Blood Clots*

Although rare, blood clots are one side effect of some hormonal therapies, such as tamoxifen. Check with your doctor if you notice unusual redness or swelling, especially in your arm or leg. Other symptoms to check out are pain (especially behind the knee or in the calf), distended veins, sudden shortness of breath or anxiety, chest pain, and cough with spitting up of blood.

## *Blood Clotting, Impediment of*

Anticancer drugs can impede the bone marrow's manufacture of platelets, blood cells that make your blood clot. Without sufficient platelets, you can bleed or bruise more easily than you usually do. Your doctor will check your platelet count often during chemotherapy and can prescribe medications to increase your count if it falls below normal.

## Signs of Blood Clotting Problems

- Unexplained bruising.
- Reddish or pinkish urine.

- Black or bloody bowel movements.
- Small red spots under the skin.
- Bleeding from gums or nose.
- Headaches or changes in vision.
- Warm or hot feeling in an arm or leg.
- Vaginal bleeding not associated with a monthly period.

## Behaviors for Low Platelet Count

- Use an electric shaver instead of a razor to avoid nicks.
- Be careful not to burn yourself while ironing or cooking or cut yourself while using knives, needles, scissors, or sharp tools. Be careful while gardening to avoid stickers and scratches.
- Ask your doctor whether to avoid sexual activity or alcohol.
- Avoid contact sports and other activities that might cause injury.
- Use a soft toothbrush and don't brush too hard.
- Check with your doctor before ingesting any vitamins, minerals, herbal supplements, or over-the-counter medications. Products containing aspirin can affect platelets.
- If you must blow your nose, blow gently into a soft tissue.

### *Blood Count, Low*

White and red blood cells are produced in the bone marrow. As an area of rapid cell division, the bone marrow is susceptible to temporary damage by chemotherapy because many of these drugs attempt to interfere with runaway cell division that characterizes cancer. Many women in chemotherapy will experience a drop in their white blood cell count (called neutropenia) or a drop in their red blood cell count (called anemia) within seven to 14 days after a treatment. If this is a possibility with your drugs, your doctor will test your blood at the appropriate time.

If your counts are low, your doctor will probably give you bone marrow stimulants such as Neupogen (for white blood cells) or Epogen (for red blood cells) and advise you to isolate yourself from other people (outside the family) until the count is back in the normal range. This will be determined by another blood test.

## Precautions if Your Blood Count Is Low

Low blood cell counts leave you very vulnerable to infection. Without the support of your bone marrow to fight off the germs, an infection could be life-threatening. Though your mental attitude can be a positive influence on your coping with cancer, it is your body that must fight off any germs, so do not have a cavalier attitude about your vulnerability during low blood counts. Save the brave face for another time and use sensible precautions (see "Infections," page 129).

## Symptoms to Tell Your Doctor About

- If you bruise easily. Apply an ice pack or package of frozen food to the wound with slight pressure for three minutes to minimize bleeding. Then massage glycerin (in the first aid or skin section of most drug stores) into the area.

- Bleeding from gums or nose. Avoid bleeding by not picking your nose or by not inhaling saline (salt water) mist in dry conditions. If your nose does bleed, pinch the bridge of your nose just below the bony part for at least five minutes.

- At the first sign of a fever (usually defined as more than 101°F), which is a sign that your body is fighting an invader. Be aware that your temperature is often slightly higher in late afternoon or early evening, but do not hesitate to inform your doctor if your temperature rises. She may prescribe antibiotics or other medication such as Tylenol, and it is important to start those as soon as possible to minimize problems.

- If you develop chills, sweats, burning sensation when you urinate, cough, sore throat, diarrhea, or tiny red spots under the skin.

## What to Do if You Develop Fever While Your Blood Count Is Low

Ask your doctor in advance if you can take any over-the-counter medication for fever, what temperature he considers a fever, and what to do if your fever does exceed his limit. Some doctors will tell you to proceed to a hospital. Others will tell you to try for a specified time to bring down the fever and call again if it does not go down.

### To try to bring down a fever

- Drink cold beverages.
- Suck on ice chips.
- Get into a bathtub of tepid water. Gradually add cool water to bring down the fever. Do not suddenly get into a tub of ice water.
- Relax; avoid expending excessive energy.
- Take fever-reducing medication only if your doctor has approved it.

## Constipation

Some cancer or pain medications can interfere with normal bowel activity and cause serious consequences. Constipation is having infrequent bowel movements, fewer than every 48 to 72 hours; hard, dry stools and straining during bowel movements; or abdominal bloating and discomfort. Being inactive or not drinking enough fluids or eating enough fiber can slow down bowel activity.

If you notice a change in your bowel habits, ask your doctor if a medication may be causing it. Try some of the suggestions that follow to move the bowels. Do not take any laxative, stool softener, or other medication without checking with your doctor, particularly if you have low blood counts. Some tips may not be appropriate if you have other side effects such as dry mouth, mouth sores, or nausea.

# To Help Ease Constipation
## Eating tips

- Most importantly, drink eight to 10 8-ounce glasses of water a day. Drinking prune juice, hot tea, and hot lemon water may help also.
- Work prunes, or "dried plums," into your diet. Eat from the package or mix into hot or cold cereal, pancake batter, or cookies instead of raisins. Substitute a few tablespoons of prunes for ground beef in casseroles and meatballs. Figs, peaches, carrots, cabbage, beans, seeds, and whole grains work as well. Avoid dried fruit if your blood count is low.
- Increase your fiber intake through whole grains instead of processed grains (for example, brown rice, buckwheat, quinoa, wild rice, or barley instead of white rice; whole grain breads instead of white bread; nuts, popcorn, granola, fresh and dried fruits, raw or cooked vegetables such as squash or celery—leave the skin on whenever possible, as that is where much of the fiber is). Foods high in fiber include raisins, figs, dates, prunes, peaches, or beans. Make the change slowly and increase your liquid intake at the same time. Make a sauce of equal amounts of unprocessed bran, applesauce, and mashed stewed prunes. Blend and store in the refrigerator. Eat 1 to 2 tablespoons before bed and drink 8 ounces of water.
- Add shredded vegetables, oat bran, or wheat bran to casseroles or other dishes. Substitute prune juice for water in muffins.
- Raw fruits and prune, apple, and pear juices are natural laxatives.
- Drink water or honey or molasses mixed in warm water.
- Eat beans, legumes, and vegetables in the cruciferous family (such as broccoli, bok choy, Brussels sprouts, cauliflower, cabbage, or collard greens). The gas they produce can help soften stools.

- Eat high-pectin foods such as apples, bananas, carrots, and cabbage.
- Avoid milk and cheese products, which can cause constipation in some people.
- Limit caffeine to one cup of caffeinated beverage a day. One cup in the morning may act as a laxative, but too much throughout the day acts as a diuretic and removes water from the stool.
- Drink warm or hot liquids after a meal. French tarragon tea can move the bowels.

### Activities
- Exercise lightly to stimulate the abdominal muscles and speed the removal of waste material from the intestines. Walk every day (30 minutes if you are able), especially after meals.
- Massage the abdominal muscles.
- Drink a hot beverage a half hour before you usually have a bowel movement.

## Solutions for Constipation
If a change in food intake and activity does not move the bowels, ask your doctor about any of the following aids (be sure to drink six to eight glasses of water a day while you are taking these):
- Stool softeners such as Colace, Surfak, or Senokot.
- Bulk-forming agents such as Metamucil, Citrucel, or FiberCon.
- Laxatives such as mineral oil, milk of magnesia, or Dulcolax.
- Ground flaxseed or herbs such as senna (use tablets as directed or drink 1 teaspoon of powdered senna in 8 ounces of water, followed by two more glasses of water; drink between meals; works in eight to 12 hours; use no more than twice a day);[3] cascara sagrada (a strong herb); turkey rhubarb; or psyllium (don't take if you are taking morphine or codeine-based drugs. Instead use flaxseed oil or freshly ground flaxseed.)[4]
- Castor oil.
- One-half cup aloe vera juice in the morning and afternoon helps soften stools.

## Preventing Constipation
The following healthy habits will help keep your bowel habits regular and comfortable:
- Drink more than 1 quart of fluid a day, not including coffee, black tea, or alcoholic drinks.
- Exercise a little every day.

- Eat slowly.
- Choose a multivitamin without iron.
- Reduce stress.
- Consume 25 to 35 grams of fiber a day.

## *Dehydration*

Having enough fluid in your system during treatment is important for several reasons:

- Many chemotherapy drugs do their jobs almost immediately upon entering your bloodstream. Afterwards they may seek out normal cells and organs to disrupt, so you want to flush them out of your system as soon as possible.
- If you become dehydrated, your body cannot function properly. When you feel nauseous, it is sometimes difficult to think of anything in your stomach, even ice water. But you must force yourself to drink at least a few ounces every hour or so. Choose whatever sounds good at the moment.
- Excessive dehydration can lead to constipation, which is uncomfortable, or bowel blockage, which might land you in the hospital. It can also lead to seizures, brain damage, and death.

Dehydration can result from diarrhea, vomiting, high fever, infection, or simply not drinking enough fluids.

## Signs of Dehydration

- The shakes when there is no environmental reason to be cold. Often this indicates that your electrolytes are out of balance. This can be dangerous to your heart, so don't let the condition linger. Try drinking some Pedialyte mixed with an equal portion of cold ginger ale or clear liquid or eat some banana to raise your potassium level.
- Mental confusion.
- Dry, sticky mouth.
- Decreased urine output; concentrated urine.
- Sunken eyes.
- Skin that looks loose and crinkled.
- Thick, dry secretions.
- Rapid deep breathing.
- The pinch test. Gently pinch the skin on the back of your hand over a knuckle. If it immediately collapses, you probably are hydrated. If it takes a few seconds to flatten out, you probably need more fluid.

If you suspect you may be dehydrated, call your doctor immediately. Keep a record of how many times you vomit or have diarrhea and tell your doctor. Try to keep any liquid (except alcohol) down. Sucking on ice chips may be all you can do, but do it constantly because you get such a small amount of fluid in each mouthful. You can probably tolerate small sips of fluids better than gulping down a lot at once.

Sports drinks such as Gatorade can supply needed electrolytes. You can make your own rehydration beverage by mixing 8 teaspoons of sugar, 1/2 teaspoon of baking soda, and 1/4 teaspoon of Morton's Lite Salt Mixture into 1 quart of water.[5]

## Dental Concerns

Because chemotherapy drugs can be hard on all parts of the mouth, get a professional teeth cleaning and take care of any dental problems such as cavities, poorly fitting dentures, or gum disease or abscesses several weeks before beginning chemotherapy, as even routine dental procedures can introduce bacteria into the bloodstream. Some dentists may suggest using a fluoride rinse in advance of treatment to toughen the teeth.

## Tips for Oral Hygiene during Treatment

- Practice good oral hygiene. Brush two or three times a day with a soft-bristle brush and a nonabrasive, regular-flavored toothpaste. If your gums are too sore to brush, clean around the gums with a soft, clean cloth or cotton swab. Avoid toothpaste containing SLS (sodium lauryl sulfate). A paste of baking soda and water is an alternative or mix 1/2 to 1 teaspoon of baking soda and 1/2 to 1 teaspoon of salt in a quart of warm water and swish your mouth with it four or five times a day, especially after eating. You must keep your mouth clean to avoid bacteria. Make a fresh batch each morning.
- If you can't brush your teeth, rinse your mouth with water after eating or drinking sweet foods or beverages or gargle with a 50/50 mixture of 3-percent hydrogen peroxide and water or an herbal gargle.
- Go easy on flossing because the gums are sensitive and can become infected from rigorous flossing. If your gums bleed or hurt when you floss, avoid those areas, but keep flossing the rest of your gums. Do not floss when your blood counts are low.
- Avoid mouthwashes with alcohol or sodium, which may be irritating to any mouth sores.
- Suck slippery elm lozenges.
- If dentures irritate your mouth, leave them out except when you eat.

- Rinse your toothbrush well after each use and let it dry completely before storing it in any place other than an open-air counter or shelf. Replace it often.

    (See also "Mouth Sores," page 147, and "Dry Mouth," page 110.)

## *Diarrhea*

Diarrhea (watery or loose stools) is a common side effect for some cancer medications. If you experience four to six episodes in 24 hours or have pain or cramping along with diarrhea, notify your physician.

Diarrhea can cause dehydration, which can have serious consequences (see page 106). Do not take over-the-counter medication for this condition without checking first with your physician. An ingredient in the medication might interact with or counteract your chemotherapy drug. If the diarrhea is severe, your doctor might order intravenous (IV) fluids to replace nutrients and fluids you have lost. This is usually done as an outpatient.

If your rectum becomes red or sore, substitute a commercial wet towelette without alcohol for dry toilet paper. Your doctor can prescribe a cream such as Desitin. Use only a thin layer of creams because they are hard to clean off and rubbing too hard can break down the skin. You can also use Kleenex with lanolin or lotion instead of toilet paper.

## To Help Relieve Diarrhea

- Eat smaller meals frequently throughout the day to find what you can tolerate.
- Rest and reduce your activity level, especially after eating.
- Fast two to four hours; then begin sipping clear liquids.
- Be sure to drink eight to 10 glasses of fluids a day. Drink slowly.
- Ask your doctor about taking medications such as Lomotil (prescription), Imodium, or Pepto Bismol.
- Mix 1 teaspoon of bentonite clay (found at natural food stores) with 1 cup of applesauce (to make it palatable). Eat 2 to 3 cups a day until diarrhea eases.
- Make rice water. Boil ordinary rice in a large quantity of water. When rice is cooked, strain the liquid. Save the rice for a meal and sip on the rice water.

## Foods That Can Cause or Aggravate Diarrhea

- Fat, fried, or greasy foods. Fats are poorly absorbed and often delay emptying of the stomach.
- Onions, garlic.

- High-fiber foods (whole grain breads and cereals, beans, cabbage, brown rice, oatmeal, raw vegetables, fresh or dried fruits, nuts, seeds, popcorn).
- Hot or spicy foods.
- Rich foods such as cakes and donuts.
- Milk products, ice cream, cheese.
- Caffeine (coffee, soda, strong tea, chocolate).
- Very hot or cold beverages.
- Alcohol, cigarettes.
- Carbonated drinks. (Instead try a splash of fruit juice in mineral water or let carbonated drinks go flat before drinking them.)
- Prunes; prune or pear juice, citrus juices.
- Sugar substitutes ending in "-itol" such as Sorbitol or Maltitol, found in sugar-free candies, chewing gum, and other foods.

## Foods to Eat if You Have Diarrhea

- High-calorie foods.
- BRAT—**B**anana, **R**ice (plain white), **A**pplesauce (unsweetened), **T**oast (white, dry).
- Low-fiber, bland foods such as white bread, white rice or noodles, Matzo crackers, gelatin, cereal, pretzels.
- Baked skinless chicken or turkey, baked fish, extra-lean ground beef.
- Canned or cooked fruit without the skin.
- Clear liquids (see page 93).
- Room temperature foods or drinks rather than hot or cold ones.
- Starchy liquids or foods such as oatmeal or rice porridge, creamed cereals, ripe banana, potato soup, mashed potato or baked potato without the skin, pasta without sauce, oat or rice bran.
- High-potassium foods (bananas, peaches, oranges, potatoes, apricots) because you lose that mineral through diarrhea.
- Nonfat yogurt with live cultures (friendly bacteria) or other fermented dairy products. Ask about taking 1 to 2 tablespoons of acidophilus a day to replenish beneficial bacteria in the intestines.
- Nonfat cottage cheese. The lactose in milk products may make diarrhea worse.
- Smooth peanut butter.
- Scrambled egg substitute, egg whites, eggs (not fried).
- Thicker liquids, such as orange juice or thin soups (as the frequency of bowel movements wanes).

- Ginger in ginger snaps, ginger tea, ginger ale, or ginger candy can soothe your stomach. Buy ginger tea in health food stores or steep 1 inch of ginger root (cut into tiny pieces) in boiling water for 30 minutes. Add honey and lemon juice; chill. Drink hot or cold to ease substances through the digestive tract and increase fat-digesting bile from the liver and gallbladder.[6]

## Dry Mouth

Some chemotherapy drugs will leave your mouth feeling as if it is full of sawdust. This is more than an irritant. Saliva protects our mouth and throat from bacteria, viruses, and fungal growths and breaks down our food so we can taste it. Lack of saliva can therefore lead to weight loss, bleeding gums, dry throat, cracked tongue and corners of mouth, mouth pain or infection, or tooth decay. Mouth dryness usually stops once treatment is finished.

If you consume any of the liquid nutritional supplements such as Ensure, be sure to drink water, rinse your mouth with water, or brush your teeth (even without toothpaste) afterwards. These drinks have high quantities of sugar that can erode tooth enamel.

For relief, try:

- Drinking as much water as you can, at least eight to 10 glasses a day. Carry a sports bottle of liquid wherever you go. Try adding 1/4 teaspoon of glycerin (sold in drug stores) to 8 ounces of water for longer-lasting relief.
- Rinsing your mouth with water often.
- Eating a soft or pureed diet. It will be easier to swallow than crisp, dry foods. Moisten dry foods with butter, margarine, olive oil, gravy, sauces, or broth.
- Eating canned fruit with the juice instead of fresh fruit.
- Eating cheese, which produces saliva.[7]
- Avoiding spices or acidic foods, which can irritate your mouth.
- Experimenting to see what temperature food is easiest to swallow. Many people prefer cold foods for a dry mouth.
- Sucking on ice chips, Popsicles, or sugar-free candies or chewing sugar-free gum or drinking tart or very sweet beverages such as lemonade to stimulate your saliva glands.
- Asking your doctor about artificial saliva to moisten your mouth.
- Placing a humidifier in the room where you sleep to moisturize the air when you are not drinking.
- Avoiding mouthwashes and toothpastes containing alcohol, sodium, or peroxides, which will dry your mouth.
- Using Biotene products for dry mouth or Salivart.

- Using water- or lanolin-based lip moisturizers if your lips become dry. Petroleum-based lip balms may foster the growth of microbes. Burt's Beeswax lip balm or Lansinoh are two good brands with lanolin. You can also break open a vitamin E capsule and apply the contents to your lips.
- Applying sunscreen such as Zilactin-Lip to your lips to prevent sun blisters.

  (See also "Mouth Sores," page 147.)

## Fatigue

Fatigue or extreme malaise is an unfortunate but common side effect of cancer treatment. In fact, it is the most common side effect, with 76 percent of all cancer patients reporting it. However, its presence (or absence) or severity has no direct connection with how sick you are or how effective your treatment is. So far, no one is able to predict who will experience fatigue. If fatigue strikes, it may last only during active treatment or it may last for months or years after treatment ends.

Fatigue can be a result of chemotherapy, radiation therapy, the cancer itself, surgery, lack of sleep, low blood counts, stress, depression, changes in activity levels (the less active you are, the more fatigued you can feel), pain, poor nutrition, or other factors. Just the mental stress of dealing with cancer and related disruptions of your daily life can cause fatigue. If you do develop this side effect, tell your doctor. He may want to monitor your white and red blood cell counts to determine whether your immune system is depressed.

Medical personnel who deal regularly with cancer patients should recognize the difference in cancer fatigue and routine tiredness. However, your family may not. When patients tell someone they are "exhausted," it is not uncommon for the hearer to respond, "Oh, you're just not as young as you used to be" or "Me too!" You will soon learn to accept that such statements come from ignorance about cancer, not from insensitivity. Talk to your family about the reality of cancer fatigue to help avoid resentment, guilt, or communication problems from developing.

Cancer fatigue is very different from the tiredness you may have experienced previously at the end of a hard day. It does not improve with a good night's sleep or a day of rest. Symptoms may include:

- Extreme tiredness that a period of rest does not eliminate.
- Heaviness of arms and/or legs.
- Being too exhausted to perform routine tasks.
- Difficulty in concentration or problem-solving.
- Forgetfulness (names, words, schedules, and so on).
- Inability to focus on the conversation or task at hand.

- Shortness of breath or heart pounding after light activity such as making the bed or walking between rooms.
- Loss of appetite.
- Crying or depression.
- Paleness or shaking.

## Describing Your Fatigue

The most important thing to remember about fatigue is to report it to your physician. It may mean something is lacking in your body or treatment that needs to be corrected. Being tired is a barrier to your healing, so be sure treatable causes are eliminated or handled. Also, fatigue may interfere with your schedule of chemotherapy and potentially reduce its effectiveness.

Some people do not mention fatigue because they:

- Are afraid their doctor will take her focus off the cancer and dwell upon a "lesser" problem.
- Don't want to "complain."
- Don't understand that it could be a symptom of a serious or curable problem.

In relating your fatigue to your medical team or your family, be specific so they will know exactly how tired you are. Do not exaggerate. Just be as clear as possible. Say, "I was so tired I couldn't stand up to brush my teeth" or "I was so tired I could work only half a day."

### Helpful ways to describe your fatigue

- Use a rating scale. Rate your energy from zero to 10, with zero being ready to run a marathon and 10 being not able to get out of bed.
- Keep a chart of your activity levels and fatigue levels during different parts of the day.
- Tell what difference the fatigue made in your daily routine.
- Tell when the fatigue began and how long it has been a problem.
- Tell what makes the fatigue worse.
- Describe the feeling in your own words—wiped out, exhausted, drained, weak, and so forth.
- Tell what you have tried to make it better and what worked or didn't.

## Ways to Combat Fatigue

Your mantras for combating cancer fatigue will be "conserve, restore, and balance." Do whatever is necessary to conserve energy, know what restores energy, and balance your energy resources and demands. Forget Superwoman. Think Queen Bee.

Conserve energy by prioritizing what is important to you. List your responsibilities (and don't forget to include a few pleasures too). Rank the top three things you value the most and focus your energy on accomplishing those.

Next, delegate. Divide your responsibilities into four lists: what must be done, what should be done, what would be nice to have done, and what does not have to be done. Choose what you must do or want to do. Think carefully about who can handle the other tasks. Does it really matter how the task is done? What resources are available (friends, paid services, alternatives)? Match the task to the resource and ask for help.

When you ask for help, be specific. If there is a way something must be done or a deadline, say so up front, but be flexible and allow for the other person to take ownership of the task if possible. Confirm that the person is able and willing to take on the task. Don't assume that just because you have mentioned the need, it will be done.

Be sure to follow up with gratitude and praise. Thank the person next time you see her, send a note or e-mail, or call. If she forgets or doesn't follow instructions, give her a second chance. If another disappointment results, rethink your requests or try another resource next time.

Other actions that will help fatigue are managing your pain (see "Pain," page 156), improving sleep (see "Insomnia," page 132), learning to relax (see "Anxiety," page 99, and "Relaxation," page 241), and seeking counseling to manage stress. The following actions may also be helpful.

## Scheduling

- Incorporate a time for rest into your daily schedule, just as you would any other appointment.
- Schedule fun into your week. Just anticipating it is energizing.
- Prioritize your responsibilities and start with the most important. Realize that you may very well not get to everything on the list—and make that okay.
- Find the time of day you feel best and do your most important tasks then.
- Ask for help for everything possible—childcare, meals, shopping, housework, yard work. Save your energy for what only you can do and for a few fun activities.
- Accept any help that is offered. Keep a list of things others can do for you. When someone says, "Let me know if I can help," you'll be ready to respond. Get over your embarrassment of receiving help. Remember the times you have helped someone else and the good feelings you had from being of service. Let someone else experience those good feelings for a change.
- Consider hiring out some jobs. Take the clothes to the Laundromat for washing and folding. Order food (groceries or prepared meals) delivered to your home. Hire a maid service or a high-school student to babysit.

## Mobility

- Maintain good posture. Poor posture uses up more energy. Stand on both feet and bend your knees slightly. Leaning forward or backward uses more energy than standing tall.
- Move somehow every hour for just a minute. Stretch, reach for the ceiling, roll your shoulders, arch your back, twirl your feet—anything to get your muscles in a different position.
- Make rest stops while walking or shopping. Place chairs around the house (in halls, and so forth) for convenient rest stops.
- Apply for a handicapped parking sticker, usually at a county office where you purchase license plates.
- Carry a cane seat, a device that looks like a cane and folds out for an instant seat, or use a cane for balance.
- Use door-to-door bus service or ask about wheelchair-accessible services.
- When driving, use cruise control if possible.
- Use a wheelchair for long trips.

## Shopping

- Consolidate shopping trips. Pick one or two days a week to run errands. Unless that makes for too long and tiring a day, you may save time and effort.
- Shop at smaller stores where you can park closer and get out faster.
- Make a list, organized by departments or aisles.
- Shop at less-busy times of the day.
- Shop with a friend.
- Use the shopping cart for support or use the scooter some stores provide.
- Accept help to get your packages into and out of your car.
- Let someone else shop for you if possible.

## Childcare

- Tell your children about your fatigue and ask for help in specific ways. Make a game of the task so it will be fun. Be sure to thank them for their cooperation and reward them in a small way if they are doing more than they usually do.
- Plan activities with them where you can lie down or sit (table or computer games, reading, art projects).
- Teach toddlers to climb into your lap or the highchair so you don't have to lift them.
- Rest when they rest.
- Ask friends or family to pitch in with childcare.

## Housework

- Schedule tasks throughout the week, not all at once.
- Decide what tasks can be done less frequently and what can be delegated.
- Allow plenty of time for the tasks you choose so you don't feel stressed if you don't finish and add to your fatigue.
- Stop working before you become exhausted, even if you are in mid-task.
- Sit for as many tasks as possible.
- Carry supplies in a carpenter's apron or on a cart with wheels.
- Drag or slide objects rather than lift them. Bend your knees, not your back, when you lift something heavy.
- Buy or borrow a lightweight vacuum cleaner for the duration.
- Hire help. Some long-term care policies provide for housekeepers. Check your policy for this benefit.

## Bathing/hygiene

- Keep moist towelettes in the bathroom for quick hand-cleaning.
- Use warm instead of hot water for baths and showers. Hot water uses more of your energy as your body tries to maintain a comfortable temperature.
- Install a grab rail or apply safety strips in the bottom of the tub.
- Take a shower sitting in a chair or on a stool. An aluminum outdoor folding chair works fine. Use a handheld nozzle.
- Use a long-handled brush to reach your back and feet to avoid stooping.
- Take sponge baths. Have someone run a sink full of warm water. While sitting near the sink, soap a washcloth and rub all over. Then rinse the washcloth and rinse off little by little. You can also use Comfort Personal Cleansing Bath disposable washcloths, which can be heated in the microwave for a luxurious quick cleanse.
- Wear a terrycloth robe instead of drying off, or sit to dry off.
- Wash your hair in the shower instead of leaning over the sink.
- Use an elevated toilet seat.

## Dressing

- Organize your clothing before starting to dress. Ask someone else to lay things out for you.
- Sit down to dress.
- Avoid bending over as much as possible (for example, bring your foot to your knee to put on socks instead of bending to slip them on).
- Wear loose-fitting clothing and front-closing garments instead of slip-ons.
- Fasten your bra in front; then turn it around.

- Wear clothes that won't need ironing.
- Wear slip-on, low-heeled shoes.
- Use a long-handled shoehorn and sock aid.

## Kitchen organization
- Move frequently used items to chest level to avoid bending or reaching.
- Line ovens and drip pans with foil for easier cleanup.

## Meal preparation
- Sit on a stool or bar chair with a high back while preparing meals and washing dishes. A drafting chair is ideal.
- Prepare simple recipes, not ones with 10 steps.
- Use small appliances instead of arm muscle whenever possible. Use ergonomically designed utensils and a jar opener.
- Use mixes and prepackaged, frozen, or canned food.
- Buy chopped frozen onions or green pepper, grated cheese, frozen fruit (for baking), and minced garlic and onion. Buy fresh, cut, and prewashed vegetables such as carrots, celery, broccoli, cauliflower, slaw vegetables, salad greens, fruits, and mushrooms.
- Use rotisserie chicken from the deli for recipes that call for cooked chicken.
- To quickly cut an apple or pear: Hold fruit upright on a cutting surface. Slice off one edge close to the core, turn fruit and slice off another edge until all that's left is the core. The slices won't be even, but you'll have spent less time than if you cut the fruit in half and cored it.
- Ladle food from the stove instead of lifting heavy pots.
- Double the recipe and freeze half.
- Accept offers of prepared meals or let this need be known among your support team. Some communities have resources that deliver prepared meals. Ask your healthcare team.
- Order take-out meals.
- Go out to eat and buy an extra meal for the next night.
- Keep an ice chest next to your bed with favorite drinks and foods so they are readily available.

## Quicker cleanup
- Cook and serve in the same container.
- Move dishes to and from the table on a rolling cart.
- Soak dishes until food is easy to remove instead of scrubbing immediately after eating.
- Let dishes air dry or use a dishwasher.

- Ask family members for help with cooking and cleanup, including loading and unloading the dishwasher.

## Eating/nutrition

- Drink plenty of fluids and eat as healthy as you can.
- Avoid foods such as alcohol, large amounts of refined sugar and flour products, unhealthy fats, and caffeine that rob your body of nutrients.
- Eat more fruits and vegetables, nuts, legumes, and whole grains.
- Eat "heme" iron: lean red meat, lean poultry, fish.
- Consume adequate calories and protein. A registered dietician can help determine your levels.
- Snack on nutritious foods such as light cream cheese on bagel or nut bread, hard-boiled egg, hummus on pita bread, a milk shake or fruit smoothie, custard or pudding, cottage cheese with fruit, instant breakfast drink, or peanut butter or cheese on crackers.
- Don't overeat. A full stomach diverts blood from your muscles, leaving you fatigued. Stabilize your blood sugar by eating small meals/snacks every two to four hours.
- Ask your doctor about taking a multivitamin or food supplements. Do not take megadoses of any vitamin or mineral without his approval because some doses of even "good" substances can be toxic or can interfere with your treatment protocol. If your doctor is not trained in nutrition, visit with a dietician or nutritionist. Just as medical doctors may not be familiar with the intricacies of nutrition, most dieticians have not been trained in cancer treatment and possible conflicts of supplements and cancer medications, so find one at a cancer center if possible. People who have studied nutrition in college may refer to themselves as nutritionists. The term also refers to scientists who have graduate degrees in the field. A registered dietitian (RD) has trained in nutrition, food chemistry, and diet planning; completed an approved clinical experience; and passed an examination by the American Diatetic Association.

## At bedtime

- Get at least eight hours of sleep at night, and nap during the day if you feel tired. The need for naps may cycle in and out for months. You will only delay your healing and feeling better if you resist your body's message to rest.
- If at all possible, go to bed the same time each night and sleep until you wake up.
- Take a warm bath or read a few minutes before bed to relax you.

- Waking up at 2 or 3 a.m. is not uncommon for women in treatment for breast cancer. If your mind is racing with things you are not able to do, jot them on a pad next to your bed, try prayer or meditation, or turn on soothing music or nature sounds to help you go back to sleep.

  (See "Insomnia," page 132, for more tips.)

## Working
- Go to work during your peak energy times.
- Talk with your supervisor about modifying job responsibilities temporarily.
- Sit when possible. Take occasional breaks.
- Use rolling carts to move things.
- Eat nutritious foods and don't skip meals.
- At lunch, buy an extra meal for the evening.
- Put a living plant in your office such as Boston fern, peace lilies, or Chinese evergreens. Some studies show they perk up the people around them.
- Apply the theory of traditional Chinese medicine that the ear is ripe with pressure points that, when stimulated, increase your blood circulation and thus your energy. For a minute, rub your ears vigorously with your fingers. When they feel hot, you'll know the blood is indeed circulating and you may feel more alert.

## Leisure
- Save some energy for activities you enjoy. They will boost your mood and ward off depression.
- Balance energy levels and specific activities.
- Use a wheelchair or golf cart.
- Invite friends to join you as a way to keep connected and maintain your self-esteem.
- Don't tire yourself with fun pursuits any more than you would with responsibilities.
- Manage your stress (see page 231). Relax (see page 241).
- Get outside about 20 minutes a day if possible or at least open the blinds. When sunlight enters your eyes, it releases serotonin, which boosts energy and mood.[8]
- Walk barefoot through the grass.

## Lifestyle
- Join a support group or share your feelings with friends.
- Don't dwell on what you cannot change. Be grateful for what you can do. Negative beliefs zap energy; positive affirmations boost energy and mood.

- Keep a journal (see page 194). In addition to venting, each day include three things you are grateful for.
- Find new hobbies that are less demanding than former ones.
- Rest during the day as often as necessary, preferably 20 to 30 minutes each time. Take short naps or breaks rather than one long rest. Power naps are no more than one hour.
- Work up to some mild exercise (30 minutes a day for four to five days a week), with your doctor's permission, of course. Contrary to popular thought, exercise will give you more energy. Just don't overdo it at first, and don't be discouraged if you can't do as much as you want. I remember days that sitting up in bed for 10 minutes or walking the 12 feet to my bathroom was an accomplishment, and I celebrated that. Later, walking across the house to the kitchen was another milestone, and I applauded my progress. If walking around the block is not even on your radar screen, pick something you might reasonably do and make it a goal. When you have mastered that, pick another, slightly more challenging goal and work up to it. Reward yourself when you fulfill each goal and enjoy your improvement.
- Practice easier or shorter versions of activities you enjoy.
- Yoga, meditation, prayer, guided imagery, visualization, or water aerobics may help with fatigue and stress.
- Alcohol and caffeine can repress REM sleep, the restorative kind, so avoid caffeine within four to six hours of sleeping and alcohol within three to five hours of bedtime.[9]

## Energizing tips
- Mental stimulation improves your physical energy level. Engage in stimulating conversation, do a crossword puzzle, or play a competitive board game to get blood flowing to your brain.
- Energize yourself with an herbal bath. Place 1 tablespoon each of rosemary, patchouli, sage, strawberry leaf, woodruff, geranium leaf, mint, and orange leaf in a clean cotton sock or muslin bag and drop into your bath water.
- Energize yourself with an invigorating foot soak. Boil mint leaves in water and steep for 10 minutes. Remove leaves. Pour minted water into a foot basin and add enough cool water to make the temperature comfortable. Soak your feet and feel the rest of you revive also.
- Light an orange, clove, or tea tree aromatherapy candle for stimulation.
- Place 1/4 teaspoon of safflower or sunflower oil in your palm and add a drop of rosemary or peppermint essential oil. Rub your hands together, cup them over your nose, and breathe deeply for a quick perk-me-up. Or place a few drops of peppermint or rosemary oil on a tissue and inhale the fragrance. (These essential oils may cause skin irritation on some people.)

- Fill a spray bottle with 4 ounces of filtered water; four drops each of lemon and peppermint essential oils; six drops each of nasturtium, cosmos, and peppermint flower essences; and an emulsifier such as macadamia nut emulsifier, grain alcohol, or unscented liquid soap. When you need a pick-up, mist lightly around your face and inhale the aroma.[10]
- Splash your face and the back of your neck with cold water; then gargle with cold water for a few seconds. The shock diverts blood to your brain and all your muscles, resulting in clearer thinking and more energy.
- Hold the acupressure point between your eyebrows with your right pointer finger for one to three minutes to combat fatigue.

Vitamin and mineral supplements, improved nutrition, lifestyle modifications, psychological counseling, and antidepressant or antianxiety medications also may help in some cases.

## Report These Symptoms to Your Doctor Immediately
- Sudden increase in the severity of your fatigue.
- Changes in the way your fatigue feels.
- Dizziness or fainting.
- Inability to manage the fatigue.

(Because fatigue is sometimes caused by pain, insomnia, anemia, or depression, see those sections in this chapter for ideas on coping.)

### Fluid Retention
If your feet, arms, legs, abdomen, or face becomes swollen or puffy or you have a sudden increase in weight, you may be retaining fluid as a result of your treatment or hormonal changes. Let your doctor know so he can prescribe a diuretic to help you pass the fluid or evaluate other options such as decreasing salt intake, gentle exercise, elevation of limbs, and so on.

### Flu-Like Symptoms
After taking some chemotherapy drugs, you may think you have the flu. You may have a slight fever, achiness, tiredness, joint or muscle pain, headache, nausea, chills, and not much appetite. These symptoms could be from medication or they could indicate an infection or be caused by the cancer itself. Check with your doctor.

### Frozen Shoulder
As if surgery weren't enough, you want to be on your guard to avoid what is called "frozen shoulder" (adhesive capulitis), a restriction of movement of

the arm on the side of your lymph node dissection. You probably won't be swinging a tennis racket with that arm for a while because of the stiffness, pain, and the need to protect the incision. Also you may have been cautioned not to traumatize the arm or lift heavy objects so as to avoid the risk of lymphedema.

Unless you are a physical therapist, you probably won't know how to balance the various goals you are trying to accomplish. And it's very likely that none of your doctors will take the responsibility of monitoring your range of motion to see if it is returning at an acceptable pace. The American Cancer Society's Reach to Recovery program sends volunteers to new breast cancer patients to show them exercises to do. However, it does not always offer in-person follow-up to see if additional help is needed.

Ask your physician or oncologist to refer you to a physical therapist just as soon as the surgeon says the incision has healed and gives you permission to start exercising your arm. (You must be referred by a doctor; you can't just go to a physical therapist on your own.) By all means, request a visit if you feel pain and/or severe stiffness in your arm, shoulder, or chest when you reach into a high cabinet, stretch behind you, or move in any other direction.

An initial session will determine if you are progressing satisfactorily or if you need exercises for specific muscle groups. Some pain, unfortunately, is normal in the area of surgery, but pain in other areas means the muscles are tighter than they should be or that nerves are being pinched and may cause trouble later, so you will want to avoid that sensation. Only a trained physical therapist can tell what your pain means.

You can jump-start your healing by moving your arm the day after surgery. Although health professionals tell you to prop your arm on a pillow after a mastectomy, they may forget to tell you to move that arm. Gently and carefully, raise and lower your forearm, move the arm from side to side, try to straighten it lengthwise—anything to challenge the range of motion. A week or so after surgery, gently knead the pectoral muscles (those on your chest just above the breast area) and those under your arm. Just moving the skin in those areas will discourage scar tissue from forming that might have to be worked out through therapy.

Though the area will be tender, see if you can gently press on the muscle with your fingertips and slowly move the tissue up and down, from side to side, then around in a circle. Move the skin to the point you feel tautness or tightness; then apply gentle pressure into the tightness.

Studies have shown that connective tissue begins to deteriorate with just seven to eight weeks of disuse, making movement difficult and painful. Also, three to five days after surgery, fibroblasts begin migrating to the incision in increased amounts. These are the cells responsible for forming connective tissue. Decreased movement of the arm and shoulder, combined with the proliferation of connective tissue formation, is a recipe for tissue tightness. Through therapy, you probably can regain the ability to move, but this is a slow, painful process that is best avoided by early detection. Unfortunately, the process can take months or several years, and even then not everyone regains all their range of motion.

When your surgeon gives permission, consider water aerobics, overhead pulleys, dance movements with your arms over your head, or gentle exercises (see page 77) for a gentle stimulation of muscles.

## *Gas*

Your digestive system can be impacted by several forms of cancer treatment. If you develop gas, try these strategies. If they do not give relief, mention the problem to your doctor.

## To Relieve Gas

- Gently massage your abdomen or apply pressure on the acupressure point three finger-widths below your navel.
- Suck on peppermints or drink peppermint tea.
- Papaya in any form may help. For instant relief, chew papaya tablets from a health food store. If indigestion is a frequent problem, drink unsweetened papaya juice or eat fresh papaya on a regular basis.
- Walk and drink plenty of fluids, especially hot tea, throughout the day to keep your digestive system in good order.
- The more you eat beans, the less problem they pose for your digestive system,[11] but certainly don't begin eating beans if you are not used to them! Beano can help with gas from beans.
- Simethicone chewable tablets can help relieve trapped gas.
- Chew 1 teaspoon of raw coriander or cumin seed after a meal or 2 tablespoons of fresh cilantro during a meal. Drink tea made from 2 teaspoons fennel, coriander, or cumin seeds steeped for 10 minutes in a cup of water and drained.

## Some Causes of Gas

- High-fiber foods.
- Cruciferous vegetables (broccoli, cabbage, cauliflower, collard greens, bok choy, kale).
- Beans, legumes. Split peas, lentils, and anasazi beans are low in gas-forming sugars. Use plenty of water (9 cups water to 1 cup dried beans) to soak beans; then drain, rinse, and cook them in fresh water. The soak water

contains the indigestible natural sugars that cause gas. Drain and rinse canned beans for less gas. Add a pinch of baking soda and chunks of carrots while cooking. Discard the carrots before serving.

- Lactose intolerance (inability to digest milk sugar). Use lactose-reduced milk or take Lactaid tablets.

## Hair Loss

Hair loss is probably the most dreaded side effect of chemotherapy. Not all chemotherapy drugs cause hair loss, and not all women lose all their hair even if they are taking the drugs that commonly cause this (particularly Adriamycin, Cytoxan, Taxol, and Taxotere). Hair loss is caused when the chemotherapy drugs destroy hair follicles. Sometimes hair just becomes thinner, limp, dull, or dry instead of falling out.

In some European countries women use an ice cap to freeze the scalp and prevent blood flow to the hair follicles. Besides being slightly uncomfortable, ice caps are not recommended by some oncologists because they fear the freezing may prevent the drug from reaching the cells in the scalp and, theoretically, missing some cancer cells. Seek your doctor's advice if this possibility interests you.

## Before Chemotherapy

Ask your doctor if and when to expect hair loss from your particular drugs. Sometimes hair loss begins right away. Other times it does not occur until your third or fourth treatment. Remember: Not all chemotherapy drugs cause hair loss!

Consider cutting your hair short before chemotherapy begins. Then the loss is not so dramatic. Also, your hair will appear thicker. You will feel more secure if you visit a wig shop or order your wig before you start your chemotherapy or have a favorite cap/hat or some scarves on hand. You can get a close match to your own hair and you are prepared no matter when the shedding begins. At least save a lock of your hair if you want to keep your same color and decide to wait until the loss begins before purchasing a wig.

Some women use this experience as an excuse to try a completely different color or hairstyle. You can have several wigs and experiment with several looks. Make the most of an unpleasant situation and live it up!

## Coping with Hair Loss

Sometimes hair will fall out slowly for a few days; then it starts to come out in clumps. You will find handfuls of hair on your pillow in the morning and in the shower or tub after you bathe.

Patients often go through a cycle of thought about hair loss. With the first few strands they find, they think, "Oh, this won't be so bad. I'll keep what I can for as long as I can." If you do not have a wig or headpiece yet, now is the time to purchase it. All your hair can fall out within just a few days and you want to be prepared.

After a few days of finding hair on the floor, the pillow, and your clothing, the messiness of it all becomes irritating. Women realize that the inevitable is happening. All of their hair—everywhere on their body (yes, pubic hair, eyebrows, eyelashes, and underarm and leg hair)—is going to come out. Their attitude changes to, "Why put up with the mess when what's left doesn't look very glamorous anyway?"

Often your scalp will become tender about 48 hours before the hair turns loose. Don't panic. The hair is falling out because the cycle of protein production for the follicles was interrupted. Once that area of the hair grows outside the scalp, it is brittle and breaks off. Once the interruptions from chemotherapy stop, your hair will grow again as usual.

Hair loss is a good situation for practicing taking charge of your life. When the hair starts to fall out, many women choose to shave it off to get the agony over with and to reduce the cleanup. Because cancer is a family affair, some women let their husbands or older children shave off their hair as a way of participating. Some family members even go so far as to shave their heads at the same time in a gesture of support! Others let kids draw on their bald heads with watercolor or tempera paint to lighten the atmosphere.

Some women find that the horror of hair loss is somewhat mitigated by donating their hair to Locks of Love (*www.locksoflove.org*), Wigs for Kids (*www.wigsforkids.org*), or a similar organization that donates wigs to children who have lost their hair. If you are interested, check the Website before your head shaving for specific instructions on hair donations. Others ease their grief by gathering all their lost hair and burying or burning it (do it outside; it can smell bad!) in a ritual of forgiveness and farewell.

Be aware that your head may be tender, so caution the shaver to be gentle. If you have a beautician shave your head, take along your wig or headpiece for the trip home. Also take some tissue with you. Seeing yourself for the first time with a bald head can be a shock. Feelings of anger, horror, sadness, and depression often well up even though you know that the chemotherapy causing this loss may also curb your cancer. See the hair loss as a guarantee that the chemo is working at least to some degree.

Your feelings will settle down eventually. Honor those that do come. Acknowledge them and deal gently with them. As you look into the mirror without your headpiece, try to think kind and accepting thoughts. This is your body for now, so you may as well love it. Hopefully the people around you love you for who you are and not for how you look and they will adjust to your temporary look also with time.

The American Cancer Society offers a free Look Good...Feel Better program that describes makeup techniques to compensate for hair loss and offers free wigs and cosmetic samples for participants.

## To Slow the Rate of Hair Loss

Although hair loss cannot be prevented with certain medications, you may be able to slow the rate at which you lose your hair. Treat your hair gently with these tips:

- Wash hair only as needed.
- Do not pull on hair or use rubber bands or scrunchies.
- Use gentle shampoo.
- Do not color or perm your hair during chemo.
- Avoid hair dryers, curling irons, or other hair appliances that use heat.

## Practical Tips for Hair Loss

- Sleep in a hair net so your pillow is not a tangle of hair in the morning.
- Use satin pillowcases, which are soothing to a sore scalp.
- Place a metal screen over your bathtub or shower drain to catch hair that comes off while you bathe (and it will come off—in bunches!).
- Keep a plastic bowl or trashcan in or near the shower to discard hair as it comes off.
- Be sure to keep the water warm, not hot, while your scalp is sensitive.
- Wear a bit more makeup or eye shadow to give you color and contrast that your hair normally supplies.
- Wear big or dangly earrings to give the movement of hair and soften your look.

## To Cover or Not to Cover

Some women are bold about their hair loss and don't bother with wigs or headwear. Others decide that they feel better and that others are more comfortable around them with the softening effect of a wig, scarf, cap, or turban. Seeing their bald head is an unwanted reminder of the cancer. Some work environments require a certain image. Only you know what makes you and the people around you feel best. Ask your family to support you in whatever choice you make about your hair covering while you are at home.

(See Chapter 8 for tips about choosing a wig or other headwear and for makeup tricks to compensate for missing eyebrows and eyelashes.)

## Scalp and Hair Care during Chemotherapy

Some women complain of a sensitive scalp before their hair falls out. If that describes your head, take the following precautions:

- Use a mild shampoo.
- Use a soft hair brush or plastic comb with rounded edges.
- Don't use brush rollers to set your hair.
- Don't dye, perm, or relax your hair during chemotherapy.
- Use low heat to dry your hair.
- Cover your head with a sun screen, scarf, or hat when out in the sun.

## When Hair Grows Back

Your hair may begin to grow back during treatment or several weeks afterward. Sometimes it takes up to three months to begin growing again. When it returns has nothing to do with the effectiveness of your treatment. Hair grows at about half an inch per month and it grows unseen under your scalp for several weeks before that welcome peach fuzz begins to appear on your scalp. Eyelashes, eyebrows, and pubic hair usually grow in faster than hair on your head.

Some women find that their hair grows back thicker and fuller than it was. Some even have a different texture (oftentimes curly) or different color hair (more or less gray, darker or lighter)! Usually after a few months your hair will generally return to its former weight and color, although some women's new look remains.

To speed up hair growth after treatment is over, some women have found success with taking brewer's yeast or wheat grass tablets or massaging their scalp with conditioner. Because your hair will be weak for about six months after it grows back, use gentle shampoo and avoid chemicals of perms, coloring, or straighteners. A few women confided they used Mane 'n Tail, a shampoo to make horses' manes silky, because their hair grew in so coarse.

### Hot Flashes

One of the most irritating side effects of chemotherapy is its triggering menopause in pre- or perimenopausal women. With that often come hot flashes—a feeling that someone has turned on a space heater deep inside you. Some women actually feel as if they are toasting and break out in perspiration. Everyone's hot flash experience is different. Some have long flashes whereas for others they last only a few seconds. Some have flashes all day;

others have just a few. Some feel hot all over, whereas others feel the flush in only their face, upper body, and neck. Fifty percent of women will have hot flashes for about a year, 30 percent will experience them for up to two and a half years, and the rest may have them for many years, some for the rest of their lives.[12]

Changing levels of hormones and the increase of the neurotransmitter norepinephrine are believed to be the cause of hot flashes. They affect the part of the hypothalamus that regulates temperature. You are suddenly hot enough to strip off all your clothes; then just as suddenly you are cold and clammy. Some women perspire with their hot flashes; others flush or feel dizzy or their heart races.

Although hormone replacement therapy (HRT) has been proven recently to be dangerous to many women, breast cancer patients whose tumors are estrogen-receptor–positive have long been advised not to take estrogen products because it is believed they can nourish any remaining cancer cells. Because estrogen and progesterone are often given to relieve symptoms such as hot flashes, this leaves a number of women at the mercy of menopausal side effects.

Supplements some women have used successfully for relief from symptoms (and that do not seem to stimulate breast cancer cells) are B vitamins, oil of evening primrose, gotu kola, dong quai, black cohosh root,[13] soy products (see page 309), and vitamin E. Be sure to ask your doctor before taking any herb or supplement because some contain natural plant estrogens that may not be wise for your particular type of breast cancer. Also work with a trained herbalist who should know the dangers and effects of the many other supplements taken for hot flashes, such as calcium, vitamin C, ginseng, vitex, fennel, spearmint, red raspberry, red clover, anise, and fenugreek.

You can ask your doctor about Effexor (venlafaxine), Wellbutrin, Bellamine S, Inderal (propranolol), and Catapres patch (clonidine)—medications that sometimes give relief from hot flashes. Bellergal is another prescription drug used to control hot flashes, although some physicians use it only as a last resort because of its powerful ingredients. The antidepressant Zoloft has shown some promise also.

Acupuncture and homeopathic compounds have helped some women with hot flashes. If you investigate these options, consult with someone well trained and check with your oncologist.

## Other Tips for Hot Flashes

If you are lucky, you can identify what triggers your hot flashes. Keep a journal for several days. Record when a hot flash occurs and what you did in the hour preceding it. What did you eat? What were you doing? What emotions were you feeling? Do you see a pattern? If so, eliminate as many of the triggers as you can and see if your hot flashes diminish.

## Nutrition/eating

- Keep a sports bottle of cool water by your bed at night (freeze it, take it out just when you retire, and it will stay cool most of the night) and sip a little when a hot flash comes. Or fill an insulated cup with ice and it will remain cool most of the night. Drink cool water through the day.
- Avoid caffeine and alcohol as well as hot, spicy foods, sugar, and smoking.
- Eat mints or hard candies as nocturnal snacks to cool you off.

## Activities

- Open the freezer door and stand in the cold air for a quick cool-down.
- Keep something handy to fan yourself with or a handkerchief to pat off the perspiration.
- Turn down the thermostat. The cooler the room, the fewer hot flashes you may experience.[14]
- Try literally to keep your cool, as stress seems to aggravate hot flashes.
- Exercise regularly—in air conditioning and at the coolest part of the day if possible. Sweating helps your body cool down, but use common sense.
- Try meditation, visualization, deep breathing, or relaxation methods. Especially think about something cold: snow, ice cream, polar bears.
- Avoid hot tubs, saunas, and sunbathing. Instead step into a cool shower, immerse your hands and feet into ice water, or place ice cubes on your wrist or chest (wrap in a washcloth).
- Layer in bed also. Wear light gowns and cover with light blankets that can be peeled off. Avoid electric blankets and flannel or silk sheets.

## Dressing

- Dress in layers so you can remove a jacket or vest when a hot flash hits.
- Wear cotton, silk, or other natural, breathable fabrics rather than synthetics. However, if you sweat profusely with your hot flashes, don't wear cotton next to your skin. It will absorb the moisture and you'll be stuck in a wet garment. Try to find athletic clothing that wicks the moisture away from your body.
- Avoid high necklines, which can make you feel trapped when a hot flash hits.

## *Indigestion*

Indigestion is heartburn or discomfort in the upper abdomen, a sour taste in the back of the throat, or reflux. It can be caused by eating spicy or greasy foods or by going to bed right after a heavy meal. Caffeine, alcohol, and tobacco can make indigestion worse. Take Tums or an antacid for relief. (See "Gas," page 122, for more tips on coping.)

## *Infections*

If you have chemotherapy, you want to be particularly careful to avoid infections because your immune system has been compromised. The length of this compromise is uncertain, so it is best to take precautions for the rest of your life. Seven to 10 days after chemotherapy is the typical time when white blood cell counts drop the lowest and you are at greatest risk of infection.

Hand-washing is the most basic and most ignored practice for avoiding infections. A recent survey showed that only one in three adults washes her hands after using the bathroom. Another survey of nurses showed that more than three-quarters did not wash their hands properly. To wash your hands, use warm, running water and soap. Lather 15 to 20 seconds, being sure to scrub between your fingers and under your nails. The longer you lather, the better. Rinse thoroughly.

## Hygiene

- When you receive a scratch, insect bite, or other abrasion, immediately wash the area with soap and apply an antiseptic ointment. If red streaks radiate from the wound, see your doctor immediately.

- Wash your hands when returning from a public place such as medical offices, grocery stores, shopping malls, even church—anywhere you could come in contact with germs. Be especially cognizant of touching shopping carts, escalator or stair railings, and doorknobs. Wash your hands also after using the bathroom, before eating, and after touching an animal or handling garbage.

- Soap and water are fine for hand washing. Preferably use liquid soap because germs can live on the bar of soap. To prevent this, wash the bar of soap in your hands, rinse the bar, and put it in the soap dish while you finish rinsing your hands. If you want to go to the next level of sanitation, choose alcohol washes over antibacterial soap, which germs can become immune to. Many of those soaps do not contain enough of the germ-killing ingredient, triclosan, to outperform soap or they require washing, rinsing, and washing again.[15] Instead select a "hand sanitizer" such as Purell with "ethyl alcohol 62%" as an active ingredient. Wash your hands first with soap; then apply a dollop of sanitizer the size of a dime in your palm. Rub your hands together until dry. Most brands include a moisturizer, as the alcohol is drying.[16] This is especially handy for travel.

- Dry your hands with paper towels. Germs love to live in soggy cloth towels.

- Do not share towels, utensils, cups, or dishes with anyone. Don't share a pillow or bed with anyone who is sick.

- Avoid being near people who are sick. If you can't avoid sick family members, keep face masks for them to wear around you.
- Avoid having your nails done commercially or be sure that all equipment is sterilized before it is used on you. Do not cut or tear your cuticles and create grounds for infection.
- Shave with an electric razor or use a depilatory instead of razor blades to avoid cuts if your underarm is numb.
- Clean your rectal area gently but thoroughly after every bowel movement. Wipe from front to back. For rectal discomfort, use witch hazel astringent or comfrey ointment (Country Comfort Herbal Savvy Comfrey-Aloe Vera). Check with your physician before using enemas, douches, or suppositories.
- Practice good oral hygiene (see page 107).
- Do not squeeze or scratch pimples.
- Bathe or shower with soap every day. Pat your skin dry instead of rubbing hard. Dry your genital area thoroughly after bathing or swimming. Bacteria love moist, dark areas.
- Avoid contact with animal litter boxes, birdcages, or fish tanks, or wear a facial mask to avoid inhaling dust and dander.
- Avoid standing water such as in birdbaths, flower vases, or humidifiers.
- Replace all makeup every four to six weeks to avoid bacteria.

## Eating

- Do not eat raw foods such as fish, seafood, meat, or eggs. (See also "Eating during Chemotherapy," page 55.)
- Cooked or canned fruits are fine, but avoid fresh, frozen, or dried fruit.
- Do not use unprocessed honey. Use molasses instead.
- Avoid uncooked herbs, spices, and salsa.

## Lifestyle

- Avoid crowds (stores; special events; yes, even church or synagogue) to limit your exposure to germs. Go shopping or to events when the facilities are least crowded.
- Avoid children who have recently received "live virus" vaccines such as chicken pox, oral polio, or nasal flu vaccine. They may be contagious to people with low blood counts.
- Wear insect repellant when insects are biting.

- Wear long sleeves and protective gloves when gardening or doing other work that might result in scratches. Sewing stores have special gloves with Kevlar in them to protect from cuts. There are also special guards for home sewing machines to protect from needle pricks that are common among quilters.
- Support your body with healthy foods, adequate liquids, and plenty of rest.
- Keep your stress level low because stress undermines your body's ability to fight off infection. When you get upset, ask yourself what difference the situation will make in 10 (or 100!) years. Or ask yourself if the situation is worth risking your health. (See also "Stress," page 231.)
- Ask your doctor about receiving a flu shot each year and a pneumonia shot (usually once every 10 years or once in a lifetime).
- Do not have blood drawn from the arm on the side where you had lymph nodes removed (see "Lymphedema," page 137).
- Use moisturizer or oil to soften your skin and prevent or cure it from being dry and cracked.
- Avoid vases of fresh-cut flowers, which can carry bacteria.[17]

## Dressing

- Do not share towels, underwear, pantyhose, or bathing suits.
- Wear underwear with a cotton crotch, which allows air to circulate and moisture to evaporate or wear underwear from the new fabrics that wick moisture away from your skin.
- Remove wet bathing suits promptly. Bacteria love warm, moist environments.
- Avoid public hot tubs. The high temperatures evaporate the chlorine, so germs can be transmitted.

## Signs of Infection

Call your doctor if you notice any of these symptoms, which might indicate an infection:

- Fever of more than 101°F or 38°C. This is an emergency if your white blood count is low.
- Hot, flushed skin.
- Loose bowel movements.
- Chills, especially combined with shaking.
- Rapid heart rate.
- Sweating when you have not been exerting yourself (not hot flashes, either).
- Severe cough or sore throat.
- Frequent, burning, or urgent urination; cloudy or foul-smelling urine.

- Unusual vaginal discharge or itching.
- Sinus pain or pressure.
- Earache, headache, stiff neck.
- Blisters on lip or skin.
- Mouth sores.
- Redness, swelling, or tenderness around a sore, wound, catheter or port site on your affected arm, on your rectum, or near a pimple.

## Infertility

Chemotherapy drugs and radiation may affect the ovaries' ability to produce hormones and therefore your ability to become pregnant. This infertility may be temporary or permanent and depends on many factors. Remember that *you can get pregnant during chemotherapy.*

If you might want to get pregnant later, ask about harvesting and freezing some eggs before treatment in case you do become infertile. (See "Pregnancy," page 265.)

## Insomnia

Nighttime, when the rest of the household is asleep, can be a very lonely or frightening time for an ill person. Also, it is a time when you are most vulnerable to your emotions.

Lack of sleep can have health repercussions as well. Sleep gives your body a chance to restore and repair itself and is essential for keeping your immune system in top form.

## Effects of Sleep Deprivation

Most adults need about eight hours of sleep, and cancer patients in treatment may need more. When we sacrifice sleep to squeeze more into our day, we are inadvertently making ourselves vulnerable to these effects of inadequate sleep:

- Impaired memory.
- Difficulty concentrating.
- Decreased ability to learn.
- Hindered coordination and reflexes.
- High blood pressure, obesity, diabetes.
- Decreased ability to process carbohydrates, manage stress, fight infection, regulate hormones.
- Headaches, depression.

# Overcoming Insomnia

Avoid sleeping pills except for short periods, such as a week or two. They produce side effects such as excitability, confusion, anxiety, and loss of memory the next day. To help you sleep at night, try some of the tips offered here.

## Eating/drinking tips

- Eat turkey, tuna, banana, or warm milk before bedtime. They all contain tryptophan, which promotes sleep. Carbohydrates such as bread, cereal, cheese with crackers, or hard-boiled egg or yogurt with fruit are other good choices. Just don't overeat or drink a lot just before bed.

- Avoid caffeine (that includes chocolate!) four to six hours before bed.

- Avoid alcohol two hours before retiring. Although it may relax you at first, it disturbs sleep after several hours and acts as a diuretic.

- Don't eat a heavy meal within two or three hours of going to sleep.

- Snack on proteins and complex carbohydrates (whole-grain bread with almond butter) about 45 minutes before bedtime. Often people wake at about 3 a.m. from a drop in blood sugar. A protein/carbohydrate snack can stabilize your sugar levels.[18]

- Place one of the following mixtures of herbs into a teapot, cover with boiling water, steep for 10 minutes, strain, and drink. If you use a tea infuser, just place the herbs inside and remove the infuser after 10 minutes. One mixture is 1/4 teaspoon of lavender flowers and 1/2 teaspoon each of lemon balm leaves, linden flowers (or lime blossoms), and chamomile. Another is 1/2 teaspoon each of valerian root, passionflowers, chamomile, and vervain.[19]

- Sip chamomile tea with crushed rosemary or French tarragon tea. (Steep 1 teaspoon dried leaves in 1 cup boiled water for five to 10 minutes.)

- Herbalists recommend motherwort, and melatonin supplement has proven its usefulness for insomnia in some randomized clinical trials.[20] Consult a trained herbalist and your doctor before consuming any herb.

- Vitamins B3 and B6 help your body make melatonin, a hormone that helps regulate your internal clock. Sources of these vitamins are salmon, tuna, sunflower seeds, and wheat bran. Chicken, turkey, peanuts, and apricots are rich in vitamin B3. Avocados, bananas, carrots, rice, and shrimp are full of vitamin B6. Foods high in melatonin are cherries, oats, rice, bananas, barley, ginger, tomatoes, and sweet corn. As an added benefit, melatonin is an antioxidant.

## Daytime activities

- Avoid long naps during the day if they prevent you from sleeping at night. Set a timer so you won't nap more than 45 minutes.
- Avoid strenuous exercise for four hours before retiring, but do exercise during the day. *Harvard Health Letter* says that exercise is "the only proven way for adults to prolong deep sleep."[21]
- Get outside during the day. Light exposure even in midday influences the release of melatonin, a hormone that induces drowsiness.
- Find ways to be around people. Dissatisfaction with your social life can hamper your sleep patterns.[22]

## Nighttime activities

- Take a warm bath or shower up to two hours before bedtime. Add five to 10 drops of valerian (it is effective although some people don't like the smell) or lavender essential oil to relax you. Mix 2 ounces of honey with five drops of lavender essential oil and an emulsifier such as unscented Ivory liquid soap. Place the container in warm water if it's too thick. Add 1 to 2 tablespoons of this mixture to your bath to calm you.

  (See also "Stress," page 231, and "Relaxation," page 241.)

## Timing

- Keep a regular bedtime and bedtime ritual. Include some unwinding time (reading, stretching, yoga, meditation, prayer, listening to soothing music) before you try to sleep.
- Take your medication for pain, nausea, or diarrhea an hour before bedtime so it has time to begin working and provide some relief before you try to sleep.
- Avoid stimulants such as caffeine, some pain relievers, appetite suppressants, nasal decongestants, and sinus or cold medicine at bedtime. Some antidepressants should not be taken at bedtime although others are supposed to be. Ask about your medication.
- Avoid television, computer work, complex projects, bill paying, or anything work related or stressful at least an hour before bedtime. Spend that time doing something relaxing such as reading, working a crossword puzzle, or doing stitchery.

## In-bed activities

- Pamper yourself with extra-soft sheets. Try all cotton with at least 200-thread-count.
- Change your sheets at least weekly, more often if you are sick and in bed during the day.

- Keep your feet warm with socks.
- Use a wool blanket, which will regulate body temperature better than acrylic or nylon.
- Breathe deeply or imagine a soothing scene to bring on sleep more effectively than counting sheep.
- Get out of bed if you are not able to sleep.
- If you begin worrying about an issue in your life, write it on a pad by your bed and let it alone.

## Environment

- Listen to soothing music or recordings of nature sounds.
- Avoid light in your room, including a nightlight. Use a rheostat (dimmer switch) or nightlight in your bathroom.
- Make the room as dark and quiet as possible. If you live in a noisy neighborhood, use a table fountain or white noise generator, run a fan, or wear earplugs.
- Ensure that the temperature is comfortable, not too cold or hot. A slightly cool room, about 68°F, is about right for most people.
- Put pets in their own bed, not in yours. They can disturb your sleep.
- Reserve the bed for sleep and sex. Climaxes are a natural sedative.
- Remove distractions, such as television and computers, and clutter such as dirty clothes or stacks of magazines or mail. All these cause anxiety and keep you awake. If you can't remove them, turn off the electronics and cover the stacks with a sheet.

## Sleep pillow

Make this easy pillow to ease your transition into dreamland. If you are too tired, ask a friend to make it for you. Place a few drops of clove oil on a tissue. Place into a muslin bag with 2 ounces of rose petals and 1 ounce each of mint and rosemary. Sew the bag shut or pin or tape it securely. Lay your head on this when you have trouble sleeping. Another soothing mixture includes 2 ounces agrimony; 1 ounce each woodruff, crushed cloves, crushed and dried orange peel, and orris root powder; and two drops orange oil.[23]

For a quicker calm, place a few tablespoons of dried lavender in a small cloth bag and tuck it under your pillow.

If insomnia persists after trying some of these ideas consistently for six weeks, consult your physician. You may have a sleep disorder. (See "Relaxation," page 241, or "Stress," page 231, for other suggestions.)

## *Intravenous (IV) Reactions*

Usually you will be in a medical office or hospital while you receive an IV, so any discomfort or symptom can be reported easily. Some drugs could cause tissue damage if they leak out of the vein. Bring to the nurse's attention any swelling, flushing, redness, itching, burning, or pain at the IV site or in the vein. Typically you feel nothing after the needle stick, so any strange feeling should be reported.

## *Itching*

If your skin begins to itch, especially at the site of an IV or port, notify your doctor before using any topical ointment or cream.

If itching occurs during radiation treatment, prescription creams or a light sprinkling of cornstarch may provide relief. Use only a light, water-based lotion. A heavy lotion may leave a film on your skin that might interfere with treatment or cause further irritation to the skin.

If you develop vaginal itching, wear only cotton underwear and avoid soap, toilet tissue, and vaginal douches that are scented.

## *Kidney or Bladder Problems*

Temporary or permanent damage to the bladder or kidney can result from some chemotherapy drugs such as cyclophosphamide or Platinol. If you are taking a drug with this possibility, your doctor will probably ask for a 24-hour urine sample and a blood sample to check your kidney function before you begin chemo.

Other drugs can change the color of your urine. Adriamycin, for example, gives urine a red or orange tint.

Drinking plenty of fluids will help pass these drugs out of your body quickly and prevent problems. Fluids can be water, fruit juice, soup, Popsicles, broth, soft drinks, or even ice cream, sherbet, or gelatin.

## Symptoms to Report to Your Doctor

- Not being able to urinate.
- Pain or burning when you urinate.
- Having to urinate frequently.
- Feeling you can't wait to get to the toilet.
- Bloody urine.
- Fever.
- Chills or shaking.

## Lifting

Your surgeon may caution you not to lift heavy objects until your incision has healed or to avoid heavy lifting forever with the arm on the side of lymph node removal. This is to reduce the risk of lymphedema, a swelling of the arm.

"Heavy" is defined differently by different medical personnel. It can mean anything heavier than a gallon of milk or about 15 pounds, depending on the source. Does that mean you can never again pick up your toddler? Not necessarily. If possible, pick him or her up with your other arm or sit and let the child crawl into your lap.

## Lymphedema

After lymph nodes have been removed, you will always be at risk for swelling of the arm on the side of surgery, a condition known as lymphedema. Always. It is not life-threatening, but it can be uncomfortable, permanent, and inconvenient. It can be caused by pressure or infection in the arm, and it may appear immediately after treatment or 20 years later. Though about 5 percent of breast cancer patients develop lymphedema the first year after treatment, about 15 to 20 percent report it during their lifetime.

The lymph system is part of your immune system that removes impurities and maintains fluid balance in the body. Lymph nodes are pea-sized bodies that act as the filters of the lymph system; lymph vessels distribute and remove lymph fluid, similar to the working of the blood vessels. Lymphedema is an impairment of this drainage function because of removal of lymph nodes and lymph vessels during surgery and the resulting limitation of how much fluid can be removed. Women who have not had lymph node dissection are not at risk for lymphedema.

No one can predict who will develop lymphedema, so you should take precautions the rest of your life. It is possible that older women and those with poor nutrition may be at more risk than others.[24] Caught early, lymphedema is manageable. By all means, alert your doctor if you notice even slight swelling of your arm, hand, fingers, or chest wall. Left untreated, lymphedema can progress to a more severe stage that is at increased risk for bacterial infection or even loss of limb function.

Some physicians dismiss the precautions because no scientific studies exist to support them per se. However, the National Lymphedema Network says that anecdotal evidence firmly supports your being careful to keep the affected side scrupulously clean and avoid even moderate pressure on the affected side. Factors that affect the lymphatic transport capacity and lymphatic load do not lend themselves to rigorous controlled studies due to the wide number of precipitators, cumulative effects of alleged triggers, variations in degree of lymphatic impairment and anatomy, and the lifetime risk factor for the condition. Be your own health advocate and take these precautions. If, for example, you plan to fly and your doctor won't prescribe a compression sleeve because you don't yet have lymphedema, ask another doctor. You are the one who will suffer the consequences if his judgment is incorrect. Most doctors, however, are willing to prescribe a sleeve if you ask.

## Before Surgery

Ask your doctor about doing a sentinel node biopsy. If that important lymph node is benign, perhaps further sampling of lymph nodes during surgery can be avoided and the risk of lymphedema will be reduced considerably.

Record measurements around your palm, wrist, forearm, and upper arm for baseline comparison later as you watch for swelling.

## After Surgery

Postsurgical swelling of the breast area on the side of surgery is normal and will usually disappear in two to three weeks. Swelling under the arm is not common and should be checked with your doctor.

### To relieve normal swelling

- Do not favor your affected side. Use it for your normal activities (hair care, bathing, dressing, and so on) as pain permits.
- While lying down, elevate your affected arm on pillows for an hour two or three times a day. Have your elbow slightly higher than your shoulder and your hand higher than your wrist.
- While your affected arm is raised above the level of your heart, open and close your hand 15 to 25 times three or four times a day (you can use a rubber ball). This moves lymph fluid out of the arm through undamaged lymph vessels and reduces swelling.
- When your doctor or physical therapist gives permission, begin exercising your affected arm to regain range of motion.
- If you have radiation, continue range of motion and stretching exercises as a daily routine.

### To avoid dangerous pressure

- Avoid having blood pressure or blood samples taken or an IV or injection given in the arm on the side of your surgery. The extra pressure or invasion can upset the lymph system of the arm and cause swelling. Therapists trained in lymphedema recommend avoiding acupuncture needles; acupuncturists do not feel there is a threat from the tiny needles. If you have had bilateral surgery, have blood pressure checked or blood drawn from your nondominant side (if you are right-handed, have it drawn from your left arm) or from your thigh or leg. If you have had a modified radical mastectomy on one side and a simple mastectomy or lumpectomy on the other, offer the side of the simple mastectomy or lumpectomy for blood pressure or blood draws. In an emergency, of course, allow whatever is necessary to stabilize you.

- Do not wear tight cuffs, armholes, or restrictive clothing or jewelry on the affected arm. If your hand swells, you may need to wear a special compression glove.

- Avoid carrying heavy (more than 15 pounds) suitcases, bags, or even children with your affected arm. Do not use shoulder straps for purses, briefcases, or bags on your affected side. If you had a bilateral mastectomy, lift groceries, children, or other loads with both arms.

- Avoid vigorous, repetitive movement against pressure such as scrubbing, pushing, and pulling with the at-risk arm.

- Avoid extreme temperature changes such as when bathing or washing dishes. Avoid saunas, steam baths, whirlpools, and hot tubs, as heat can increase fluid buildup. Protect the affected arm from the sun always.

- Do exercise with the affected arm in moderation. If the arm begins to ache, lie down and elevate it immediately. Ask your doctor or physical therapist whether weight-lifting exercises are appropriate for you and whether you should wear a compression sleeve during strenuous activities.

- If using an exercise band, wrap a washcloth or other padding material around the handle to avoid putting too much pressure on the body part involved.

- Tennis, racquetball, and golf are considered risky sports for people at risk for lymphedema.[25]

- Wear light breast prostheses because heavy prostheses put pressure on the lymph nodes above the collarbone. You may need soft padded shoulder straps for your bra. Be sure your bra is well fitted, is not too tight, and preferably has no underwire.

- Use a lambskin pad (attaches with Velcro) to keep your seat belt from rubbing the affected area.

- A rare complication from tamoxifen is blood clots, which can lead to lymphedema of the leg.

- Avoid leaning on your armpit area, say with your arm draped over a hard-back chair.

## To avoid infection

- Keep the at-risk arm extra clean and moist. Dry carefully and use lotion after bathing.
- File your nails instead of cutting them to avoid breaking the skin. Also avoid hangnails to avoid infection.
- Avoid having your nails done at a salon unless the personnel sterilize scissors, files, and other equipment between customers.
- If you get a paper cut, insect bite, or scratch, wash the area with soap and water and apply an antibacterial ointment immediately. Always carry individual packets of antibacterial ointment and bandages in your purse and car.
- Wear gloves when you garden (to avoid pricks or scratches), wash dishes (to avoid dry skin and extreme temperature changes), or perform chores using steel wool or chemicals. Wear a thimble when sewing or doing needlework and oven mitts when handling hot dishes.
- Keep your hands moisturized to avoid cracked, dry skin that is susceptible to infection.
- Avoid insect repellants with significant amounts of alcohol (any ingredient ending in "-ol") that dries out the skin. A good substitute is Avon's Skin So Soft.
- Use an electric razor or depilatory to remove hair under your arm to prevent danger of nicks. Keep the razor clean.
- If you are diabetic, control your blood sugar levels to minimize the danger of small blood vessel damage and infection.

## Other suggestions

- Use soaps that are pH-balanced or glycerin soaps.
- Try substituting cornstarch, witch hazel, lavender oil, or rose water for antiperspirants.
- Add drops of comfrey, calendula, or poke essential oils to glycerin emollient (sold at drug stores) or almond or olive oil. (An emollient is necessary to help the oil diffuse through the water.) Test on another part of your body. If you have no reaction, rub the mixture into your affected arm *if you have been trained in the proper technique for lymphatic drainage.* Otherwise, add the mixture to bath water. Pink grapefruit, cypress, geranium, and juniper berry oils also promote lymph drainage. You can use unscented Ivory soap or unscented bubble bath as an emollient.

## Symptoms of Lymphedema

Seek immediate medical attention if you notice any of the following in the affected arm:

- Heat, redness, inflammation, or red streaks. If signs of infection in the arm are associated with flu-like symptoms, immediate medical attention is warranted.
- Bursting pain.
- Skin that looks shiny or has fewer folds than normal.
- Your arm is feeling full, stiff, achy, weak, heavy, or swollen.
- Watch, ring, or bracelet is feeling tight.
- Decreased flexibility in hand, fingers, wrist, or elbow.
- Difficulty fitting an arm into the sleeve of a garment.
- Feeling of pins and needles in your arm, hand, or shoulder area.
- New area of numbness under the arm (this area is often numb right after surgery) or new swelling anywhere.
- Pressing an area of skin and the indention stays.
- Tissue that feels spongy.
- Sudden discoloration anywhere on your body, which could mean a hematoma, or pooling of blood beneath the skin.

Any of these could mean the beginning of infection or lymphedema and need immediate attention. If you notice symptoms at night or on the weekend, call your doctor's office rather than waiting for Monday or morning. Infection is the only irreversible cause of lymphedema and can be stopped with antibiotics before it gets serious.

## Precautionary Actions

- Carry a card in your purse or wear a medical alert bracelet (National Lymphedema Network, *www.lymphnet.org*, 1–800–541–3259) stating "No IV, blood draws, or blood pressure" in your affected arm.
- If you have lymphedema, wear a compression sleeve during all waking hours. Have it checked by your physical therapist or sleeve salesperson every four to six months for proper fit.
- Maintain your ideal weight by eating a high-fiber, low-sodium, well-balanced diet. Lymphedema is a high-protein edema, but reducing your protein intake will not improve the disease. In fact, too little protein may worsen the condition.[26]
- Restrict your salt (less than 2,400 mg/day) and sugar intake to reduce the amount of fluid your body retains.

- Drink lots of water to remove excess fluid from your body. Diuretics offer only temporary relief because they remove only water and not protein, which draws fluid back to the affected area to swell again.[27]
- Avoid alcohol and smoking. Alcohol makes blood vessels dilate and leak extra fluid into the tissues. Smoking constricts small blood vessels and interferes with fluid flow in the arm.
- Attempt new physical activities slowly. Your muscles pump the lymphatic fluid through your system. Overexercising can pump more fluid than your impaired system can cope with, and swelling may result. Monitor yourself by measuring your arm in several places. In weekly intervals after beginning the new activity, measure again until you are confident your lymph system has adjusted. If you work with a personal trainer, inform her that you are at risk for lymphedema.

## Treatments for Lymphedema

If you do develop lymphedema, there are several treatments your doctor may recommend. It is very important to find a physical therapist or massage therapist who is certified in treating lymphedema because the skin is more sensitive and the risk of infection is higher than normal. Treatment may include:

- MLD (manual lymph drainage) compression bandage, an elastic sleeve custom fit to hold the proper amount of pressure on the arm. It is best to be measured for a sleeve by a trained specialist rather than buy one off the shelf. Once a limb has swollen, the lymph vessels are stretched and more susceptible to swelling another time. Bandaging attempts to stop the vessels from refilling with fluid. Compression sleeves are not the same as Ace bandages; they are short-stretch bandages. A compression sleeve expands very little as muscles push against it. Do not wear the sleeve at night, although it is acceptable to wear bandaging at night as long as it cannot wrinkle and restrict circulation in a way that is not planned. Have a qualified therapist train you in how to apply a bandage. Most insurance companies pay for a compression sleeve with a prescription from your doctor.
- Manual lymph drainage, to move the lymph fluid into areas where it can be absorbed, where the rest of your lymph system is working well. The therapist moves the skin with a pumping motion from the hand to shoulder; then wraps the arm to provide gradient pressure and may assign exercises for you to do. Ideally, therapy would consist of one or two sessions a day, five days a week for three to six weeks; however, most insurance plans do not cover twice-daily sessions. Each session lasts about an hour. Many insurance plans cover MLD with a letter of medical necessity.

- CDP (complete decongestive physiotherapy) combines MLD, bandaging, and exercises in one session a day for one to four weeks. Trained therapists teach self-care techniques. The exercises encourage the body to develop new pathways to drain lymph fluid.
- Pneumatic compression pump. This specialty device moves the fluid from your hand to your shoulder in sessions that last about two hours. Be sure your pump exerts gradient pressure (more to the hand and less to the shoulder to move the fluid in that direction) and sequential pressure (rhythmic squeezing). Rent your pump from a physical therapist, rehabilitation center, or doctor who provides trained personnel to monitor your care. Misuse of the pumps can worsen lymphedema. Many insurance plans cover this expensive device.

Though surgery and benzopyrone medications are used in Europe, these are not recommended in the United States.

# Travel Precautions

Most women are able to resume most normal activities after cancer treatment. However, if you had surgery for breast cancer, you will want to take extra precautions against lymphedema.

## Before you go

- Schedule any required vaccinations over several weeks. Do not have them in your affected arm.
- Be sure you have extra medications. Take prescriptions with you in case of delays or customs inquiries. Ask your doctor for a prescription for antibiotics as a precaution. Fill it before you leave.
- Take a sunburn cream with an SPF of 20 to 30-plus, moisturizing lotion, and an oil-based body wash (rather than drying soap).
- Consider travel insurance that covers treatment as well as luggage. You may have to state, and have your doctor sign the statement, that you have a preexisting condition to claim payment if you need treatment while away from home.
- Pack insect repellant, something for insect bites, and an antifungal powder.

## Luggage/clothing

- Carry your medications and travel documents with you in case your luggage is delayed. Minimize whatever else you carry on the flight. Aim for one small bag so you don't have to carry one on your shoulder. Don't carry hand luggage with your affected arm. A case with wheels or a small backpack is advisable. Ask a traveling companion to manage your luggage or pay for a porter.

- Don't remove luggage from a luggage carousel or overhead bin with your affected arm.
- If traveling by automobile, have someone else move your luggage and heavy packages in and out of the car or trunk.
- Wear loose and nonconstricting clothing and avoid tight belts or jewelry. Layer to avoid temperature extremes.
- Wear "sunblock" clothing if possible. (This is clothing made with sun protection built into the material.)

## During travel

- Wear a compression sleeve or wrap with bandages on flights. Some women have had swelling in their hands from the compression bandage. Realize that in some countries air pressure in aircraft is not the same as international standards. If you travel on local airplanes, consider bandaging as well as wearing a sleeve. Periodically run your hand with slight pressure from the wrist to the shoulder of the affected arm.
- Move every 30 minutes or so on an airplane ride. Move any muscle and as many muscle groups as you can. Flex your feet; rotate your shoulders or ankles. If you feel awkward exercising in your seat, seek privacy in the restroom or place a blanket over you.
- If you have lymphedema, take a rubber ball to squeeze or clinch your fists and wring out an imaginary towel with your arm above your head.
- Keep your seat belt loosely fastened except during takeoff, landing, and real turbulence.
- Increase fluid intake, preferably water, while in the air.
- For bus travel, choose a schedule with many stops. Get out and walk at each one. If driving, stop every hour or so and walk around. Protect your affected arm from sun through the car or bus windows.

## Upon arrival

- Do not remove your compression sleeve for several hours after arriving. Then have a cool shower and rest with the affected arm elevated. Use an oil-based cleanser and a moisturizer on the affected arm.
- Do some mild exercise after your rest.

## On vacation

- Remember that you can get sunburned through a compression sleeve.
- If your compression sleeve becomes hot to wear, wet it by putting your arm under a shower or faucet with the sleeve already on. It will cool as the water evaporates.

- Use the antifungal powder as a preventative, between your toes and in your shoes. Athlete's foot can easily spread to the groin area and the folds under your breasts, especially if you have lymphedema.
- Realize that lowered atmospheric pressure in ski areas or mountains can trigger or exacerbate lymphedema. Take the same precautions as if you were flying and wear a compression sleeve.
- Avoid sunburn, insect bites, scratches, and bruises on your affected arm.
- Avoid exercise more strenuous than you normally do.
- Coral infection can cause lymphedema in people with normal limbs, so don't dismiss the risk of a scratch from the sharp edges of a reef.

A key factor to remember about lymphedema is balance. Be aware of precautions to take, but don't become so paranoid that you can't enjoy living.

## *Memory Loss/Mental Confusion*

Although some breast cancer survivors joke about "chemobrain" or "chemonesia," it is a very real side effect that frightens women who are unaware of its usually temporary nature.

Chemotherapy drugs can affect the brain and the central nervous system and cause depression, confusion, and memory loss. Also, a drop in estrogen production affects cognitive function. The effects usually stop once chemo is finished. However, sometimes they last months or even years after treatment.

You may notice difficulty with something that has been routine for years such as balancing the checkbook or recalling your neighbor's name. Organizational skills seem to be particularly affected. Your brain can't handle as much information at a time, so there is a decline in focused attention. Also, rapid retrieval of stored memory, concentration, and spatial perception can be impaired during chemotherapy. The extra effort it takes to be as efficient as you used to be can contribute to cancer fatigue.

If any of these conditions develop, tell your doctor and know that they will probably disappear in time. In the meantime, try to accept them as part of the new you and try to laugh about them. They are a very handy excuse sometimes!

## Tips for a Sharper Memory
- Write everything on one calendar.
- Put a list to music or pick words that begin with the same letter.
- To find a missing item, retrace your steps mentally or physically.
- To recall details you have forgotten about a topic, begin by writing down what you do remember. Use as many senses as you can.
- Tape notes around the house to remind you of things to do.

- Practice relaxation.
- Repeat several times what you want to remember. Memorize whatever you can.
- Read as much as you can and write often, perhaps in a journal.
- Play games and do crossword puzzles to hone strategic skills.
- Get enough sleep.

## Early Onset of Menopause

Some drugs given during chemotherapy affect the ovaries' production of hormones and may change your monthly periods. Some women, usually those close to natural menopause, go into medical menopause (meaning the condition was brought about by conditions outside your own body) and their periods cease. About 30 percent, often those in their 30s or 40s who were still producing hormones when treatment started, may resume their periods after treatment is over.[28]

If your periods continue through chemotherapy, the flow may be heavier or lighter and you may experience cramping.

Women in medical menopause experience the same range of symptoms as women in natural menopause, but their changes are immediate and often more severe.[29] Symptoms may include hot flashes, night sweats, depression, anxiety, irritability, mood swings, loss of libido, vaginal infections or dryness, dry skin, joint pain, fatigue, heart palpitations, significant weight changes, headaches, disrupted sleep, poor memory, decreased attention and concentration, bladder infections, and incontinence. You will not experience all and may not experience any of these. Although some medications and natural remedies may help, do not take any (even over-the-counter supplements) without asking your oncologist first. Some substances can impact the effectiveness of treatments. You may have to put up with some irritating side effects until treatment is over.

Though the cessation of the menstrual cycle can be devastating for a woman who wanted to have more children, it should pose no problem to other women. You will want to discuss with your oncologist and your gynecologist ways to prevent osteoporosis and enhance heart health, tasks that rely at least partially upon the hormone estrogen. Hormone replacement therapy (HRT) has become very controversial recently after a study was canceled early because of an increase in breast cancer among participants. Discuss this with your doctor and read up on the issue yourself before you decide whether HRT is for you.

(See also "Hot Flashes," page 126, and "Sexuality, Changes in," page 162.)

## *Mouth Sores*

Because the cells lining the mouth divide rapidly, they are sensitive to drugs used to kill rapidly dividing cancer cells.

If you notice any sores or white bumps or patches developing in your mouth, notify your doctor, who can prescribe or recommend medication to get rid of them before they become a problem. Sores typically occur seven to 10 days after a treatment. If they are left untreated, dealing with them can delay your cancer treatments.

If mouth sores make it hard to swallow pills, dab a little Biotene Oral Balance Gel on the pill to help it slide down easier or put the pill in a spoonful of applesauce or pudding.

(See also "Dry Mouth," page 110.)

## Symptoms of Mouth Sores
- Swelling.
- Bleeding.
- A sticky, white film in your mouth.
- "Pimples," ulcers, or "bumps" in your mouth.
- Red patches.

## Tips during Chemotherapy
- Examine your mouth once a day for symptoms.
- Suck on ice chips.

(See also "Dental Concerns," page 107.)

## Tips for Eating to Avoid Mouth Sores
- Avoid spicy, acid/tart, or salty foods that may irritate the sores. Stay away from curry, chili powder, nutmeg, or cloves; condiments containing pepper; vinegar-based salad dressings; and citrus (orange, lemon, or grapefruit) or tomato juices.
- Avoid dry, scratchy, or rough foods such as raw vegetables, dry toast, crackers, chips, nuts, popcorn, or dry cereal. Dunk dry food in a soup or beverage before eating it.
- Eat foods at room temperature or cool. Do not eat hot foods that may burn the irritated tissue.
- Cook food until tender. Many foods can be pureed for easier swallowing. Soups are especially useful at this time.
- Do not drink alcohol or use tobacco. They can increase mouth pain.

- Use a straw, which may help liquids go down easier.
- Add gravy or sauce to make food easier to swallow.
- Suck on ice chips.
- To make swallowing easier, tilt your head forward or backward.
- Eat foods high in protein to help your body rebuild tissue.
- Ask about taking a multivitamin that contains zinc and vitamin C to promote healing of mouth sores.

## Rinse Your Mouth with

- Antiseptics.
- One teaspoon salt, 1 tablespoon baking soda, and a cup of warm water. Mix just before using. Rinse with this especially after vomiting. Otherwise gargle with it three to six times a day.
- Buttermilk.
- Ice chips.
- Oral anesthetics such as Benadryl elixir, Ulcerease, viscous Xylocaine, Hurricaine Topical Anesthetics (benzocaine), or Cepacol lozenges before a meal, or apply directly to the sores with a Q-tip.
- The contents of a capsule of vitamin E. Swish it around in your mouth before swallowing.
- A mixture of liquid Benadryl and milk of magnesia.
- Cold chamomile tea.
- A rinse of 1 tablespoon cherry Maalox, 1 teaspoon Nystatin, and 1/2 teaspoon Hurricaine Topical Anesthetic liquid. Swish 2 to 3 teaspoons in mouth for one minute. Or ask your doctor for a prescription of equal parts of Xylocaine (or viscous lidocaine), Maalox, and Benadryl. Swish 1 teaspoon around your mouth and swallow. Use every four hours as needed for pain.[30] If these stop working, ask about a prescription for Diflucan tablets to get rid of the fungus overgrowth. Or ask about taking L-lysine (available in the vitamin section of pharmacies and health food stores).
- Swish your mouth with Carafate (sucralfate) liquid, a prescription medication. Use it with each chemo cycle before mouth sores start.

## To Relieve Mouth Pain

- If your mouth is so sore you cannot eat, tell your doctor. He can prescribe a local anesthetic (such as Gelclair, Cepacol, or Xylocaine) to numb the sores so you can eat. Ask if you may use acetaminophen (Tylenol), ibuprofen, or other pain medication for the discomfort.

- Spread Orabase, Orajel, or Zilactin on the sores. Orajel also offers mouth swabs for easy application.
- Take a pain pill a half hour before meals to allow you to eat.
- Squeeze the contents of a 500-unit vitamin E capsule onto the mouth sores three times per day.
- Suck on ice chips, Popsicles, frozen juices (not citrus), or sugar-free candy, or chew sugar-free gum.
- Three times a day, open and close your mouth as far as you can without pain to relieve stiffness in your chewing muscles.

## Muscle Effects

See "Nerve and Muscle Effects," page 154.

## Nail Problems

Chemotherapy can sometimes result in grooving, increased sensitivity, or a change in growth rate in your nails. Nails may also develop vertical lines or bands or become dark, yellow, brittle, or cracked during chemotherapy. They also can fall out.

Notify your doctor if your cuticles become red or painful or you notice other signs of inflammation.

Some precautions to observe during treatment are:

- Use nail-strengthening products with caution as they may irritate your skin.
- Wear gloves for housework or gardening to protect your nails from infection of the nail bed. Excessive exposure to water can result in fungal infections.
- Don't cut your cuticles. Use cuticle removers instead.
- Use nail polish to harden your nails and protect them from the environment.
- Use an oily polish remover to keep from overdrying the nails, which are prone to brittleness.
- Avoid glue-on nails during chemotherapy. The adhesive may worsen the condition of your natural nails.
- Soak your hands in ice water during chemotherapy to reduce nail problems.
- If nails do become brittle or unattached to the finger or toe, check your local feed store for Rio Vista Hoof Manicure, use Vick's VapoRub, or rub a strong moisturizing cream into the nail bed to keep cuticles supple.
- Keep nails filed so they are less prone to catch on something and tear.

If the base of your nails becomes infected, soak your hand in warm, salty water.

## *Nausea*

One of the most common side effects of chemotherapy is nausea, but other factors involved in breast cancer treatment such as stress, pain, or medications can cause it also. Because about half of cancer patients experience nausea or vomiting, ask your doctor if your particular medication might cause nausea and what she will do if it develops. Knowing solutions exist may ease your mind.

Chemotherapy drugs are targeted at rapidly dividing cancer cells. Unfortunately, they also affect other rapidly dividing healthy cells such as those lining the gastrointestinal tract. The result can be loss of appetite, nausea, vomiting, and sore mouth. Radiation and chemotherapy drugs also may cause the body to manufacture substances that enter the bloodstream and reach the areas of the brain that control nausea and vomiting. Once these areas are stimulated, you begin to feel sick and want to throw up.

People react differently to the same drug, and not all drugs for breast cancer cause nausea. In fact, some women get nauseated *before* their chemotherapy because of anxiety. If you do get sick, it may last a few hours or a few days. The feeling will be similar to how you felt when you had the flu or morning sickness or when you traveled in a car or boat. It's no fun, but it doesn't last forever.

Ask your anesthesiologist about antinausea medication you can take before surgery as a preventive measure. Your doctor can prescribe medication to take before or with chemotherapy or to take after you develop nausea or vomiting. These antiemetic medications may be given intravenously, by mouth, by injection, under the tongue, as a patch, or as a rectal suppository. If one medication does not work, ask your doctor for another.

Other techniques that have been used successfully to control nausea are self-hypnosis, progressive muscle relaxation (PMR), biofeedback, guided imagery, acupuncture, and systematic desensitization.

Be sure to communicate with your doctor or nurse about this concern and follow his recommendations for your particular drug. It is important not to let nausea continue because your body needs nutrients from food. It is helpful to record the time you began feeling sick, what you ate and drank, and what activities you participated in. These may give your doctor a clue about controlling the nausea.

In general, the following suggestions will help.

## Tips to Minimize Nausea

- Avoid heavy meals two hours before or after a treatment.
- Cold or room-temperature foods usually cause less nausea than warm ones, partly because they do not have the strong odors that hot foods do.

- Eat sitting up and stay upright for 30 minutes to two hours after a meal if you can. If you are lying down, food can back up into your esophagus. If you can't manage to sit that long, prop your head up with pillows.
- Keep mealtimes pleasant and stress-free.
- Stay away from strong cooking odors by having someone else cook or by using an odor neutralizer (such as a pet odor remover) that does not leave a heavy perfume smell. You also can prepare and freeze small portions of food ahead of time.
- Eat small amounts every 30 to 60 minutes instead of three big meals to keep your stomach from feeling too full.
- Keep something in your stomach. Starving yourself worsens nausea.
- Eat and drink slowly to help your digestion. A smaller fork will help slow your speed of eating. Sip liquids through a straw.
- Chew your food well to aid digestion.
- Distract yourself from the meal with TV, music, reading, or interesting conversation.
- Rinse your mouth with lemon water after eating to get rid of unpleasant tastes.
- If you are nauseated in the morning, nibble dry foods such as cereal, toast, or crackers before you get up.

## Foods to Minimize Nausea

### Avoid, especially right before treatment
- Greasy or fatty foods, butter, oil, red meat, whole milk and cheese, salad dressings, chips, nut butters.
- Sweet, sugary foods.
- Hot (with temperature or spice) foods.
- Fried foods, junk food.
- Heavy foods such as donuts, cake, and casseroles.
- Raw food or foods with a lot of fiber such as beans or raisins.
- Foods with strong flavors or odors such as garlic or Brussels sprouts.

### Eat easy-to-digest foods
- Pasta, rice, potatoes (mashed or baked).
- Canned fruit.
- Cooked vegetables (but none with a strong smell).
- Custard.
- Ice; ice cubes made from a favorite liquid (fruit juice, for instance).

- Sorbet, sherbet, fruit ices.
- Baked poultry or fish.
- Whole-wheat toast; saltine crackers; pretzels; vanilla wafers; other dry, starchy foods; toast with honey.
- Mint sugarless gum or peppermint candy.
- Light and low-fat foods such as fruit and cereal with skim milk, angel food cake.
- Slippery elm bark balls. Mix 2 tablespoons of the powdered herb, available at health food stores, with water or maple syrup to form balls. Suck on the balls as a lozenge. Make enough for several at a time.

## Drinking to Minimize Nausea
- Drink lots of fluids, preferably water, to aid digestion. Drink small amounts frequently.
- Choose clear, cool beverages instead of hot drinks.
- Avoid liquids at mealtime. Drink them 30 to 60 minutes before a meal. You don't want your stomach filled with fluid, but with some appropriate food.
- Sip on peppermint, chamomile, ginger, or herbal tea. Dunking tea bags continuously for three minutes (instead of leaving the tea bag in the cup) or using loose-leaf tea (instead of tea bags) is reported to permit the release of five times more of the cancer-fighting and heart-protecting molecules called polyphenols.[31]
- Drink some sports drink with electrolytes if you vomit or develop diarrhea.
- Mix equal parts of lemon juice and fresh ginger (a little goes a long way!). Add sugar and salt to taste. Either swallow a spoonful like a tonic or mix into a beverage.
- Some people like carbonated beverages when they are nauseated, but others find the fizz can instigate vomiting. Stick with noncaffeinated, light-colored sodas such as 7-Up, Sprite, or ginger ale that has gone flat.
- Drink cold water or clear, cool fruit juices such as apple or grape. Freeze these juices into ice cubes and crush them for a refreshing change from ice. Suck on Popsicles.
- Freshly juiced cabbage controls nausea for some during chemotherapy.[32]

## Activities to Minimize Nausea
- Get fresh air. Turn on a ceiling fan. Open the windows. Eat or sit outside if the weather permits or take a slow walk. This is not the time to set speed or endurance records.

- Keep your mouth rinsed and your breath fresh. Keep hard candy or sugar-free gum handy if you can't brush your teeth.
- Try taking your medicine at different times of the day for nausea control.
- Sometimes mind over matter can help. Some women have found relief by not looking at the pills before swallowing them. Some visualize something pleasant as they swallow or while the IV is dripping. Distractions such as music or TV, reading, meditation, deep breathing, acupuncture, acupressure, and hypnotherapy may help.
- A few hours before treatment, place an acupressure or Sea-Band about 2 inches above your wrist. The band stimulates the acupressure point that relieves nausea. Most pharmacies carry the bands. Leave on for 24 hours.
- If you feel nausea coming on, place a cool, wet washcloth on your forehead, neck, or throat.
- Breathe deeply and slowly from the abdomen, not the chest. As you breathe in, feel your abdomen balloon out. As you exhale, press your navel toward your spine. Breathe through your mouth instead of your nose.
- Buy unscented toiletries and cleaning products to avoid the strong odors. Avoid cooking smells, perfume, smoke, or other odors that bother you.
- Wear loose-fitting clothing.
- Try to relax after eating by reading a book, listening to soothing music, or practicing meditation, yoga, biofeedback, or self-hypnosis.
- If you generally get sick at a certain time of day, try to sleep then.
- Notice whether nausea is worse if you stay in bed for an hour or so after taking medication or whether you walk around.

Whatever works for you is best. If you crave pizza and it does not make your nausea worse, then enjoy!

## Tips for Treatment Days to Minimize Nausea
- Be sure to have a little something in your stomach. Eat a light, low-fat meal before your treatment with such foods as peach or pear nectar, cereal or oatmeal, toast with apple butter, grits, or fruit cocktail.
- Drink lots of fluid 24 hours before a treatment.
- Avoid any food for two hours before or after a treatment. For 24 to 48 hours after a treatment, stick with bland foods such as liquids, soups, or puddings.
- If only one or two foods appeal to you, eat only those until you feel like eating something else.

## To Settle an Upset Stomach

Try:

- Toast with honey.
- Hard candy, mints, or ice chips.
- Sniffing the scent of peppermint, spearmint, basil, ginger, lavender, or mandarin essential oil.
- Small sips of ice water, ice beverage, iced tea (peppermint or herbal), ice chips, or fruit sorbets.
- Clear or salty liquids rather than sweet ones.
- 550 mg ginger root, three times a day. (It will not stop vomiting once it has started.)
- Ginger tea (use a tea bag or simmer two thin slices of gingerroot in 8 ounces of water for 20 minutes) or ginger candy.
- Keeping crackers or hard candy by your bed.
- Drinking lemonade before getting out of bed and throughout the day.
- Distracting yourself with pleasant music or sitting on the patio and watching the dogs or garden.
- One tablespoon of olive oil on an empty stomach.

The brain is as involved as the stomach in nausea and vomiting. It receives signals from the sensory receptors in the stomach as well as from the bloodstream about possible toxins that need to be expelled from the body. It remembers those substances and can initiate the same reaction the next time they enter the body. This is why you are told not to eat your favorite foods around the time of chemotherapy treatment. If the treatments make you nauseated, your brain may associate the nausea with that food and cause you to react negatively to it for years.

## Nerve and Muscle Effects

Some chemotherapy drugs (such as Taxotere, Platinol, or Oxaliplatin) can affect your nerves and muscles. They can cause peripheral neuropathy, which is tingling, burning, weakness, or numbness in your hands or feet. They can make your muscles ache or feel weak.

Many of these problems will disappear when chemotherapy stops. However, some can last up to a year or forever. Ask your doctor whether your medication might cause such side effects. If they develop, mention them because there are many remedies to try and some neuropathies can be reversed at an early stage but not later. Some antidepressants have been used with good results for nerve pain (and the doctor is not saying the pain "is all in your head"!).

## Symptoms to Report

- Tingling, burning, weakness, or numbness in hands and/or feet.
- Pain or difficulty while walking.
- Stomach pain.
- Constipation.
- Hearing loss.
- Tired, achy, sore, or weak muscles.
- Loss of balance.
- Shaking or trembling.
- Jaw pain.
- Difficulty with small motor coordination (buttoning clothing, picking up objects).

## Coping with Nerve or Muscle Problems

- If you experience any pain, ask your doctor for pain medication.
- If your fingers are numb, be careful picking up objects that are hot, sharp, or slippery.
- If your feet are numb, your gait is unsteady, or your muscles are weak, use handrails on steps, a cane or companion for walking, bath mats in the bathroom, and rubber-soled shoes to help prevent falls.
- If feet or hands become red and blister, use Bag Balm, a moisturizer for cow udders, on hands and soles of feet several times a day.
- Some patients with nerve problems in their feet have found relief using magnetic insoles in their shoes.
- If your feet are numb, inspect them every day before bed. You could have a sore or blister that could develop into an infection if not treated.

### Night Sweats

If chemotherapy sent you into early menopause, you may wake up during the night drenched in sweat. This too will pass, as they say, but in the meantime, what do you do?

For one, dress cool. That means all-cotton bed linens and nightclothes. Turn down the thermostat to the high 60s F. Keep an extra pillow near your bed to replace one that gets wet. Or keep a few wet washcloths in the freezer during the day and place them in a cooler by your bed at night. If you have the sweats, take out a cloth to cool you down.

Try visualization or affirmation. Visualize lying in a shallow stream of icy water or tell yourself, "I am cool and comfortable." (See also "Hot Flashes," page 126.)

## Numbness

Some chemotherapy drugs can affect nerve endings and cause numbness in fingers and toes. The sensation is usually temporary, but do mention it to your doctor.

Following a lymph node dissection, you may experience numbness under your arm where nerves were cut. This lack of sensation may correct itself in a few months; however, it does not return in some women. If that is your situation, it is safest to shave with an electric razor there to prevent nicks that you might not feel or use Magic Shaving Powder or other depilatory.

## Pain

One fear that surfaces with a cancer diagnosis is the fear of pain. However, many women with breast cancer will not experience significant pain during any part of their treatment. Many others will experience temporary pain, such as after some surgeries. Even though metastasized disease brings more possibility of pain, there are many remedies, including medication, surgery, radiation, cortisone, and relaxation techniques, that can help you cope. Cancer does not guarantee a painful existence.

The pain from cancer comes usually from nerve compression, bone damage in metastatic disease, or infiltration of the cancer into soft tissue or organs. Only a small percent of cancer pain results from treatment, although some drugs can result in muscle pain, mouth sores, stomach pain, nerve damage, or tingling or numbness in fingers and toes. Patients feel pain after some surgeries. Most of the time it goes away, but sometimes a tenderness or sensitivity lasts many months. Radiation can result in local pain and is usually short-lived. Some pain felt during cancer treatment results from unrelated issues such as injury, overactivity, or other situations experienced by persons without cancer. Because the brain produces endorphins that help regulate pain, techniques such as biofeedback, self-hypnosis, imaging, or meditation that help stimulate their production may be useful.

Fear of pain can bring on the feared pain, just as some women get nauseated on the way to a chemotherapy treatment from the anticipation alone. Everyone's pain threshold is different, so the same stimuli will affect different patients differently. Whatever you can do to relax and enjoy as many hours of the day as possible will bolster your natural pain-blocking mechanisms.

## Assessing the Pain

An important first step in pain management is determining the reason for the pain. You can help by keeping a record of your pain and by telling your doctor as soon as the pain appears. Do not wait until your next appointment to inform her.

Then be your own advocate. You have the right to have your pain addressed adequately. Unfortunately, not all pain can be erased completely, but keep trying. Don't give up until you have exhausted all of the many remedies.

Your physician will prescribe medication based on the location and severity of your pain and the other medications you are taking. Most pain medications are not habit-forming. In fact, addiction is very rare in cases of cancer pain management. If you are afraid of becoming dependent on the medication, discuss this with your doctor. Doses can be adjusted.

The most common side effects of opiate pain medications are constipation, nausea, and oversedation. If you experience any of these or other side effects, inform your doctor so you can get relief. Often, as your body gets used to these medications, the side effects will lessen or disappear.

## Why Control Your Pain?

Besides the fact that there are no medals for enduring pain, there are very good reasons for reducing pain:

- Pain can elevate your blood pressure.
- Your body can work more efficiently on other functions if you control those responses that you can and leave your limited physical resources for other matters.
- You can't eat right, sleep well, exercise adequately, or participate in regular activities such as sex when you are in pain.
- Pain introduces the side effects of stress into your body.
- Pain management often means shorter hospitalizations, reduced costs of treatment, and better quality of life.
- Pain can build a barrier between you and your caregivers if it makes you angry, tired, worried, lonely, or grouchy.
- Pain may cause you to feel depressed, afraid, helpless, or inadequate. Any of these feelings can interfere with your healing process and your quality of life.
- Pain can cause you to miss work and trigger financial concerns.

## Describe Your Pain Clearly

Help your healthcare professional understand how you feel by keeping a record of your pain and describing it clearly. Include such things as:

- Exactly where is the pain?
- What does it feel like (sharp, dull, stabbing, achy, tight, throbbing, steady, burning, tingling, deep)?
- When did the pain start?
- Has the pain changed in any way since it started?
- What time of day or night is the pain better or worse?
- How long does the pain last?
- What triggers the pain?
- What relieves the pain?
- Does a change in your mood affect the pain?
- How bad is the pain on a scale of one to 10, with 10 being unbearable? It may help to draw a line and label one end "0" and the other end "10." Now mark on the line how bad your pain is.

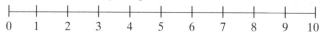

- What daily activities does the pain interfere with?

## Types of Pain

All you know is that you hurt and want to stop, but a doctor will need to know more about your pain to help you. Begin by helping her determine which type of pain you are experiencing:

- Acute pain may be severe and lasts a short time.
- Chronic or persistent pain may be mild or severe and lasts a long time.
- Breakthrough pain is moderate to severe and surfaces while you are taking medication for chronic pain. Sometimes breakthrough pain occurs at the end of a cycle of medication for chronic pain. Medication for this type of pain can be given before activities that usually cause pain.

Usually you can take medications for chronic pain and for breakthrough pain at the same time because they work on different schedules, but check with your doctor.

## Barriers to Pain Management

Patients fail to seek help for pain for various reasons. The most common are:

- They or their family members are afraid of their becoming addicted to the medication. Addiction rarely happens.

- They don't know options exist for controlling pain.
- They are afraid what the pain may mean.
- They don't want to "complain" or distract the doctor from treating the cancer.
- They fear the side effects so they take less pain medication than is prescribed. Most side effects can be prevented or managed. For instance, drowsiness may last the first two to three days and often subsides after that.
- They want to save strong painkillers for "later" when the pain may be worse. Pain has a better chance of being relieved if treated early. It is not common in cancer patients for their body to become so used to a medication that it stops working. If that should happen, there are many other drugs to use.
- Some cultures think that mentioning pain is "weak." Pain is real, and there is no good reason to suffer from it.
- Their insurance does not cover prescription medication or the particular drug the doctor prescribed. Ask about another drug or a free drug program.

## Pain Control

Most cancer healthcare professionals take pain very seriously. When they have a clear picture of your pain, they can choose from a variety of methods to relieve it: medications, surgery, physical therapy, radiation, chemotherapy, nerve blocks, or nonmedical therapies. These may include biofeedback, imagery, massage, distraction, acupuncture, music therapy, heat and cold therapy, hypnosis, positioning for comfort, emotional support, or relaxation techniques. Although these are effective in the majority of cases and most pain can be reduced, sometimes pain cannot be eliminated totally. Usually this is in advanced stages of the disease.

An easy technique you can try on yourself is simply applying pressure with your hand to the area of pain. Hold for about 10 seconds. Apply as much pressure as you can without causing more pain. Sometimes you have to find a point near the painful area to press. The relief can sometimes last for several hours.

Another technique for pain control is a TENS (transcutaneous electric nerve stimulation) unit. A mild electric current is applied to the skin where the pain is. The pleasant sensation relieves some of the pain.

With varying degrees of pain medications, there is no need to suffer in silence. Pain medications are long lasting or immediately effective to combat chronic or temporary pain. There are pills, patches, injections, IVs, and suppositories to dispense the medications. In some cases, patients are hooked to a patient-controlled analgesia (PCA), or computerized pump, through a thin tube. The pump dispenses a set dose of medication when the patient pushes a button. Breakthrough pain can also be treated with Actiq oral transmucosal fentanyl citrate. This medication saturates a swab at the end of a stick that is rubbed onto the inside of your cheek. It works quickly and is easy to use.

Some pain can be prevented. Some can be controlled. You can help with either outcome by:

- Taking your pain medicine regularly if the pain is chronic. Staying on top of pain is better than letting it get really bad. If you wait longer than recommended between doses, the pain can get ahead of the medication or will require larger doses and/or a longer time before you experience relief.

- Practicing relaxation techniques such as deep breathing, meditation, or visualization when you take your medicine. These exercises can sometimes reduce tension and anxiety that make pain worse.

- Asking to see a pain specialist or asking your doctor to consult with one, if your doctor cannot control your pain. There are many different methods of pain management. Keep working with your health professionals until they find what works for you.

If you are taking a narcotic pain medicine and have no other contraindications, increase your fiber intake. Such medicine can slow the normal contractions of the bowel and cause constipation. Extra fiber, non-prescription stool softeners (such as DSS or Colace), and fluids can help.[33]

## Rice bag relief

To ease sore muscles and surgical incisions, make a cloth bag, fill it with spices and rice, and heat in the microwave.[34] Use a piece of all-cotton fabric (all-cotton flannel feels good in the winter) 44 inches by 12 inches, or two fingertip towels. Fold the material in half lengthwise (to make a 22-inch × 12-inch piece) or lay one towel on top of the other. Sew the bottom and long sides with double stitching for strength. Fill the bag with a mixture of 6 cups long-grain white rice (not instant), 1 tablespoon of ground cinnamon, and 1 teaspoon whole cloves or use 2 to 3 pounds of uncooked rice and 1 cup of dried herbs such as lavender, marjoram, or rosemary. Fold in the fourth side and double stitch or pin. To use, heat the bag in the microwave approximately three minutes. It will retain the heat for about 45 minutes. Give it a one-minute boost after a while if you want longer relief.

A quick alternative is a cotton sock. Fill with 2 cups of rice and 1/2 cup dried herbs. Just tie a knot at the end.

When either bag begins to lose its fragrance (after about three months), snip a few stitches or untie, replace the mix or sprinkle a few drops of your favorite essential oil on the old mix, and refasten the bag.

Some people find that cold relieves sore muscles better and find relief from a chemical cold pack, ice bag, or, in a pinch, a bag of frozen food.

## Finding Help

If you are not getting the pain support you need from your doctor, contact one of these for recommendations on a doctor to visit:

- Local large hospital.
- Local hospice.
- State and county medical societies.
- Local chapters of American Chronic Pain Association, American Society of Pain Management Nurses, American Pain Society, or American Academy of Pain Medicine.
- National Cancer Institute's Cancer Information Service.
- A clinical trial for pain management that you might qualify for. (Ask your doctor if there is one.)

## Radiation Recall

Some women experience blistering, reddening, itching, burning, or peeling of the radiated area several months after radiation ends. This reaction is called radiation recall. It is usually temporary, but do report it to your doctor so he can advise you on the type products to use on the area and rule out an infection.

## To Soothe Irritated Skin

- Place a cool, wet cloth over the area.
- Wear soft, natural fabrics such as cotton or linen.
- Wear loose-fitting clothing.
- Wash clothing and bed linens in mild, hypoallergenic detergent. Rinse twice to be sure all detergent has been removed.

## Restricted Movement in Arm

A very rare side effect of lymph node removal is a clotted vein in the inner side of the upper arm. It may feel like a taut cord and may restrict your movement of the arm. Heat treatments and gentle stretching will help.

(See also "Frozen Shoulder," page 120.)

## Scars

Breast cancer treatments can leave physical as well as emotional scars. Both are important to address and deal with.

Most physical scars will fade in time although they will always be visible. If they seem infected, inform your surgeon. Some women are prone to keloid scars, which are overgrowths of scar tissue that leave a discolored scar. They can often be reduced by steroid shots.

Emotional scars take longer to heal. The majority of women who have had surgery or radiation for breast cancer have strong, usually negative reactions when they look at their chest in a mirror or touch that area. Many feel hate, revulsion, anger, or depression. All of these are valid emotions that need to be expressed. Something has been taken away; there is a void even if you were indifferent about your breasts before.

It is in your best interest to confront your emotions and deal with them rather than try to ignore them. They will rise up in unexpected and inappropriate moments unless you acknowledge them and put them to rest. Just as a child wants an adult to kiss her "boo-boo" and "make it well," nurture your scar and learn to accept, even like it.

You can do this by looking at it daily and saying kind things to it, touching it lovingly, massaging lotion into it, or gently stretching it (after the first month). Your scar is a part of you now, and making peace with it is important to your emotional healing. Some women get a large tattoo over the scar area of an unreconstructed breast to add an artistic flair to their new body. Check with your doctor about timing.

The same is true if you choose reconstruction. You need to "accept" your artificial breast.

This may sound crazy to you, but, believe me, your reaction to seeing your changed chest will affect your attitude toward your spouse and other areas of your life. Certainly grieve over your lost part; then determine to move on.

If you have difficulty accepting your new look after six or eight months, consider professional counseling. The emotions of cancer are overwhelming. You cannot heal an emotion until you feel it. It is not a weakness to seek help to identify and handle the emotions.

## Sexuality, Changes in

A difficult side effect of breast cancer that many women do not anticipate is sexual change. This can include lowered libido or sex drive, vaginal dryness that makes intercourse painful, or difficulty becoming aroused or reaching orgasm. It is hard enough to redefine your sexuality without one or both breasts or your hair. Then medications, fatigue, depression, and self-esteem play havoc with your interest in sex. Chemotherapy or even tamoxifen alone can throw you into chemical menopause ("chemopause"), a sudden onset of menopause brought about by disruption of hormone production due to chemicals. If you were in perimenopause before your diagnosis, the double or triple hit can be overwhelming.

Some women find that, even after treatment is complete, their sexual drive is not what it used to be. If vaginal dryness is a problem, ask your doctor for a lubricant that does not have estrogen in it or a vaginal suppository with a very low level of estrogen.

Some areas of the body that brought sexual pleasure may be numb. Some women who opt for breast reconstruction are surprised that the lovely shape on their chest does not have the ability to carry pleasurable sensations the way their breast did. Even with lumpectomies, the radiation that follows can eradicate tactile sensitivity in the breast, and the nipples that brought sexual pleasure cannot continue that role. However, reconstruction often enhances a woman's self-esteem with a more normal appearance. The lips have an erotic connection to your genitals, so perhaps kissing can become more a part of foreplay.

One big fear among patients as well as lovers that interferes with sexual activity is that cancer is contagious and can be transmitted sexually. This is not true! You need have no fear about hugging, kissing, or having intercourse. In fact, it is important that you keep touching, kissing, and hugging. Remember to think of your husband as a lover as often as you see him as a caretaker. The emotional benefits are many.

Most women are embarrassed to ask their physicians about lowered libido. Fortunately, some of these issues will take care of themselves in time, and there are alternatives for others. Approximately half the women who receive long-term treatment for breast and gynecologic cancers report some sexual dysfunction. There is no guarantee that you will feel the same sexually after treatment as before, but you can still enjoy your partner—even if in new ways. Close personal relationships are a factor in coping with a breast cancer diagnosis and recovery, so don't shy away from discussing this issue. Unspoken distance in a relationship will produce stress and prevent the benefits the relationship could be providing for both partners.

Remember that sexuality is not just intercourse. It begins with feelings of closeness. If you are anxious about your first post-treatment sexual encounter, arrange other times of intimacy before you attempt intercourse. Talk ahead of time about your feelings, fears, and worries. Studies show that men are not as turned off by the sight of a missing breast as women have feared. They focus on the pleasure of the experience instead and are just glad their spouse is alive.

In most relationships, for both married and dating women, it boils down to this: If you can accept your new situation, your partner can also. Love bears all things. If your partner can't accept you, don't blame breast cancer on killing the relationship. There was probably a major flaw in it before the cancer came along.

## Ways to Work around Sexual Limitations
### Medical interventions

- The same Kegel exercises that help other women stop "leaking" urine can strengthen your pelvic muscles and enhance sexual sensation. They can be done almost anywhere without others knowing you are doing them. Simply contract the muscles that control the flow of urine. Hold for a count of 10. Release. Do a set of 10 contractions a few times a day. For a variation, contract the muscles in rapid succession up to 100 times.

- Vaginal cones can be used to enhance Kegel exercises. A cone is placed in the vagina for a few minutes like a tampon. You contract your muscles to hold it in place. Over time you gradually increase the time you hold the cone in place and the weight of the cone. Work with your doctor for proper fit and instructions.

- Once treatment is completed, ask your gynecologist about taking a small dose of testosterone. Also inquire about herbs such as panax ginseng, ashwagandha, or licorice root, which some cultures have found to have positive effects on libido. Do not take them unless you are under the care of a qualified herbalist.

- Eating lozenges made from aloe vera juice and slippery elm may help moisturize dry mucous membranes in the vagina. (See also "Vaginal Dryness," page 171.)

- Ask your doctor about the medication Wellbutrin SR, which can increase libido.

- Ask your doctor if any of your medications could be causing depression, lowered libido, or fatigue and whether you could try a substitute.

- Inquire about using an estradiol vaginal ring, such as Estring, for vaginal dryness.

### Relationship issues

- Talk, communicate, share. Communication is the most important factor in restoring or maintaining intimacy at any time, and especially during cancer treatment. The shock of diagnosis can send spouses withdrawing into themselves to handle the crisis. Misunderstandings arise, and any areas of tension in the relationship fester and may explode. Do not assume that either person knows how the other is feeling. Say what you really feel, not what you think you should say. It may take months for you to be ready to be seen naked even if you had a healthy relationship before surgery. Of course you will want to keep your husband's needs in mind, but accept that your needs are paramount for now—and that's okay. Show him that you love him in other caring ways and tell him often how much you appreciate him and all he is doing for you.

- Redefine sexuality. It does not have to include intercourse. Just skin-to-skin contact brings pleasure to couples in love. Try "mapping" each other's bodies. Take turns gently running your hands over the other's body to find places that bring pleasure.

- Remember that men are attracted to features of a woman's femininity other than her breasts. Hips and legs also excite some men.

- If you are afraid your husband will stray to a more attractive woman, gently express your fear. If you don't get instant reassurance, perhaps marriage counseling is in order. Energy and caring are much more important ingredients in a satisfying sexual life than physical appearance. If issues are interfering with your relationship, take this opportunity to iron them out with professional help.

- Consider professional counseling to surface and handle any underlying psychological or interpersonal factors that could be hampering your interest in sex. Inquire to find someone specifically trained in sexual issues. Someone at a major cancer center is a good choice because she would be familiar with particular issues related to breast cancer.

## Foreplay/environmental issues
- Wear a sports bra to bed if you are uncomfortable with how you look.
- Wear attractive lingerie. This will help you as much as it does your partner.
- Spend time looking at yourself and loving your new appearance. It may take determination more than anything else. What you see is likely not what you want to see, but it is what is. Force yourself to look and affirm your health and your survivor status. Learn to love your different healthy body. In time you will accept what you see.
- Your erogenous zones change after treatment. What aroused you before may not now. In private, maybe in the shower or bath, gently stroke yourself in different areas of your body and see if any new area provides a pleasant sensation. If so, guide your spouse's hand to that area the next time you are intimate.

- Begin your sexual encounter with a warm, relaxing bath with scented candles and mood music. Steep a few handfuls of dried or fresh lavender, rose, and jasmine in a quart of cold water for a few hours. Pour into your bath water along with three drops of each herb's essential oil. Soak for 20 minutes.
- Try a massage with oils that have aphrodisiac properties. In a small container mix two drops each of neroli, sandalwood, jasmine or rose, ylang-ylang, and spikenard essential oils. Close and shake until blended. Add 2 ounces of sunflower or safflower oil and shake again.
- Incorporate soft materials, good wine, romantic movies, incense, perfume, music, and creativity into your time with your special someone.
- Use the back of your hand, your palm, feathers, or silk for arousal. Have fun and be creative. Remember that the biggest sex organ is your mind.
- Realize that stimulation will take longer than before. You might even consider masturbation, as the more you use your sexual muscles, the stronger they become. Some people substitute oral sex.
- If hot flashes accompany you to bed, install a ceiling fan over the bed to help reduce their longevity and interference with intercourse.
- Consider erotic videos or sex gadgets. Even perfectly healthy couples use them. Some doctors will write prescriptions for dildos (rubber vaginal dilators that mimic an erect penis). Use with a lubricant. Vaginal dilators are another option, although many women feel they are too hard and straight for comfort. One doctor even suggests using a lubricant on a candle or vegetable such as a zucchini wrapped in a plastic bag.
- You may feel less self-conscious if your spouse is behind you rather than on top of you during intercourse.
- If you have pain in your chest or arm, support it with pillows during intercourse.

## Scheduling issues
- Schedule sex at the time of day you have the most energy. If possible, schedule medications so side effects are least at that time.
- Plan your sexual time in advance and anticipate it the way you used to look forward to a big date.

## Lifestyle issues
　　Some simple lifestyle changes can enhance your sexual desire. Again, exercise comes into the picture. Sexual drive and performance can be affected by impaired circulation. A 20- to 30-minute walk every day can help.

Load your diet with nutrient-rich fruits, vegetables, and whole grains. Too much red meat or saturated fat can make you sluggish and quash sex drive. Consuming flaxseed (4 to 6 tablespoons a day) or flaxseed oil (1 to 2 tablespoons a day) helps moisturize the vagina and other tissues, but consider the cautions for breast cancer patients.

Sex is really a cycle. When you make changes to take care of yourself, you feel cared for. That brings out a confidence, an inner vitality, and joy that are sexy. You'll have more energy and feel more energetic, and your spouse will respond.

In good relationships, the loss of a breast, though being a source of sadness, is not a permanent catastrophe. Talk through your feelings and listen to your partner's. He may have grief or other emotions to share also. Believe whatever he says. You may be surprised that he is not as bothered about your changed appearance as you are.

Your attitude may be a bigger factor in your sexuality than you realize. If your spouse is not initiating sexual intimacy after your treatment, it may not be because he finds you unattractive. It may be because he is afraid of hurting you or because he feels you have placed distance in the relationship and doesn't want to rush you into something you are not emotionally ready for. Be sure to verbalize what feels good and what you want to wait on. For a while you may want just to hug and cuddle. Then you need to give notice when you are ready to explore other sexual activities.

Take your time. It is hard for some women to bare their changed chest to their spouse even if he is supportive and says the changes don't matter to him. There is no time table for being comfortable being seen with your new body. Some women ease into the transition of exposing their new body by wearing to bed a gown or camisole that holds a soft prosthesis.

If your sexual feelings or sensations do not return to their former state within a year or so, seek professional counseling. Talking with a trained professional can help distinguish your fears and hesitations from physical reasons for disinterest in sex. Possibly you would feel more comfortable talking with a female counselor. Also share your feelings with your spouse. Of course, it would be best if you both talk to a counselor together.

Try to balance the hope you derive from your treatment against this loss. Most husbands prefer your life over your breasts.

## Dating Concerns

Single women most often ask, "When should I tell the man I'm dating about my breast cancer?" Breast cancer does not define who you are. It looms large in your mind, but it may not matter that much to your dating partner.

Treat your cancer as you would any other very personal information. Reveal it as you develop trust in the other person. His reaction to your information, whenever you discuss it, may tell you volumes. If he runs, perhaps he would not have been the supportive life partner you had hoped anyway. Be prepared for rejection, but consider rejection as saving you grief on many other issues later on.

## Skin Problems

Skin irritation such as redness, rash, hives, sudden or severe itching, dryness, acne, peeling, and sun sensitivity can be the result of some chemotherapy drugs. Some drugs given intravenously can result in a darkened area along the vein, especially in people with very dark skin. Although most skin reactions are merely uncomfortable, some indicate serious problems, so inform your doctor.

Temporary color changes (redness or tanning) sometimes occur during radiation treatment. If they bother you, your doctor can recommend a cosmetic concealer.

## Coping with Acne

Keep your face clean. Ask your doctor if you can use over-the-counter medicated creams or soaps or whether she can prescribe something.

## Coping with Itching and Dry Skin

- Avoid cologne or perfume that contains alcohol.
- Keep your skin moisturized. Apply creams or moisturizers while your skin is moist. Use a moisturizing soap (such as Dove) or gel or cleansing cream instead of drying soap.
- Use cornstarch instead of dusting powder.
- Take a quick shower or sponge bath instead of a long, warm bath. Go European and bathe every other day. Wash only sweaty areas such as underarms, feet, and genitals.
- Avoid dehydrating activities or foods such as dry air, saunas, alcohol, caffeine, and diuretics.
- Use a humidifier.
- Drink eight glasses of fluids a day.
- Use oil-based cosmetics.
- Because exercise improves circulation to the skin, move every day.
- Get your eight hours of beauty rest each night.
- Quit smoking.

# Coping with Sun Sensitivity

Even people with dark skin need to protect themselves from the sun's rays during chemotherapy and radiation. Follow these tips:

- Avoid direct sunlight as much as possible, especially between 10 a.m. and 4 p.m. when the sun's rays are strongest.
- For sunscreen, use zinc oxide to block the sun's rays completely. You can buy it without a prescription. Or wear a sunscreen with an SPF (sun protection factor) of at least 15. Sunscreen allows some rays to penetrate your skin whereas sunblock does not. If you will be in the sun more than 20 to 30 minutes, consider sunblock.
- Apply lip balm with SPF.
- Wear long-sleeved clothing. Cotton is best to keep you cool and avoid any skin reactions.
- Wear a hat with a wide brim for maximum protection. If you have lost your hair, be sure to keep your head covered from the sun or apply sunscreen.

## Smell

Chemotherapy can intensify your sense of smell. As it targets other rapidly dividing cells, the treatment also can affect smell receptors and cause loss of appetite or nausea. This should disappear when treatment is finished.

## Sores, Mucous Membranes

Mucous membranes are the mucous-secreting lining of bodily passages that are open to the air, such as nose, sinuses, and genital areas. These areas, in addition to areas of rapidly dividing cells, such as the digestive tract from the mouth to the rectum, are especially susceptible to the effects of chemotherapy.

Your body is most vulnerable to producing sores in these areas 10 to 14 days after receiving chemotherapy. The best way to keep the mucous membranes moist is to drink at least two quarts of water a day.

Your doctor can prescribe rinses, topical applications, or even systemic treatment if sores develop in the genital area. If you develop sores in the rectal area, avoid tampons, rectal thermometers or suppositories, and intercourse until they heal. Sitting in 2 to 3 inches of warm water for 10 minutes may provide temporary relief.

## Swelling in Arms

If you notice a tightness or swelling in the arm on the side where you had lymph nodes removed, see your doctor at once. It may be lymphedema (page 137). The sooner you begin treatment, the better chance you have to control it.

## Taste, Changes in

Drugs used in chemotherapy can affect the nerve endings in the mouth and cause a temporary change in the way you taste. Some women have described the new taste as bitter, metallic, or muted. If foods have a metallic taste, consider using plastic utensils instead of metal ones and, if you can tolerate spices, use more than normal to overcome the disagreeable taste. Sweet tastes are unaffected by chemotherapy so are good choices during this time. Usually your taste returns to normal quickly after treatment stops.

If chemotherapy causes a change in your taste buds:

- Suck on a peppermint, tart candy, or lemon drops during treatment. Low-sugar varieties are a better choice because tooth decay is heightened during chemotherapy. Chewing gum or peppermint Altoids are other options.
- Suck on a slice of dill pickle before meals to stimulate taste buds.
- Avoid beef and soy sauce if food tastes bitter. Get your protein from fish, legumes, poultry, ham, eggs, dairy products, cottage cheese, tofu, yogurt, or milk. Marinade beef in wine, fruit juice, beer, barbecue sauce, or Italian salad dressing. Also try eating meat with something sweet such as applesauce, cranberry or mango sauce, or jelly.
- Increase the flavor of food with spices, marinades, sauces, herbs, and extracts. Onion and garlic are two good strong flavors.
- Eat cold or room-temperature foods or beverages, as they may be more palatable than hot ones because they do not affect the taste buds.
- Keep your mouth and tongue rinsed and your teeth clean to eliminate any bad tastes. Brush your teeth at least twice a day, and rinse your mouth with lemon water after meals or snacks. Commercial mouthwashes with alcohol or sodium, however, may dry out your mouth.
- Drink filtered or bottled water instead of tap water, most of which has some taste to it.
- Try lemonade, which is tart.
- Make meals pleasant. Vary food textures, colors, and smells to make up for lack of taste. Celebrate meals the way the French do. Decorate the table in new linens or colorful paper napkins. Add a bowl of potpourri (unless you are experiencing nausea). Get out the good china (if you have someone to wash it for you!). Keep the conversation light and pleasant.
- Select foods that smell good to you.
- Drink fluids with your meal to rinse away bad tastes.
- If you discover a white coating on your tongue, it could be a common fungus that can grow in the mouth during treatment and change your taste. Ask your doctor for a prescription to cure it.

## *Vaginal Dryness*

Another common symptom women experience in menopause is dryness of the vagina, which can make sexual intercourse painful or uncomfortable. Many women are embarrassed to mention such symptoms to their physician and suffer needlessly. Some things that can help are to:

- Use water-soluble lubricants such as K-Y Jelly, K-Y Liquid, Lubrin Inserts, Summer's Eve Lubricating Jelly, Women's Health Formula, Wondergel, Surgi-lube, Astroglide, plain yogurt, vaginal gels, canola oil, or water- or mineral oil–based vaginal lubricants at the time of intercourse. Avoid using petroleum jelly or oils because they are difficult for the body to absorb or dispose of, so the risk of infection increases. They can also break down the latex in condoms. Avoid those with spermicide unless you are using the lubricant for birth control. Spermicides can increase vaginal irritation.

- Use moisturizing gels such as K-Y Jelly Silk-E, Replens, Silken Secret, Summer's Eve, and Vagisil several times a week, not just before sex. Do not use Vaseline, which is petroleum-based. When dry, the walls of the vagina stick together and can tear or itch. Use the gels as you would a hand lotion.

- If possible, avoid antihistamines, which can lead to vaginal dryness.

- Pop open a vitamin E capsule and spread the contents on the vagina. Do this daily for a week, then once or twice a week.

- Ask your physician if you can try supplements of evening primrose oil, gotu kola, or black cohosh root or soy products to see if they bring relief. Ask an herbalist about taking motherwort tincture or dong quai by mouth.

- Try to find a moisturizer without hormones. The estrogen in vaginal creams can be easily absorbed into the body and may interfere with your treatment or stimulate cancer cell growth. New slow-release vaginal inserts are being tested to give only a minimum amount of estrogen. Ask your doctor if this is an option for you.

- Ask about a vaginal dilator if intercourse continues to be painful.

- Have sex more often. Sexual activity increases the amount of lubrication your vagina produces and stretches the muscles, so more is better.

- Drink adequate water during the day to keep your vagina, as well as your whole body, hydrated.

- Avoid douching.

- Do not wear underwear at night. Keep the area dry and open to the air as much as possible.

## *Vomiting*

If nausea progresses to vomiting several times in a day, inform your doctor. Antiemetic drugs can prevent or lessen nausea or vomiting. Many of these can make you drowsy and throw off your sense of balance, so be careful when getting out of bed or performing any activity requiring coordination and reaction time, such as driving.

Dehydration from not being able to keep down liquids is a concern. Sip on clear, caffeine-free liquids every half hour or so. Try water, Popsicles, soda pop that has gone flat, ice, or apple juice. Salty food is also a good choice, but don't try anything heavy or rich.

The National Institutes of Health recommends acupuncture as an effective means of treating chemotherapy-induced nausea and vomiting, and some insurance companies now pay for it.

Gargle with salt water after vomiting to rinse away the bitter aftertaste and rinse away stomach acid, which can erode tooth enamel.

(See also "Nausea," page 150.)

## *Weight Loss/Gain*

There is no way to know if you will gain or lose weight during your breast cancer treatments—or you may see no change at all.

If women lose weight during breast cancer treatment, the most common time is during chemotherapy (because nausea or a change in taste or mouth sores make eating less pleasant). Also, cancer can change the way our bodies process proteins, fat, and carbohydrates. Fats are broken down at a higher rate but are not stored for energy. Fewer proteins are stored, and more are broken down. Carbohydrates are processed differently so it's harder for them to get into the cells for energy. What does get in is less efficient. A no-carbohydrate diet is not recommended for a cancer patient. Increasing calories alone cannot reverse cancer-induced weight loss.

However, the majority of women gain weight during chemotherapy or while taking hormone therapy (such as tamoxifen). One study from the University of South Florida, Tampa, showed that women on chemotherapy craved high-fat foods and reported fatigue, which curtailed their activity level. Chemotherapy may also lower one's metabolic rate, making weight gain more likely. Other factors that have predicted weight gain in recent studies are being premenopausal upon diagnosis, having positive lymph nodes, and receiving multi-agent and higher dose chemotherapy for longer durations. One study concluded that cytotoxic agents may influence thyroid function in breast cancer patients and suggested a thyroid function review if weight gain occurs.[35]

While in active treatment, try to maintain your weight and concentrate on eating healthy—fruits and vegetables, grains, and legumes rather than processed foods, sweets, and pastas or breads from white flour. Red grapes and purple grape juice, for instance, are packed with the same antioxidants as red wine and without the alcohol.[36] (See "Diet," page 305, for suggestions on changing your eating habits.)

The main help you can give your body, besides completing your prescribed treatment, is to supply nutrients for it to repair itself and assist in overcoming the cancer. Because radiation and chemotherapy damage healthy cells as well as cancer cells (although not to the same degree), your body will need high-quality fuel (food). Calorie and protein needs may increase.

Obviously, if you are nauseated, only certain foods will sound good to you. Eat what you can. A few days of any kind of diet won't make a huge difference in the whole scheme of things. It's better to eat something, even if it's less than the best, than to eat nothing.

Once treatment is over, it is wise to shed excess pounds because excess body fat may contribute to relapse of breast cancer.[37]

A registered dietician or nutritionist can help determine your particular needs. Avoid appetite suppressants. You need a long-term solution, not a quick, and maybe dangerous, trick.

## To Reverse Weight Gain

A number of studies of different breast cancer populations show that obese women are more likely to die from breast cancer than their thinner counterparts with similar characteristics.[38] A small study of breast cancer patients in New York found that patients who ate the most meat, butter, and margarine and drank the most beer were twice as likely to have a recurrence than those who seldom ate these foods.

If you notice a few extra pounds, do not immediately go on a diet. Check with your doctor in case a medication or some other part of treatment is causing fluid retention. Also, you may be eating higher calorie foods than normal. Remember that your intake of nutrients is the most important goal during treatment. If you can switch to foods with less fat, that's good, but don't reduce your calorie intake without consulting a registered dietician.

Healthy habits generally include:

- Emphasize fruits, vegetables, cereals, and breads.
- Cut the fat. Eat lean meat and low-fat dairy products.
- Use low-calorie methods of cooking (steaming and broiling instead of frying).

- Reduce consumption of "little extras" such as butter, sauces, and sweets.
- Exercise to the extent you are able. Strength training helps build muscle. The more muscle mass you have, the more efficiently your body burns calories to offset what you eat.[39] Strength training is easy to do at home with resistance bands, exercise balls, or free weights.
- Avoid crash diets. You must make healthy eating a habit for excess weight to stay off.
- Don't keep fatty, forbidden foods in your house. Then when you are hungry, you'll have to eat something healthy.
- Eat slowly. You'll end up eating less.
- Don't eat out of a package. Measure out the amount you want to eat and stop there.
- Fill up on water rather than calorie-dense foods.
- Eat a balance of protein, fat, and carbohydrates for breakfast to prevent hunger and fatigue mid-morning.
- Don't eat carbohydrates by themselves for any meal.
- Don't eat while watching TV or reading. You lose track of how much you have eaten.

## Choose to Lose

Almost anyone who has tried to lose weight will tell you that discipline and denial are not the keys to weight loss. You must find a way to change your habits and stick with those changes.

New habits should include low-calorie, nutrient-dense foods such as vegetables and fruit, not low-calorie versions of cookies and ice cream. In case your weight gain is due to fluid retention, reduce your salt intake. And most of all, monitor your portion size. You can still enjoy some of your old favorites but in smaller quantities. Have the fattening foods as side dishes, not the main dish.

I have found success with changing my eating habits through a technique I call Future Factor. Keep in mind your ultimate goal (fit into a special dress again, prance around in a skimpy bathing suit, hit a certain weight, help your body fight the cancer, and so forth); then identify behaviors that will bring that about. Stay with your vision of what you want to happen or what you want to look like. Make choices based on that vision. Psychologically this is much different from telling yourself you can't enjoy a fudge sundae. Instead, your goal empowers you to choose the strawberry and raspberry combo and not feel deprived.

## To Reverse Weight Loss

- Drink fluids between meals instead of with meals so you will fill up on food, which generally has more calories than liquids. If you cannot tolerate solid food, by all means get nutrients from soups, juices, or other fluids. Add powdered milk, yogurt, honey, or prepared liquid supplements to drinks for added nutrition.
- Eat foods you like. This is not the time to worry about balanced nutrition.
- Keep small portions of foods handy for snacking—individual-size cans of fruit or yogurt, soups, frozen dinners, commercial liquid supplements—so you can eat any time you are hungry.
- Have a snack before bedtime, especially milk or a dairy product.
- Eat dried fruits or nuts, which are calorie-dense and full of nutrients. Add them to salads or cereal.
- If you are on pain medication, take it 30 minutes before a meal. The medicine as well as the pain can interfere with your appetite.
- Mix canned soups with half-and-half or milk instead of water.
- Exercising 30 minutes before a meal may increase your appetite.
- Try to eat your meals in a different place from where you have spent the day (such as in bed). The change of scenery can stimulate your appetite.
- Surround yourself with pleasant meal mates. If that is not possible, turn on music or a radio or TV to distract you from your food.
- Have your doctor explain to well-meaning family members who urge you to eat even if you are not hungry that you should eat when and what sounds good. There will be a time later to resume regular mealtimes and foods.
- If you don't have the energy to cook, check with the American Cancer Society or Meals on Wheels for carry-in services. Order from nearby restaurants that deliver. Ask friends to set aside one serving of their meal for you.

## To Supplement or Not

Anticancer activity of a whole food comes from a variety of molecules in that food, not just the well-known micronutrients such as vitamins and minerals. Research into the important function of other micronutrients called phytochemicals such as lycopene (and the other phytonutrients with anticancer activity in tomatoes, such as polyphenols and flavonoids) will continue to expand, particularly how various aspects of food cooking or processing will maximize their beneficial contributions through our diets. Because much of the benefit of foods lies in their combination of ingredients, supplements are not as reliable a source of essential nutrients as foods that contain them. Many nutrients have not yet been identified and combinations of nutrients are just now being studied. Research is finding that often nutrients are more beneficial in combination than alone. This is another reason to skip the supplements and push the whole foods whenever possible.

## Better Choices

Think about every bite you put in your mouth. Is it the best choice at the moment? If you are at a party, perhaps the mushroom stuffed with cream cheese is a better choice than the triple-chocolate brownie. Of course, you can splurge occasionally—and probably should to keep your goal obtainable. Just don't splurge at every meal.

A good way to monitor your calorie intake and make better choices about portion size is actually to measure how much your cereal bowl or serving spoon holds. Also, serve yourself a typical meal and, before you eat, place each item into a measuring cup to see how many servings you actually have. You may be surprised at how much you really eat each day. To make your smaller portions seem adequate, serve them on a smaller plate.

Remember that almost every side effect of breast cancer treatment has a solution. Tell your healthcare team what is troubling you and be persistent until you find what works for you. There are usually numerous options to alleviate a problem. If the first one does not work, inform the doctor and try the next. You need to eliminate as many distractions for your body as possible so it can concentrate on the work at hand: stemming the cancer.

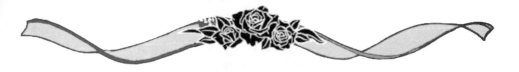

*Chapter 4*

# What Else Can I Do?
# Complementary/Alternative Therapies

Every day you can see advertisements for or news stories on unconventional methods of treating diseases. Such approaches, outside the standard Western care choices, are referred to as complementary or alternative medicine (CAM), or sometimes holistic medicine. *Alternative* means taking the place of. *Complementary* means working in conjunction with. CAM therapies are any that fall outside the conventional practice of Western medicine (as practiced by holders of M.D., medical doctor, or D.O., doctor of osteopathy, degrees. Other terms include *traditional, mainstream, orthodox,* or *allopathic* medicine). As therapies become used more, they drift into the realm of traditional medicine and are no longer thought of as CAM.

The most recent numbers available show that 42 percent of Americans (that's 83 million) use some form of CAM. Patients in general paid more out of pocket for CAM than they did for all hospitalizations.[1] By the late 1990s there were 243 million more visits to CAM practitioners than to primary care physicians.[2]

A study reported in *Alternative Therapies in Health and Medicine* in January 2004 found that two-thirds of the participants who had completed treatment for breast cancer had used at least one CAM treatment in the last 12 months. Most of their doctors had not recommended the therapies. The most commonly used therapies were relaxation/meditation, herbs, spiritual healing, and megavitamins. Younger age, some college education, and private insurance were predictive factors for using CAM.

Interestingly, use of CAM did not reflect negative thoughts toward their conventional medical care. So why did the women turn to CAM? The main reasons given were to enhance overall quality of life, to feel more in control, to strengthen the immune system, and to reduce stress.

Western medicine is gradually beginning to acknowledge treatments and approaches that differ from its technological, measurable focus. In 1993 Congress formally established the Office of Alternative Medicine at the National Institutes of Health. Five years later the office was expanded into the National Center for Complementary and Alternative Medicine (NCCAM) to "explor(e) complementary and alternative healing practices in the context of rigorous science." Significantly the budget increased from $2 million in 1992 to $68.3 million in 2000.

The medical establishment is slower to embrace CAM therapies. As of 2000–2001 no U.S. medical school required a course in CAM, although 91 included CAM as part of a required course and 64 offered elective courses.

If you become frustrated with your treatment plan, investigate other techniques that may enhance what you are doing. Do not quit your treatment plan for a therapy that has catchy advertisements and heart-rending testimonials. Check the validity of the method and, if your healthcare team does not object, try it in addition to your conventional treatment. In fact, try it several times before you decide it doesn't work. Some techniques such as imagery or progressive relaxation take practice to derive the maximum benefit. A trial of two months should be sufficient to know if the therapy will help your condition.

If you do choose to participate in a complementary therapy, inform your doctors, particularly if you are ingesting an herb, vitamin, or supplement. Some substances are believed to interfere with treatment (for instance, too much vitamin A or C is feared to offset the effects of radiation or chemotherapy, and folic acid may interfere with methotrexate, sometimes used in chemotherapy).

Realize also that there is a difference between curing the cancer and improving your quality of life. Many people have found relief from pain, stress, or fatigue from a wide variety of complementary treatments. This is a valuable addition to your treatment plan and to your general well-being and should not be ignored. However, investigate carefully any unconventional treatment that promises to "cure" you. If breast cancer could be cured, that treatment would be standard. If it's not, there may be a good reason.

## Separating Hype rrom Help

Some alternative medicine approaches have been proven to have value in the healing process, so don't automatically avoid them. In fact, it has been estimated that about a quarter of all prescription drugs come from trees, herbs, shrubs, or plant extracts. Aspirin was first made from the bark of the willow tree (*Salix* species), digitalis from foxglove, and penicillin from a mold.

The World Health Organization points out that, of 119 medicines made from plants, about 74 percent are used in ways that correspond to their use by native cultures, so not all beneficial ideas originate in a laboratory.[3]

Keeping in mind the historical use of plants in medicine, look carefully at what is being claimed, who is claiming it, and what proof there is that the claim is sensible and true.

How do you make sense of the many claims for impacting disease? Evaluate them the same way you would if someone offered you a chance to "make a quick buck." Don't let your emotions and fears override your ability to weigh information thoughtfully.

Here are some questions to begin your investigation:

- **What exactly is the claim—a cure? remission? "healing"? What specific kinds of cancer are claimed to be helped?** There are hundreds of kinds of cancer, and the cancer cells work in different ways. One treatment cannot cure all cancers.

- **Is there scientific evidence that this treatment is successful?** Unfortunately, companies can sometimes get away with making outlandish claims for some types of products. Regulations for herbs and dietary supplements, for instance, apply after the fact, so manufacturers might use misleading words or make unproven claims on their labels or in their advertising before the FDA or FTC catches up with them. On the other hand, just because a treatment or activity has no proof does not mean it is useless. Not everything can be proven (can you prove scientifically that you are in love?) and not even everything that Western medicine knows is useful has been tested. The overwhelming experience of thousands of physicians supports the use of many procedures that have not been subjected to laboratory examination. Two questions to ask about unproven techniques or products are how many researchers are studying it and how many companies or health professionals are making similar claims. There may be strength/truth in numbers.

- **Has any traditional medical organization endorsed the treatment?** An endorsement gives credibility although a lack of one may not necessarily discredit the approach. It may mean that it has not been studied thoroughly.

- **What rate of success is claimed?** If no percentages are given, only "testimonials," possibly the company is sharing only its success stories and you don't know what percentage of people has been helped. Ask about measurable results such as measurements of tumor response rates (how the tumor reacted to the substance), overall survival times (how long patients lived after the treatment), and how a diagnosis was determined in the first place (is there evidence of a medical biopsy?).

- **Does the material/Website/article give documentation or sources of the claims it makes?** Be leery of programs or articles that claim a specific health benefit but do not quote related information from a recognized expert or organization or study. If studies are quoted to back up the claim, see if the studies are (in order from best to worst evidence): randomized clinical control trial, case control trial (prospective, retrospective), case report or study, or observational study. One ploy used by some food and supplement manufacturers is to "bind" a legitimate claim to their product. For instance, a food package may boast, "Calcium makes healthy bones. Our cereal contains calcium. Our cereal makes healthy bones." There is more science behind healthy bones than the presence of a measurable amount of calcium in one selection in your diet. You would want to find out how much calcium is recommended for a person of your age, size, body structure, activity level, health condition, and so forth. And you would want to know how much calcium and what kind of calcium are in the cereal. It would be even more helpful to know whether there is a maximum amount of calcium recommended for you and whether you are ingesting it in other foods or supplements. Even if someone with initials after his name is quoted, learn who that person is, where he works, what his training is, and whether he has a financial interest in what he is promoting.

- **How much will the treatment cost?** Although you cannot put a value on human life, most decisions must be weighed through the filter of costs. When considering a treatment, learn up front what it will cost, the duration of the treatment, if any special equipment is required, where you have to go for treatment, and whether it will impact your ability to work or perform services that would have to be hired out if you could not do them (such as childcare, yard work, cooking, ironing, and so on).

- **Who will pay—you or your insurance company?** Get in writing from your insurance company whether a particular treatment is covered before you commit to it. If it is not covered, you of course may choose to participate in it, but you will want to weigh the out-of-pocket costs in your decision. Sometimes an insurance company will deny access to a treatment (perhaps if it is experimental or nonstandard) and change its mind if you appeal. Don't take the first "no" as the final answer.

- **Does the person promoting the treatment stand to gain financially from it?** This does not always mean the treatment is bogus. After all, pharmaceutical companies profit from the drugs they sell. However, they are held to rigorous standards of testing and manufacturing by the Food and Drug Administration. Try to learn whether the company or physician is accountable to any group or government agency for the effectiveness of the proposed treatment. Facts from a disinterested party are usually more reliable than those from someone who will benefit from the sale of a product. Two concepts to investigate are bias on the part of the person promoting the product/treatment and disclosure, revelation of any financial ties the promoter has to the company/clinic being promoted.

- **How will the treatment affect your daily life?** For example, do you have to take six capsules three times a day or have an enema every four hours or delay eating two hours before and after a treatment? You might be able to handle a disruption of your schedule for a limited time. Be realistic about your motivation to follow through with the requirements for a long period.

- **Is the treatment available to everyone (and not an "exclusive" or available only through a certain doctor, clinic, or Website)?** Obviously someone has to be first to discover new treatments for various diseases. However, with technology as advanced as it is, one company or program could not maintain a monopoly on a radical new medicine or treatment for long. Others would quickly develop their own version. Approach any exclusive claims with some skepticism. Perhaps the treatment is so new it has not been duplicated yet or perhaps it has more publicity than scientific basis and that's why it is offered by only a few clinics or companies.

- **What are the risks associated with this treatment?** Do the known benefits outweigh the risks? What side effects are common? There are risks with any treatment. If the promoter says there are no risks or side effects, be extremely cautious.

- **Will the therapy interfere with conventional treatment?** Many CAM treatments such as massage, biofeedback, and even special diets can be used along with standard treatment to offset side effects or enhance quality of life. Consult your healthcare team to be sure the therapy does not offset gains from standard treatment.

Check out the growing number of authoritative books and Websites that are reviewing the scientific evidence for complementary and alternative medicines (see Resources).

## *Insurance Issues*

More and more CAM therapies are being covered by more and more insurance plans. Ask about your particular plan. Does it cover the treatment you are interested in? What are the requirements and limits on number of sessions? Must the practitioner be in your plan network? What costs will you be responsible for?

Some plans offer a rider that covers some areas of CAM. Others have contracted with a network of providers who will offer a discount for services. To learn about laws governing coverage of certain therapies, contact your state insurance commissioner.

## *Finding Qualified CAM Practitioners*

Check out any CAM practitioner before you rely on her advice. Some questions to ask include:

- Have you completed an accredited training program? By whom? When?
- Are you certified by a national body? What are the requirements for certification? Payment of a fee? A structured education program?
- Are you licensed by the state? Ask your state insurance board whether this type of practitioner needs to be licensed.
- How long have you been practicing?
- Have you treated any patients with breast cancer?
- What are your fees?
- How many sessions do you anticipate treatment taking? How often will sessions be scheduled? Where are you located?
- What benefits can I reasonably expect?
- Will treatment affect my daily schedule?

Most states license acupuncturists, chiropractors, massage therapists, and doctors of homeopathy. Some states also license herbalists and naturopaths.

## What Is Integrated Medicine?

As complementary/alternative techniques enter the mainstream, more and more physicians are taking notice—and taking classes in these nontraditional methods. The term *integrated* (or *integrative*) *medicine* refers to medical care given by physicians or other healthcare providers who are trained in both nonconventional or other traditions and Western medicine, and routinely integrate concepts from both systems into their practice or to healthcare providers trained mainly in Eastern or other systems who work closely with Western-trained physicians.

A doctor of integrated medicine can give you the best of both worlds: the focus on subtleties and the interconnectedness of Eastern or other medicine and the precise diagnostic and technological abilities of Western medicine. When your doctor says, "The test results were normal," and you still have symptoms, perhaps you will want to consult with a doctor of integrated medicine to see if there are other approaches to your condition.

## Types of Complementary/Alternative Therapies

There are several ways to categorize CAM therapies, and some therapies could fit into several categories in any particular system. The descriptions in this section are just a small percent of available therapies and are necessarily limited. What is important is to know techniques exist so you can investigate further any that appeal to you. As always, ask your doctor if there is any reason you should *not* participate and inform him of any you choose to participate in. Keep in mind that his lack of exposure to these therapies may color his attitude. Be wise as you try to separate knowledge of real harm to you from prejudice against unconventional approaches in general.

## Sensory

Sensory therapies incorporate the five senses—taste, touch, sight, smell, and hearing—with the body's energy.

**Acupuncture** is a system of healthcare begun in China more than 5,000 years ago. It works on the premise that fine needles, just one-tenth of the size of needles used for blood draws, placed along meridians in the body can remove blocks and restore balance in *qi* (pronounced *chee*), the life force energy. Meridians are 12 theoretical energy pathways that crisscross the surface of the body and contain points, or specific locations that are tied to the functioning of parts of the body. Where an acupuncture needle is inserted may seem unconnected to the source of your problem, but the relationships of points and their corresponding areas of influence have been developed over thousands of years.

Acupuncture is believed to encourage the release of endorphins, natural painkillers that can also increase well-being. The proper stimulation of points produces a response in which the body is believed to correct, strengthen, and heal itself. Some patients have found this an effective way of controlling nausea, vomiting, pain, and hot flashes. Some practitioners recommend avoiding acupuncture during radiation treatment and for two days before or after a chemotherapy treatment whereas others recommend acupuncture during active treatment to boost immunity and relieve nausea.[4]

One component of traditional Chinese medicine (TCM), acupuncture is practiced as mainstream medicine in most hospitals in modern China along with Western medicine. The World Health Organization cites numerous conditions that can be treated successfully with acupuncture, although few of them have been substantiated with scientific studies. This technique will not cure cancer; it is used to alleviate side effects and to tune the body for optimum efficiency in fighting the cancer.

Some insurance companies and Medicaid programs in some states cover acupuncture treatments.

Thousands of years ago soldiers and their horses were given acupuncture treatments before battle to boost their stamina and performance.[5] Today more than 10,000 physicians in the United States are trained in acupuncture and about 80 percent of those use it in their practice. That's about four times as many as 10 years ago. Acupuncturists who received training as physicians within Asian countries such as China and Japan will have had an average of six years of training in medicine and more training and experience with acupuncture. Other acupuncturists are not medically trained but are licensed with more than 2,800 hours of education and training. Always consult a medical doctor first to get a diagnosis and rule out any emergency. After several acupuncture treatments, evaluate your progress.

When a needle is inserted, you might feel a slight sting akin to a mosquito bite, a sharper sting similar to an injection, or nothing at all. Needles are usually left in for up to 30 minutes to hold open the pathway. Although an individual session might offer benefit, usually several sessions are recommended to complete a treatment. The number of sessions needed is related to the severity and type of condition and your overall health and response to the treatment.

**Acupressure** is a system in which the same acupoints as in acupuncture are stimulated by hand or laser. This technique should not be used near the site of wounds or sores. Patients with brittle bones or who bruise easily should inform the practitioner so pressure can be applied accordingly.

**Aromatherapy** is the therapeutic use of oils. Essential oils, fragrances distilled from plants, are absorbed into the body either through the pores of the skin during massage or by inhalation. The scents released by the oil act on the hypothalamus, a part of the brain that influences hormones, and the limbic system, the emotional seat of the brain. Thus, in theory, a smell might affect mood, metabolism, stress levels, or libido.

Fragrant oils have been used as medicine and aphrodisiacs and to promote a sense of well-being for about 5,000 years. The Romans and Greeks washed down their walls with rose oil. The Egyptians placed solid cubes of fragrances under their wigs to release pleasant scents as they melted. People of many cultures have understood for a long time that fragrances can affect mind, body, spirit, and emotions.

Clinical research into claims for the effects of essential oils on medical conditions is not extensive, but the psychological effects of smell have been studied more. There are conflicting reports regarding the properties and uses for oils, and responses to smells are highly personal. A few voices have raised concerns about the safety of aromatherapy in cancer patients, especially during chemotherapy, because essential oils are powerful chemicals and chemotherapy can sometimes affect a person's sense of smell.[6]

Essential oils can be added to steaming water, nebulizers, or diffusers to spread the oil molecules into the air. They can be diluted in vegetable oils such as grapeseed or sweet almond oil and added to a bath or used in massage. They should never be ingested because some are poisonous, and they should never be used full strength.

Seven toxic oils that should be used only under the direction of a qualified herbalist or aromatherapist are calamus, camphor, pennyroyal, tansy, wintergreen, wormseed, and wormwood. Some oils such as rose, gardenia, vanilla, and jasmine are rare and precious (and expensive!) so are sometimes falsely presented for sale.

Some essential oils that have traditionally been found to be appropriate or pleasing for various cancer-related conditions are presented in the chart on page 186. Combinations will bring out different properties of the essential oils.

## Ways to incorporate aromatherapy into your day

Fresh herbs are not as concentrated as essential oils and may be a better choice for people with sensitive skin.

- Spray a handkerchief lightly with a mist of an essential oil or place a few drops of oil onto a piece of cloth. Tuck the cloth into a lingerie drawer, car, briefcase, purse, or desk or between your sheets or inside your pillowcase. Don't place oils directly on your clothing because some stain.

- Place two drops of your favorite essential oil on a terra-cotta ring. Rest the ring on a lightbulb and turn on the light. The heat will infuse the scent throughout the room. A car diffuser plugged into the cigarette lighter works the same way.

- Hang a cotton bag of lavender in your car for a calmer driving experience.

- Burn fragrant grasses in your fireplace. Test with a little grass to see your reaction to the smoke.

- Put a few drops of an essential oil on the defrost vents in your car and turn on the fan.

- Add herbs to your bath. Place them in a clean cotton sock or muslin bag. Tie the bag to the faucet and let the water run through it as it fills the tub or float the bag in the water. You can also place the herb in a quart of water, bring to a boil, simmer for 15 minutes, and strain. Pour the liquid into the tub. Wrap the remaining solid residue into a washcloth and rub your body with it.

- Soak in an aromatherapy bath for 10 to 20 minutes (it takes this long for the oils to reach the bloodstream). Mix five to 10 drops of essential oil to 1 teaspoon of almond oil or apricot kernel oil. Add when the tub is full and step right in. Close windows to keep the aroma in the room.

- Keep a bottle of essential oil at your desk and sniff as needed.

Find essential oils at health-food stores or stores that carry natural cosmetics. Books on aromatherapy usually include sources in the back.

| Condition | Essential oil |
|---|---|
| Anxiety | Lavender, neroli, sage, thyme, lemon balm, rosemary, geranium, pine, peppermint, chamomile |
| Aphrodisiac | Cedar, clary sage, gardenia, jasmine, patchouli, vanilla, sandalwood, rose bulgar, rose maroccan, Egyptian rose, geranium, ylang-ylang, cucumber and licorice allsorts[7] |
| Concentration | Rosemary |
| Constipation | Basil (dilute with oil and massage into abdomen) |
| Depression | Basil, benzoin, bergamot, clary sage, gardenia, grapefruit, jasmine, lavender, lemon balm, rose, neroli, patchouli |
| Energy | Patchouli, geranium leaf, juniper, spearmint, mint, orange, sage, lemon, lemon balm, rosemary, lime, bergamot |
| Fatigue | Rosemary, citrus, eucalyptus, mint |
| Fever | Lavender, peppermint, spearmint |
| Gas | Ginger, peppermint, spearmint, tangerine |
| Immune system weakness | Bay, lavender, bergamot, thyme, sandalwood, lemon |
| Infections | Bergamot, cedar, eucalyptus, lavender, lemon, sage, thyme |
| Insect repellant | Eucalyptus, citronella, tea tree, pennyroyal, orange |
| Insomnia | Chamomile, lavender, vetiver; place one or two drops of clary sage or lavender essential oil on your pillowcase or the collar of your pajamas |
| Mental fatigue, fuzzy thinking | Basil, rosemary, frankincense, myrrh |
| Muscle pain, soreness, tension | Bay, chamomile, cinnamon, lavender, thyme, rosemary, marjoram |
| Nausea | Basil, ginger, lavender, peppermint, spearmint |
| Nervous tension | Bergamot, chamomile, cinnamon, clary sage, lavender, orange, tangerine, vetiver, geranium, lemon balm |
| Pain | Rosemary, chamomile, cayenne oil, ginger |
| Stress | Neroli, lavender, chamomile, marjoram, clary sage |

**Chiropractic** involves the manipulation of the vertebrae to alleviate blockages of nerve bundles, which practitioners believe are the root of much illness. Sessions can involve deep tissue massage, heat, trigger-point manipulation, tissue manipulation, or recommended exercises. Claims include improved mental functioning, immune system, and circulation. Chiropractic is not recommended for people with bone cancer or diseases of the spinal cord or bone marrow.

A review by the National Center for Complementary and Alternative Medicine found that all studies of chiropractic treatment had found at least some benefit to the participants. In six of the eight studies, chiropractic and conventional treatments were found to be similar in effectiveness. One clinical trial found treatment at a chiropractic clinic to be more effective than outpatient hospital treatment. More study is needed, but the therapy has value in some situations, especially in relieving lower back pain.

**Massage** relies on the body's nerve endings and pressure points to promote relaxation. The most widespread techniques use a combination of five basic strokes ranging from slow, rhythmic gliding strokes to drumming hands on the body.

Massage therapy offers many benefits to cancer patients such as reduced stress and anxiety, improved mood, relaxation, and pain management. Massage at an incision site can reduce scarring, but ask your doctor about your particular case. Massage is generally not recommended for patients who bruise easily, have had lymph nodes removed, or have low platelet counts or for areas of infection, wounds, or soreness.

In some circumstances massage can be risky or the techniques need to be adjusted. For example, massage should not be given if a surgical site shows signs of infection or until an incision has healed, and it should not be used at a tumor site. The technique is not appropriate during radiation treatment because the massage, even with the lightest touch, may further irritate the irradiated skin and underlying tissues. It also should be avoided during chemotherapy cycles when patients are at increased risk of bruising. Most massage therapists require a signed statement from your oncologist that massage is not contraindicated in your situation.

**Reflexology** practitioners deliver pressure to reflexology zones on the foot that they believe correspond to particular organs of the body. The stimulation brings balance to those organs. Although there is no proof of this connection, this technique can provide a sense of well-being and relaxation. Some women find this a valuable alternative when they are too tender to be touched on their upper body.

**Therapeutic touch, healing touch,** and **Reiki** are forms of energy work based on the theory that we are all connected into one energy field. They differ in their philosophies, but, in each, the practitioner provides the environment in which the patient can self-heal by manipulating imbalances in the patient's energy field. Therapeutic touch, which is taught in dozens of U.S. universities and nursing schools and used in many U.S. hospitals, has been used to promote healing of wounds and lymphatic disorders. Studies show it helps reduce pain and stress, enhances relaxation, and raises levels of hemoglobin. Endorsed by the American Holistic Nurses Association, healing touch has reduced pain, enhanced a feeling of well-being, and accelerated wound healing. Reiki, which means universal life energy, is a form of Japanese therapy used for both physical and spiritual healing. Practitioners aim to balance the body's chakras, or energy centers, to dissolve energy blockages that they believe cause disharmony and disease. After any energy work, some patients feel relaxed and others feel invigorated.

**Craniosacral therapy** is a gentle therapy similar to chiropractic in that its goal is proper alignment and balance, but it involves the membranes and cerebrospinal fluid that surround the brain and spinal cord. Therapists very lightly place their fingertips upon the bones of the skull and spine in order to sense and to improve the flow of cerebrospinal fluid. Although no scientific studies support this theory, patients do report a reduction in both tension and headaches. Many physical therapists are trained in this technique.

The **Trager Approach** is a form of bodywork using gentle movements that release deep-seated physical and mental stress patterns a person has developed over a lifetime. The technique includes table work with a certified practitioner and Mentastics, simple movements the patient practices in her daily life to reinforce the table work. This technique is painless and enhances deep relaxation by "hooking up" a patient with a universal energy force.

The **Feldenkrais Method** teaches people to identify ways they move, often unconsciously, that lead to pain or dysfunction and shows them better ways to move. By increasing range of motion, flexibility, and coordination, the patient can experience enhanced functioning in other aspects of her life. Its deep massage technique is not recommended when platelet counts are low because of the risk of bruising. **Rolfing,** a system of soft tissue manipulation, also teaches more efficient use of muscles for better movement and posture.

The **Alexander technique** is a therapy that concentrates on body mechanics and muscle control. By improving posture and movement, proponents believe the technique allows the body's systems to perform at a higher level. Studies have shown reduced stress, pain relief, and improved breathing and posture from this technique.

**Skin stimulation** enables the skin to feel some sensations that can displace pain. Pressure, heat, cold, massage, vibration, and menthol preparations can be used. The stimulation may be at the site of the pain and redirect blood flow to it or relieve the pain by stimulating another area.

If you are receiving radiation or chemotherapy, check with your doctor before applying hot or cold packs or any ointments, lotions, or salves, particularly on treated areas of your body.

Pressure near a painful area may bring relief. Press your hand on or near the area as firmly as you can without causing more pain. Hold for 10 seconds.

A handheld vibrator or a vibrating chair or pad may soothe sore muscles or pain. Do not use vibration over raw, tender, or swollen areas or after radiation.

Cold packs may numb an area and a painful sensation. Gel packs from the drugstore that can be used and refrozen are helpful, or place ice cubes in a towel. Stop cold therapy if you start to shiver or if it causes more pain.

Heat packs may relieve sore muscles. Use gel packs from the store, a hot water bottle, a heating pad, a hot bath or shower, or a home hot tub. Do not use heat on bare skin or within 24 hours of a new injury. Always cushion heat packs with a towel. Do not go to sleep with a heating pad on.

Do not use heat or cold therapy over any place where your circulation or sensation is impaired and do not leave it on anywhere for more than 10 minutes.

Menthol rubbed into your skin via lotions or creams may bring relief for several hours. Before you use a preparation, test a small amount on the area. If no reaction has occurred within a few hours, it is probably safe to use. Taking a warm shower before application will increase the intensity of the feeling. Do not use a heating pad for this. Do not use menthol if you have been told not to take aspirin because some preparations contain an ingredient similar to aspirin. Do not use menthol in an area being irradiated and do not get menthol in your eyes, mouth, or genitals or on a rash or area of broken skin. Wash your hands thoroughly after applying it. Be aware that menthol has a strong odor, which may be an irritant to you or to others in the room with you.

**Hydrotherapy** is the use of water for medicinal purposes. Roman baths and American Indian sweat lodges are only two examples throughout history. Water is used in cold packs to reduce swelling, in hot packs to stimulate circulation, or in spas to combat stress. However, the American Cancer Society warns against any internal hydrotherapy such as colonic irrigation, which it says can perforate the colon and lead to electrolyte imbalance. It also notes reports of bacterial infection from some contaminated public bathhouses, so be extra cautious during chemotherapy.

**Light therapy** uses UV or colored light to affect circadian rhythm and lead to better health. Although light is used in Western medicine to treat jaundice in newborns and seasonal affective disorder (SAD), its effectiveness in cancer treatment is unproven. Do not use this therapy if any medications you take or other conditions make you sensitive to sunlight. A new therapy studied by the National Cancer Institute is photodynamic therapy, which injects an agent into cells to make them supersensitive to light. The agent lingers in cancer cells, which are exposed to a laser beam and destroyed.

**Music therapy** is the prescribed use of music or musical interventions by a trained music therapist to promote physical, emotional, psychological, and spiritual healing. Music causes neurons to fire faster and energizes our thought process. Studies have shown music therapy to relieve pain, reduce nausea and vomiting during chemotherapy, decrease depression and sleep disturbances, and lower blood pressure.

Music employed successfully in music therapy is soothing and simple so it is not distracting. Generally it is instrumental (acoustic instruments, harp, and flute work well) with no more than one instrument or voice at a time and not much variation in tempo or volume. Music is chosen for specific therapeutic goals. Activities may include singing, listening to music, playing instruments, composition, moving to music, and music and imagery exercises. You don't need a trained therapist, however, to play a soothing CD when you are feeling bad.

## Cognitive Therapy

Cognitive therapy uses the power of positive thinking and the mind/body connection to promote healing.

**Guided imagery or visualization** is sometimes called a "focused daydream." In this technique a patient imagines the ideal solution to a situation or a very relaxing scene. A patient may visualize getting through a diagnostic test without pain or relaxing tense muscles or avoiding nausea during chemotherapy. Studies have shown guided imagery to be effective at managing depression, pain, stress, and anxiety.

To use this technique, sit or lie comfortably. Soothing music in the background may help you relax. Put a small pillow under your knees or neck if you are lying down. Either stare at an object with your eyes open or gently close your eyes. Imagine the scene you want to influence. Walk through every detail in your mind, creating only the best outcome in every facet of the situation. Remain calm and positive throughout the exercise. If you are just trying to relax, think of a calm, peaceful scene. It may be a beach or mountain waterfall or a favorite place from your childhood. Explore this place in detail, using all your senses, to help calm you.

Another way to use imagery is to picture something that will help your body fight the cancer. It may be a dragon that flashes fire at cancer cells, a robot that plucks up cancer cells as they hide behind tissues in your body, or a white light that acts as a magnet to attract pain and dissolve it. Find an image you are comfortable with. Some people don't like the fighting images and prefer something more friendly. Whatever your image, begin your session by relaxing and concentrating on your breathing for a few minutes. Just be aware of inhaling and exhaling in a slow, rhythmic pattern. Now incorporate your image into your mental picture. As you inhale, see the "conqueror" image doing its work. As you exhale, see the results of that action. Continue this exercise for a few minutes. When you are ready to stop, concentrate again on your breath for a count of three. Open your eyes and slowly resume your activities.

Working with a trained therapist is known as interactive guided imagery. The therapist may direct your attention to the body part that is ailing and ask you to enter into a dialogue with it. This provides the opportunity for your unconscious to present knowledge that the therapist can help interpret. There are no known risks associated with guided imagery.

**Prayer** is a mystical practice that has been studied in the laboratory with amazing results. Larry Dossey, author of *Healing Words*, says that prayer's healing ability "is one of the best kept secrets in modern medicine….If any new medical therapy had been as successful…it would have been headlines around the world. Unfortunately, science, while giving us a lot of material progress in this age, has also declared immortality and belief in God as fantasy."

Study after study of prayer shows that it does have an effect on such diverse subjects as mice, humans, cells, enzymes, and algae, although some scientists question the validity of the studies. According to some theories, prayer does not work like any other known form of energy and works as well for one faith as another. It works when the subject does not know she is being prayed for, and it works across thousands of miles. Dr. Dale Matthews of Georgetown University, author of *The Faith Factor*, reports that about 75 percent of studies of spirituality show definite health benefits.[8]

Some propose that prayer brings about a sense of calm that triggers stress reduction in the body. That could be part of the explanation of how prayer works, but it does not explain the results of intercessory prayer, prayer for someone else. The *Annals of Internal Medicine* reviewed 23 studies on intercessory prayer and "distant healing" and found that 57 percent found a positive effect. In some of these studies the patients did not know they were being prayed for.

Studying prayer via a scientific method seems particularly unreliable. Does it make sense to examine a theological phenomenon with methods designed to measure the physical world? How can a researcher be sure that the control group is not being prayed for by others? However you evaluate the studies, believers will continue beseeching their God for intervention—and miracles will continue to happen without explanation.

**Relaxation and deep breathing** can reduce stress and anxiety, relieve muscle tension, and give a greater sense of control. To achieve a state of deep relaxation, sit in a comfortable chair with your legs and arms uncrossed or lie on a bed or the floor with a pillow under your head, neck, and knees. When you are comfortable, close your eyes or find an object to stare at. Begin by breathing slowly and rhythmically. Count, "In, one, two. Out, one, two." If your rhythm gets off track from your breathing, just take a deep breath and start counting over again. Each time you inhale, tense one muscle, such as your forehead or a foot. When you exhale, release the tension. When you are finished, count to three and slowly open your eyes and resume your activities.

There are several breathing techniques you can adopt, such as conscious breathing. Most techniques involve breathing from the abdomen instead of the chest. As you inhale, imagine your abdomen is a balloon filling with air. Gradually allow the air to flow into your chest. As you exhale, imagine you are flattening your abdomen against the chair or floor. Abdominal breathing circulates lymph, may be deeper than chest breathing, and may get more oxygen into the body.

You can buy commercial tapes to assist your relaxation time. Try to listen to them before you buy in case the voice grates on you. Do not listen to them while driving! If you get sleepy during this exercise, sit in a hard chair. If you get dizzy from breathing too deep, take more shallow breaths or breathe slower.

To help you relax throughout the day, think of a "trigger" that will remind you to check your breathing and slow it down. It might be when the dog barks or when you look at your watch or when an e-mail arrives. Pick something that happens several times a day so you can make deep breathing into a habit.

**Meditation** conjures up monks sitting silently or chanting in a monastery. However, ordinary people from all walks of life and religions are benefiting from this versatile practice.

Meditation is practiced by religions and nonreligious people worldwide. Some meditation practices attempt to help you clear your thoughts (Buddhist meditation, for example); others attempt to help you focus your thoughts (Christian meditation, for example).

Meditation is basically an intentional break from everyday problems and the stress they produce. It takes you to an inner place that is more peaceful than your current environment. Although there are many ways to meditate, they all involve deep concentration that produces relaxation and calm. The relaxed state that meditation can induce can lower stress and its negative effects on the body, such as suppressing the immune system. It has also been shown to reduce pain, anxiety, and panic.

For most types of meditation you sit or kneel. You can sit in a straight chair with your hands limp on your knees, palms up. You can sit cross-legged or in a yoga position or you can kneel with your thighs and buttocks resting on the back of your calves and your hands resting lightly on your thighs. Place a thin pillow or blanket under your ankles for comfort and place a pillow between your buttocks and calves to straighten your spine.

Most methods of meditation involve concentrating on your breathing. In the simplest form you inhale and exhale, paying attention only to your breathing. When the inevitable thoughts crowd into your mind, just acknowledge them and return to concentrating on your breathing. Do this frequently throughout the day as a destressor.

Another simple form of meditation may begin with a relaxed posture, concentration on your breathing for a few moments, then repeating one word slowly. Pick a positive word and focus on it. If your mind wanders (as it almost certainly will), just dismiss the thought, don't berate yourself, and focus again on the word or phrase. As one priest advised, "It's one thing to have a thought [during meditation]; it's another to have it in for coffee."[9]

An alternative form of meditation is to take a short saying or prayer and meditate on each word in turn. Squeeze every good thought out of each word before moving to the next. When you finish, focus again on your breathing for several cycles and slowly return to your normal activities.

People with a vivid imagination use imagery in their meditation. Sit quietly, focus on your breathing for a few breathing cycles, and then recall a time you felt whole, peaceful, and just happy to be alive. Relive that moment in every detail and with all your senses. Remember the good feelings. Dwell on that scene for a few minutes and gradually come back to the present.

People who are restless do not feel comfortable sitting to meditate, so they practice walking meditation. Begin by walking a normal, brisk pace for five minutes. Be mindful of the movement of your arms and legs and the connection of your feet to the floor or pavement. Deliberately cut your pace in half for five minutes. Then cut it in half again for the last five minutes. When thoughts come, kick them away gently with the next step and focus again on your movement in the moment.

A spiritual form of walking meditation uses the labyrinth, a replica from the famous Chartres Cathedral outside Paris. Participants walk a winding path that is a metaphor for their spiritual journey. With proper instruction walking the labyrinth can be a powerful spiritual experience. Most large cities have at least one outdoor labyrinth associated with a church, park, or retreat center.

By concentrating on something calming and pleasant in any form of meditation, our minds relax and our bodies slow the stress cycle.

**Biofeedback** uses a special machine with visual or other signals and a trained technician to help you learn to control specific body functions such as heart rate, muscle tension, or blood pressure. It is also used in conventional medicine for pain relief and other effects and can be used to alleviate depression.

**Affirmation** is similar to autosuggestion. It gives your mind positive feedback that is verbal instead of visual. Repeat things to yourself such as "I am well and active" or "I am a sexy woman." Use only positive statements. Say, "I have lots of energy" rather than "I'm not tired." Also make statements in the present: "I am" rather than "I will be." The goal is to fill your subconscious with positive thoughts.

**Hypnotherapy** involves inducing a state of acute concentration. This can be done by a licensed hypnotherapist, or one can teach you to hypnotize yourself. In this state you are very aware; you just don't want to open your eyes or wake up. This technique has been used with success for pain management.

When you are hypnotized, you are in control. No one can make you do something you don't want to do. Basically you are reprogramming your brain and body to respond differently to common stimuli or situations.

## Expressive Therapies

Expressive therapies encourage patients to express their feelings in a positive, creative way and thus release anxiety, fear, and other negative emotions.

Counseling (see "Choosing a Counselor," page 213) and support groups (see page 211) are commonly used by cancer patients with much success.

**Journaling/scrapbooking.** A cancer experience brings to light and creates its own wide swath of emotions. Many of us are not equipped to deal with all they entail. One technique people have used successfully to cope with overwhelming emotions is journaling. This is a private, nonjudgmental way of expressing negative and positive emotions that is healthier than trying to deny or ignore them.

Forget your high-school English assignments and give this technique a try. There are no rules or formulas to follow. Just begin writing and keep writing as fast as you can without stopping to correct spelling or grammar or reread what you have written. Your mind will guide you along paths that will surprise you. In the process you will identify some feelings you were not aware of and you will get out some feelings you are afraid or embarrassed to share with someone else.

If you have trouble getting started, pick a topic such as a feeling (fear, anger, hope), a memory, a specific incident, a person, a symptom, or a phrase that has stuck with you. Use the item as a title or the beginning sentence; then write whatever comes to mind. You may even end up writing, "I can't think of what I want to say about today's conversation with Betsy. When she called...." Every word does not have to make sense. The point is to help your mind put "skin" on elusive thoughts so you can see them and deal with them.

Another technique is to have a dialogue with another person or symptom or even an object such as your tumor. Imagine the person or problem sitting in a chair across from you. What would you say? How would he or it respond? Continue the dialogue until you have resolved your feelings.

Some people find it helpful to create worst-case scenarios. They begin writing about a stressful situation or a bothersome feeling and write it out to its logical (or ridiculous!) conclusion. Sometimes reviewing the entry later helps put it all in perspective.

## Recording your history/biography

Because cancer leads us to think about our mortality, many people find it therapeutic to record their life stories, values, or lessons learned for their families, creating a legacy. There are many ways to do this. You can write poems or stories from your life. Rather than record a tedious timeline of events in your life (although this has value), include as much detail and as many feelings as you can. Describe the tin pail you carried your school lunch in and how you felt to have dry biscuits for lunch when others were having sandwiches on store-bought bread—or other events that show the contrast of your upbringing with today's children. Although the "what's" of your life are of some interest to your family, the "why's" and "how's" can teach them about motivation, choices, determination, and other characteristics you might want to instill in them.

If writing stories is intimidating, you can also create a list of "Lessons Learned" or write a letter. You might want to tape-record the stories instead of writing them. Have someone you enjoy sit with you as you relate the events and ask questions or prompt you to add details.

Another way of recording your life story is through scrapbooking. This can include photographs slipped into sleeves or artistically laid out or simply images from magazines that illustrate points you want to record. Be as creative as you like and concentrate more on the content of your life story than the style. The point is to let someone get to know you.

**Art therapy**—including drawing, painting, and sculpting—encourages pleasure in creativity and enables people to find a way of expressing their feelings that cannot be easily put into words. Proponents of this therapy believe this release of emotions such as fear or anger reduces stress and promotes general well-being. Being involved in creating, especially in a group setting, can also be a distraction from pain and malaise.

## Physical Exercise

Exercise of any intensity and duration can have beneficial effects on a person's health. Besides relieving stress, exercise can promote positive attitudes and better body functioning.

**Dance therapy** provides the benefits of exercise as well as psychological benefits of positive thoughts, social interaction, and expression of emotions. The therapy can improve physical coordination and self-esteem, thereby increasing self-confidence. A key is to pick music that irresistibly leads your body to move.

**T'ai chi** is a form of gentle movement and breathing that is available even to those who are frail or uncoordinated. It can even be done in a chair! The exercise has been called "meditation in motion." Actually a martial art, it seeks to help *qi*, or life energy, move unrestricted and to balance yin and yang, which are active and passive principles in one's life. You don't have to believe in its philosophy to reap benefits from the graceful exercises. Those who practice t'ai chi can experience better balance and flexibility, greater muscle mass and strength, improved posture and stamina, and reduced stress and depression. Scientific studies have proved that regular t'ai chi may slow the rate of bone loss in postmenopausal women. T'ai chi is a moderate aerobic exercise on par with brisk walking and improves abdominal muscle strength. It also has been found effective for reducing the risk of falls.

**Yoga** is a form of gentle exercise involving body positioning and breathing techniques. Practiced in India for thousands of years, it has come into its own in the West as a way to relieve stress and fatigue, especially mental. Stretching can reduce muscle tension, and squeezing of various muscle groups can improve circulation while concentrating on your body can block out mental stressors and calm you.

There are numerous styles of yoga, which emphasize different aspects of the practice: breathing, fluid movement, spiritual concerns, postures, and so forth. The benefits depend on how you practice the techniques and can include improved muscle tone and flexibility, decreased blood pressure, improved posture, better sleep, increased energy, and reduced pain. You will benefit more from an experienced, trained yoga instructor.

**Qi gong** (pronounced *chee gung*; also spelled *chi-kung*) is an ancient Oriental system of movement, breathing techniques, and meditation that is designed to develop and improve the circulation of *qi* around the body. Meaning "energy work," this technique can be internal, involving intense mental concentration and little movement, or external, involving the participation of a qi gong master to direct his energy to the patient's benefit. The exercises are not strenuous so they can be used by frail patients. Studies have shown benefits of improved sleep and balance and reduced stress and number of falls.

**Nia** (the Swahili word means "with purpose" and the initials stand for neuromuscular integrated action) is a form of movement developed as nonimpact aerobics. Its movements combine pieces of martial arts, aerobics, dance, and psychology. In contrast to the carefully crafted forms of t'ai chi or other Eastern meditative movements, Nia offers students total flexibility of movement, range of motion, style, and choreography that draw from Eastern and Western philosophies and programs. It uses a combination of relaxing movements blended with the conscious use of mind and energy.

**Pilates** (pronounced *pea-la-tease*) is a body-conditioning program that uses stretching and strengthening to achieve proper breathing, balance, flexibility, middle body control, and extremity strengthening. Many of the exercises are done on a floor mat, and some special equipment may be needed. This technique can be more taxing physically than t'ai chi or qi gong, but feasible if approached slowly with an experienced teacher. Individualized sessions may be necessary if group sessions are too challenging.

## Medical Systems

Experts refer to some alternative therapies that use nontraditional medicines as medical systems. Read up on the philosophy and check the credentials of a practitioner as you would for any other CAM therapy.

### General precautions
- Consult a doctor before starting any nonconventional form of treatment.
- Do not stop taking any prescribed medication without first consulting your doctor.
- Tell your complementary practitioner about any prescribed medication you are taking and any other complementary treatments you are receiving.
- Do not start on a vigorous exercise program without first consulting a doctor.

**Osteopathy** or osteopathic medicine is a complete system of Western medical care that treats the whole person rather than the symptoms. Doctors of osteopathy focus on the interconnectedness of all body systems and place special emphasis on the musculoskeletal system, which they believe reflects and influences all other body systems. Osteopathic physicians (DOs) can prescribe medicine and perform surgery just as MDs can. They are fully trained medical professionals.

**Traditional Chinese medicine (TCM)** has developed over thousands of years. One of its supposed strengths is its ability to detect some conditions in their early stages. One saying is that "Chinese medicine can cure what is disturbed, not what is destroyed." In other words, the earlier a symptom is treated with TCM, the better the chance of its being reversed.

Another advantage is TMC's virtual lack of side effects, with the exception of occasional gastrointestinal upset. TCM includes nutritional interventions (including herbs), breathing, and exercise as well as acupuncture and other similar therapies.

TCM has been used effectively to treat side effects of breast cancer such as nausea, vomiting, pain, symptoms of PMS, and sleep disorders. In a literature review of TCM and human cancers, the University of Texas M. D. Anderson Cancer Center reported that outcomes showed increased survival times, improved recovery from surgery, reduction of side effects from chemotherapy and radiation, enhanced immune response and quality of life, and alleviation of pain with the use of TCM in conjunction with traditional therapy compared to traditional therapy alone.[10]

**Homeopathy,** which developed in Germany 200 years ago, works on the premise that we have, in essence, two bodies: our mass body, the one we can touch, and a body of energy that is a mirror image of the mass. Treating illnesses with energy work clears the way for the mass body to work more effectively on that same condition. The theory behind homeopathy also purports that less is more and that like cures like (the law of similars). Holistic practitioners use small doses of specially prepared minerals and plant extracts to stimulate the body's defense mechanisms to heal themselves. The underlying theory is that tiny amounts of substances that would cause symptoms in a healthy person will relieve those same symptoms in one who has them by affecting the energy body and allowing the mass body to heal. Homeopathy treats the whole person rather than individual symptoms.

**Naturopathy** aims to support the body in healing itself. In addition to the basic medical sciences and conventional diagnostics, naturopathic education includes therapeutic nutrition, botanical medicine, homeopathy, natural childbirth, classical Chinese medicine, hydrotherapy, naturopathic manipulative therapy, pharmacology, and minor surgery. These and other modalities are used to effect prevention as well as healing.

**Ayurveda,** the traditional medical system of India, purports that health is achieved through an inner harmony. The practice gives equal weight to mind, body, and spirit through the use of exercise, diet, herbs, meditation, massage, controlled breathing, and exposure to sunlight. The name itself means "science of life." This system's emphasis on prevention and well-being means that many of its goals are compatible with allopathic medicine. Some of its herbal therapies are being studied rigorously for confirmation of benefits claimed.

**Anthroposophical medicine** seeks to exploit the mind/body/spirit connection to understand illness. Using traditional medicine as a basis, this system includes nutrition, movement therapies, and homeopathy along with other techniques that place illness in a perspective larger than just a range of symptoms.

## Other CAM Techniques

Some other complementary/alternative medical techniques don't fit easily into a category. One is the field of energy therapies that claim to manipulate energy either within the body (biofields) or outside the body (electromagnetic fields).

Biofields are the focus of such therapies as qi gong, Reiki, and therapeutic touch.

Electromagnetic fields, including direct and alternating current fields, magnetic fields, and pulsed fields, have been used to manage pain and treat cancer. For example, in hundreds of Chinese hospitals electrodes are inserted into small tumors (including breast, lung, brain, and melanomas), current is applied, and tumors break apart. Electromagnetic therapy is also known as electromagnetism, bioelectricity, magnetobiology, magnetic field therapy, and magnetic healing. Scientists know that electricity and magnetic energy exist in the body. Practitioners of this therapy claim they can resolve energy imbalances to restore health by applying external electrical energy. The use of therapeutic magnets has been scientifically proven to reduce certain types of pain and improve physical functioning under some circumstances.

Other CAM techniques are biologically based therapies such as the use of herbs, special diets, minerals such as magnesium or hormones such as melatonin, megavitamins, or special substances such as bee pollen for therapeutic purposes. One such therapy, Essiac tea, contains some herbs that have shown anticancer activity in laboratory tests. However, no clinical tests have been done on humans to determine whether its claims of supporting the immune system or detoxifying the body are true. Another theory is Bach flower remedies, in which specific flowers are diluted many times in water and brandy. Drops of the remedies are given for various emotional problems such as fear, despondency, or oversensitivity. Anecdotal reports claim results—although no scientific evidence shows measurable results.

The variety of CAM techniques is staggering. Many claim to cure cancer. Do your research before adding one to your regimen—and certainly before substituting one for conventional treatment. Though the "cure rate" of chemotherapy, radiation, and surgery is not where we want it, at least you know the risks and possible benefits.

Obviously all CAM techniques will need to pass rigorous tests for effectiveness, safety, and optimal dosages. Until they are tested, however, what are we to do? The best we can do is to read extensively about the technique and consult with our doctors, dietitians, clinical pharmacists, professionals trained and certified in the techniques, and reliable, impartial organizations that can offer objective information. Then make an informed decision using the questions on pages 179–181 (under "Separating Help from Hype"). Western medicine does not have all the answers or you would not need this book. However, some promoters of CAM (as well as investments or real estate or a hundred other products) do not have your best interests at heart. They are out to make money and will say or do anything to that end. Let facts, not fear, drive your decisions.

## *Supplements*

It is natural to panic when a cancer diagnosis is pronounced. "Do something!" we want to scream. "Anything!"

And something "simple" such as some extra vitamins or "natural" substances certainly seems harmless enough. Perhaps this approach is helpful. Perhaps not. No one really knows. Evidence-based researchers come down dogmatically on both sides of the supplementation issue.

So what's the problem with taking vitamins or herbs? There may be several:

- Any substance that enters the body through your mouth, skin, veins, or any other way has a potential effect on your body. After all, that's why people take supplements, hoping to reap positive benefits. Just because a substance is "natural" does not mean it cannot be harmful. Remember poison ivy and toxic mushrooms.

- The term *natural* is not used in a uniform manner or regulated by law. Is the entire compound you are considering unprocessed? Was the crop sprayed with pesticides? What sanitary measures are taken in the factory? What percentage of the ingredients is covered in the claim? There are more issues than meet the eye.

- Herbs and dietary supplements are regulated by the Food and Drug Administration (FDA) in a different way than prescription drugs are regulated. Theirs is a post-marketing function. In other words, the FDA is responsible for investigating any claims of unsafe supplements. Manufacturers are responsible for accurate labeling and ensuring their product is safe before it is marketed. For information on specific herbs or supplements, go to *www.nccam.nih.gov.*

- Not many controlled studies have been conducted to learn the effects of particular supplements on humans, and even fewer have been performed on supplementation for cancer patients. Part of the reason is that laboratories or pharmaceutical companies are not willing to pay to test ingredients that cannot be patented. However, more and more research facilities are adding supplements to their agendas. The German Commission E has studied many herbs.

- Because food-based research is complex, it is difficult to isolate the components in a diet that may produce a particular effect. Just because someone ate a lot of grapes, for instance, and her tumor shrank does not necessarily mean the grapes were responsible. Perhaps compounds in the grapes worked in conjunction with other components in the diet and other people would not benefit similarly if they were not consuming the other unknown ingredient along with the grapes. Foods contain dozens of different chemicals and often results are synergistic, although the majority of research does not study compounds with this in mind. Very often a particular ingredient is isolated and studied—too often giving inconclusive results.

- A study might show that an herb or supplement had a positive effect for people with one specific condition, but that does not mean it will have the same effect on someone with a slightly different condition.

- The effects of herbs and supplements on other components of treatment such as chemotherapy are unknown in most cases.

- Long-term effects have not been studied for most supplements.

- Herbs may be ingested in several forms: tinctures (soaked in alcohol), pills/capsules, tea, or infusions (tea brewed a long time). Sometimes an herb may be effective in one form and not in another. Also, different parts of a plant (roots, leaves, flower) may have different properties.

- Although side effects are less common and often less severe than with pharmaceuticals, they do occur. Add only one herb at a time to your regimen and watch for side effects for a week or more before adding another. Common side effects might be nausea, dizziness, blurred vision, stomach pain, headache, or diarrhea. If side effects occur, stop the supplement. If symptoms persist, notify your physician.

- Do not assume that if a little is good, a lot is better. Moderation is always prudent. Follow guidelines on the container.

- Are phytoestrogens, plant estrogens that bind with estrogen receptors in your body, safe for breast cancer patients? No one knows for sure. The level of estrogen in these plants is very low: their activity is no more than 2 percent as strong as estradiol.[11] Some phytoestrogens block the growth of an enzyme important for cancer growth and others block the growth of new blood vessels in tumors. Although what we know about phyto-estrogens makes them intriguing, we really don't know enough for a definitive answer.

- Some herbs have weak estrogenic activity. If you have estrogen-receptor–positive breast cancer, you should check with a trained herbalist or your doctor before taking ginseng (Asian "red" and American), peony, red clover, licorice, angelica (dang quai or dong gui), bupleurum (cai hu), and other herbs found in menopausal or PMS formulas. Other herbs such as flaxseed and black cohosh appear to be safe for most uses but have some mixed or unclear evidence concerning safety for hormone-related cancers.

Because no government body regulates the manufacture of vitamins, herbs, or dietary supplements, consumers have to be vigilant when purchasing these. Consider all claims with a skeptical attitude. Ask yourself or the company:

- Have any evidence-based studies been done?
- Were the studies in vitro (in a test tube), on animals, or on humans?
- How many humans were in the study/studies?
- What does other research tell about this supplement? For instance, manufacturers could claim the need for supplement x to prevent a certain condition and the label may tell you to take y mg per day. You would need to know how much of the supplement it takes to prevent the condition and the upper limit after which toxicity or damage may result.
- Did the study test people with your exact diagnosis? Just because a particular antioxidant impeded growth of a colon cancer tumor in a test tube, that does not mean you necessarily should take it if you have breast cancer. Substances used effectively for one cancer may have adverse effects for another cancer.
- What are the known effects of a substance? For instance, a number of antioxidants are anticoagulants, meaning they thin the blood. If you are already on a blood thinner or anticipating surgery soon, that could be a dangerous supplement for you.
- How bioavailable is the form of the substance? Bioavailability measures how well a substance can be assimilated into the body. In other words, how much gets into the bloodstream and how fast?

- How is it metabolized? In your liver? Kidneys? If you have liver disease, you should avoid any herbs metabolized by the liver.

The National Library of Medicine (*www.pubmed.com*) contains information on dietary supplements.

## Supplement Scams

Unfortunately, there is no way to verify the claims on a supplement label because manufacturers have the first responsibility for accuracy. The Federal Trade Commission regulates advertising of dietary supplements and gives very specific guidelines on how claims can be made, then depends on the manufacturers to comply and investigates any complaints. To protect yourself, if a company boasts miracle cures, look somewhere else. Be sure the company lists the Latin and common names of the herbs used, the strength per serving, and any warnings about taking the herb.

Some things you need to understand about supplements as we know them today are:

- Some supplements don't contain the active ingredient responsible for the result in other similar compounds. In other words, one substance may depend on the presence of another to be effective.
- Some supplements contain so little of the active ingredient that they do you no good unless you take huge amounts.
- Some supplements are in a form your body cannot absorb.
- Some supplements have never been proven safe or effective.
- Some supplements contain substances such as dyes or binders that can actually be toxic in your body.
- Don't choose a brand of supplement on price alone. Research the company, the way the products are made, and studies done on the product.
- Buy only supplements for which the "sell by" date has not passed. If there is no "sell by" date, the quality is probably questionable.
- If a label on a dietary supplement claims it can cure, treat, or prevent disease, it is being sold illegally as a drug.

## Choosing a Multivitamin

A Harvard review of 30 years of supplement studies, reported recently in the *Journal of the American Medical Association*, concluded that taken daily, a multivitamin can help prevent cancer and osteoporosis; other studies have shown the opposite or unclear results. Choosing the best multivitamin is a challenge, however. Here are some guidelines to follow:

- Choose one with close to 100 percent of most important vitamins such as B6, B12, C, D, and E and folic acid.

- Many supplements will not have 100 percent of essential minerals because of their bulk. You may have to take additional minerals.

- Be wary of doses over the Dietary Reference Intake (DRI). Know the healthy upper limits on substances. Excess vitamin A, D, and E can be dangerous because they accumulate in the liver. Limit vitamin D to 400 IU and select a supplement with beta carotene instead of vitamin A.

- Usually avoid iron in supplements unless you know you are deficient.

- Reject any multivitamin that does not have an expiration date on the container.

- Choose a brand that minimizes extra ingredients such as artificial colors, binders, fillers, and preservatives.

- Choose the form that works best for you: capsule, tablet, powder, chewable, or liquid.

- Consider a product that contains a quality seal (see the next section).

When ConsumerLab.com tested 37 multivitamins for containing stated ingredients, disintegrating properly to allow absorption, and containing harmful lead content, one-third failed. For their report, visit their Website (*www.consumerlab.com*).

## Certifications for Supplements

Four organizations are recognized for testing and certifying dietary supplements. Look for one of their seals on the products you buy to assure quality:

- U.S. Pharmacopeia (USP) (*www.usp-dsvp.org*) sets the standards used by the Food and Drug Administration. Products that earn its Dietary Supplement Verification Program (DSVP) seal must label all ingredients, contain the type and amount of ingredients listed, be free of toxins (such as heavy metals, pesticides, bacteria, or other pollutants), have consistent quality in different bottles, dissolve completely in your body, contain label and dosage warnings, and be packaged in a clean, controlled environment.

- NSF International (*www.nsf.org*) awards its seal to products that clearly label all ingredients, contain what's listed on the label, are free of dangerous contaminants, and are packaged in a clean environment.

- ConsumerLab.com (*www.consumerlab.com*) also tests and approves supplements although it does not inspect the manufacturing plants and also charges a fee for a complete list of its approved products. Its seal means the product contains what its label says it does, is free of harmful contaminants, is the same composition in each bottle, and dissolves completely in the body.

- National Nutritional Foods Association (NNFA) (*www.nnfa.org*; 1–800–966–6632) is a nonprofit trade group that attests to good manufacturing practices.

## More Is Not Necessarily Better

Though some supplements can help your body strengthen itself, do not fall prey to the theory that if a little is good, a lot is better. *You can overdose on vitamins!* The Food and Drug Administration has determined upper limits on most vitamins. If you take more than that amount, you may suffer serious health consequences.

Water-soluble vitamins, such as B and C, pose less risk to the body because excess amounts are excreted. However, damage can still occur from megadoses. Fat-soluble vitamins such as A, D, and E can become toxic because they are stored in the body. High doses of vitamin C can cause diarrhea and kidney stones. Megadoses of certain B vitamins can cause nerve damage.

## Values for Food Supplements and Products

In place of the familiar Recommended Daily Allowance (RDA), supplement and food product labels now show "%Daily Value." The RDA was established by the National Academy of Sciences (NAS) in 1941 to ensure that U.S. troops around the world got adequate nutrition. In the 1990s NAS developed levels of nutrients that would optimize health instead of just prevent certain diseases. They call these new categories Dietary Reference Intakes (DRIs). These combine the former RDAs with new dietary guidelines based on diets in the United States and Canada. Daily Values (DVs) are the percentage of a DRI based on a 2,000-calorie diet. DV is measured in international units (IUs) rather than micrograms (mcg). To convert micrograms to IUs, multiply by 3.3. To convert IUs to micrograms, divide by 3.3.[12]

DRIs apply to a healthy population and refer to an average daily intake over time. Medical conditions requiring high-fiber intake or chronic illness, for example, may change what an individual needs. Variance from a normal diet for a short term should have no great effect on those needs. Intake also depends on the concentration of a nutrient in a particular food and how often that food is eaten.

Levels of DRIs are described for life stage and gender groups. There are 22 of these groups (four for infants and children, six for men, and six for women, with six more for stages of pregnancy and lactation). You can see already that supplementation is no simple matter.

RDAs for some nutrients have been replaced with a measurement called Adequate Intake (AI). Wheras RDAs were recommended amounts, AIs means there is not enough scientific evidence to set a standard for that nutrient to prevent disease.

Recognizing that excessive nutrients can be harmful, another new guideline is Tolerable Upper Intake Level (UL), the highest level of daily intake for individuals in a specified group that will probably pose no adverse health risk. Consuming more than this level may be dangerous. Different levels exist for men and women. The term *tolerable* is used to denote that this amount is not recommended; it is merely a level that is likely to be tolerated biologically by healthy individuals in the group. Some nutrients refer to ULs including food and supplementation; others refer to supplementation only. If no UL exists, that only means that no evidence exists to set one. It does not mean that there is no risk in exceeding the DRI for that nutrient.

Another new designation is Estimated Average Requirement (EAR), the amount of a nutrient that will meet the needs of half the individuals in a specified group. If sufficient evidence does not exist to establish an EAR, an AI is established, based on observation or experiment as to the requirements a healthy group of individuals needs to maintain good general health.

In choosing supplements as well as processed foods, read the label to see how the ingredients jive with the marketing spin.

## Purchasing Tips for Supplements

- Choose supplements with the least amount of artificial fillers, colors, binders, excipients, and nonessential ingredients.
- Buy no more than three to six months' supply so they remain fresh and potent.
- Keep containers tightly fastened. Do not expose supplements to excessive light. Dark or opaque bottles are best.
- Check the serving size. How much do you have to take to get the recommended amount?

## Herbs with Anticancer Properties

Herbs have been used in other cultures to prevent or treat cancer. Although you should not self-medicate with these, by all means research them and ask your doctor if you are interested in taking them. One current theory on anticancer herbs and antioxidants is to rotate several (one bottle of one, then one bottle of another) so the body does not have a chance to become resistant to a particular one. (See Resources for reliable Websites for the latest research and trials.)

## How Do Herbs or Dietary Supplements Help?

Our bodies produce unstable molecules called free radicals during normal functioning (aerobic exercise, killing bacteria, detoxifying substances like pesticides, or even exposure to chemotherapy or radiation). These molecules are able to attach to DNA and damage it. Because damaged DNA can promote cancer cell growth, modifying free radicals is a top goal in some CAM therapies.

Antioxidants are believed to be substances in food that help neutralize free radical damage or remove free radicals from the body, although even this theory is complex and controversial. Using food to combat illness is no new theory. It began about 400 B.C. in the Hippocratic School of Medicine in Greece. Hippocrates believed that air, water, and food were the cause of illness and also contained all people need for the body to heal itself.

Phytochemicals are compounds produced by plants (fruits, vegetables, beans, grains, and others) that exhibit antioxidant or hormonelike (phytoestrogen) activity. Free radicals do their damage by oxidizing cells. Antioxidants prevent oxidation. Research has isolated some individual chemicals that have exceptional antioxidant properties. Dietary supplements attempt to provide these in a convenient form. Although research does show benefits from consumption of some supplements, it is always best to get the antioxidants or other chemicals from your food if possible. We do not know how one chemical works in conjunction with others to provide its benefits. An isolated compound may not have nearly the impact on your body as the compound eaten in food.

Other phytochemicals activate liver enzymes, which help remove toxins from the bloodstream. There are so many nutrients in whole foods that science has just begun to identify or study them. Choose whole foods whenever possible. They are far greater than the sum of their parts.

The array of CAM therapies is mind-boggling—and also frustrating. Cancer patients want answers now, not 10 years from now when a study is completed. Because uncertainty describes the field of complementary and alternative medicine, you can only be diligent in your research, persistent in your quest for health, and wise in your choices. Your choices will look very different from the next person's—and that's okay. It's your body and your health—and your decision.

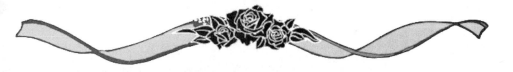

## Chapter 5

# Handling Your Emotions

Although every person will experience a cancer diagnosis differently, many go through similar phases: shock, sheer terror, denial, depression, acceptance. You may not feel these emotions in that order or even feel them all, but chances are your initial emotions will not be the same as those you feel six months into treatment.

Many women feel betrayed by their own body and are embarrassed when they find themselves angry or depressed during the cancer experience. There is no reason to be. These emotions are very normal. Depression can result from any of several things you are going through: chemical changes in your body, fatigue, medications, a life-threatening disease, lack of exercise or routine, or plain fear and lack of control over your life.

Though you can't avoid the feelings that come, you will benefit from working through them rather than trying to ignore them. Bottling up negative emotions will only weaken your immune system and use up energy you need. Fred Rogers, star of the famous children's TV series, *Mr. Roger's Neighborhood*, is credited with saying, "Anything you manage is mentionable, and anything mentionable can be managed." In other words, given the right timing and company, there are no taboo topics or emotions and they can all be handled.

If you have someone you can trust to let you talk out some of your emotions, take advantage of that gift. If not, by all means seek out a pastor, rabbi, counselor, or social worker trained in counseling or a support group. If you do not know someone who can help, ask your nurse, doctor, other health professional, cancer center, hospital, or cancer organization for referrals.

## Timing of Emotional Reactions

Your emotions will probably change as you move from diagnosis through treatment to "whatever is next." You may feel alone and afraid as you wait for treatment to begin. After a few weeks of treatment you may feel discouraged if you are not feeling well and stressed if you are still juggling your normal load of responsibilities. You may feel out of control as your life spirals on in a direction far different from your wishes. By the end of treatment you may feel abandoned by being out from under the watchful eye of your medical team, fearful about the cancer returning, and stressed from being so far behind in so many areas of your life.

At any time a professional counselor can help you sort through your emotions and help you plan the best scenario for that particular time.

## *Asking Family and Friends for Help*

As cancer patients, we must realize that we are not the only one affected by the diagnosis. Those who care for us are also frightened, feel helpless, and may want to run away from the problem.

Know up front that not every friend and family member will be supportive through your cancer experience. This has nothing to do with how they value their relationship with you. Most of the time fear and ignorance keep them at a distance: fear of catching cancer, which of course is not possible; fear of their own mortality; not knowing how to help and not wanting to show their lack of understanding of your situation; and fear of saying the wrong thing.

## How to Help Those Close to You Deal with Your Cancer

Be open about your feelings—your real feelings, not how you think you should feel. Let others know whether or not they can talk about your illness in your presence. Some people close to you will not know how to talk to you anymore. Tell them what helps you: trivialities, favorite subjects, just hearing them breathe on the phone.

Answer honestly and completely when your family and close friends ask about your treatments so others will understand what you are dealing with. Realize that your extended family is probably as uninformed as you were about cancer before your diagnosis and may have misconceptions affecting their feelings about your situation. Some people think a cancer diagnosis is an immediate death sentence and will treat you as if you are going to die the next day. Gently let them know the hope your treatment brings and that you plan to be around a long time.

If someone says something insensitive, forgive them quickly. Probably they have no idea how their comments affected you. If you can correct them without rancor, do so with as much love as you can muster. This is as much for your own good in eliminating stress as it is for their benefit.

# Helping Your Helpers

Maybe you *can* get through cancer treatment alone, but why would you want to? Let people do things for you. Most of us are fiercely independent and hate to ask for or accept help. If you are fatigued from treatment, you can heal faster by not pushing yourself. Also remember how helping others makes you feel good. Help your friends feel good by helping them help you!

When you are deep into treatment, fatigued, or sick, keep a list of things you need done: yard work, shopping, cooking, cleaning, childcare, phone calls, transportation, paying bills, and so forth. When someone says, "Let me know if I can do anything," you'll have a ready answer. Let them choose what fits their schedule. If you are not up to handling even that much, ask someone to be your designated help coordinator and give people her phone number. It's a win-win situation.

## Support Groups

Sometimes the best treatment for side effects, emotional or physical, is a good talk with someone who understands exactly what you are going through. If you know other people who have had breast cancer and are willing to talk, by all means, take advantage of their experiences. You will probably end the conversation much more hopeful than when you began it and you will probably have some guidance about whatever issue you are dealing with.

Another source of emotional support is organized support groups. Such groups are often sponsored by hospitals, clinics, cancer organizations, churches, and synagogues. Some women cannot imagine sharing their deepest fears and needs with strangers. Usually after sitting quietly in a few group sessions, however, they find that their emotions are not unusual and the other women in the group can suggest successful ways to deal with emotional or physical concerns. They also feel supported and encouraged in their cancer journey—and sometimes they make new friends for life. Participating in a group is a way of helping others, which is healing in itself. Also some studies have shown longer survival and better quality of life for those who regularly participate in a support group.

## Criteria for Successful Support Group Experiences

Before attending any support group, find out about the group:
- **What kind of cancer do participants have?** Probably the more closely the group matches your situation, the more you will gain from it. Breast cancer causes different concerns than, say, prostate or lung cancer, so a group of only breast cancer patients could get more specific regarding managing side effects or emotions you are experiencing.

- **Are participants patients or family members?** Many people find that, although it is helpful for family members to have the support of other families facing cancer, being in a separate group from you gives both you and them more freedom to voice real frustrations and needs. Your children's attending a support group can help them deal with their fears, but do check out the group first. Ideally it will be a group of others near their age and with mothers in a similar stage to yours. Watching someone deal with a mother in a terminal stage would be unnecessarily frightening for a child whose mother has DCIS (ductal carcinoma in situ). If you ask your children if they want to attend a group, more than likely they will decline, but many children find relief after a few sessions of learning that others have sick mothers too and are handling life adequately.

- **What stage are participants in?** Try to find a group with women in your same stage of disease. There is no point in frightening yourself around women whose cancer is more advanced than yours. Also, your issues will be different from theirs. Often groups are broken into newcomers, those in remission, those who are stable, and those with more advanced disease.

- **Who leads the group?** A professional can provide a wonderful balance to a group that some laypersons cannot. A professional can draw out shy members, reign in those who monopolize the floor, stimulate conversation, and keep the group on track. Many groups sponsored by cancer organizations or medical facilities are led by professionally trained counselors or trained volunteers.

- **What does the group talk about?** Some groups invite speakers on relevant topics, although most concentrate on personal sharing. Topics typically include interpersonal relations as affected by cancer, physical and emotional reactions, grief and loss, communication issues, treatment and side effect solutions, and the impact of the diagnosis on values and meaning in life.

Visit a group a few times before committing to it, especially if you have never participated in a similar group. Some groups meet for a specific number of times and can decide to continue meeting informally. Also, some groups charge a small fee.

## Online Support

The Internet is rife with message boards and chat rooms for people with specific medical conditions. Though these can be a source of emotional support, they can also breed fear and spread misinformation, especially if they are not monitored by experts. As with any other information you find, online or offline, apply critical thinking skills and discern whether the information sounds reasonable. If the site is sponsored by a credible organization, it is more likely to contain information worth evaluating. Remember also that the anonymity of the Internet can breed dishonesty. A person can pretend to be whatever he wants to be. Be cautious of connecting in person with someone you met online.

Some people find online support groups helpful at first, then begin to tire of all the e-mail. If you sign up for a group, be sure to keep the instructions on how to unsubscribe.

## One-on-One Support

Several national cancer organizations and some local groups have programs that will match you with another woman similar to you in age, stage of cancer, treatment, and so forth. Most often you will visit with the person on the phone. Sometimes she will give you her phone number in case you have additional concerns. A close match is invaluable when the person can warn of possible complications or give practical advice about an aspect of treatment. Do take advantage of several of these programs. Each volunteer will have different experiences to share.

## Choosing a Counselor

At some point in your cancer journey, the guidance and support of a professional counselor may be a wonderful resource to utilize. Trained counselors may be social workers, clergy, psychologists, or licensed professional counselors. If at all possible, find a counselor who has counseled with many breast cancer patients. Although any emotion a breast cancer patient experiences is certainly shared by many people with other issues, breast cancer has its own set of emotions and factors, some of which are difficult to verbalize. Thus many women feel more comfortable with a counselor who already knows what they may be feeling and can jump-start the healing process with some helpful questions or comments.

Consulting a counselor is not a sign of weakness. Instead it indicates that you recognize a situation that is beyond your training. Just as you consulted an oncologist for the cancer, you seek a trained counselor for the confusing emotional symptoms you are experiencing.

What good does a little talking do? If you've never visited with an effective counselor, you will be amazed. A counselor does not tell you what to think or how to feel or label your feelings in any way. She helps you express what you are really feeling and find ways to handle those emotions. Sometimes just putting a name on a vague feeling releases you from its effects. Sometimes questions the counselor asks help you clarify areas you had not thought about.

## Relationships

It is hard enough to admit to yourself that you have cancer, and telling others can be awkward. How much do you tell and how often do you update the information? Though the answer will vary considerably with each patient and each relationship, here are some guidelines that have worked for other breast cancer survivors.

## Anyone

- Be honest—even if the truth is scary. Dishonesty is a lot scarier because others don't know what part to believe the next time. Secrets are hard to keep. By being honest, you build trust.
- You decide how much to tell. Your needs are the most important at this point.
- Be aware that anyone you tell will have to deal not only with your news, but also with the awareness of her own mortality and fears. Some people will withdraw from your fellowship. Others will speak clichés at you because they have to feel, for their own comfort, that cancer is controllable. If either happens, it will mean more about what they are dealing with (or trying to avoid dealing with) than it will about your relationship with them.
- Recognize that your diagnosis introduces issues for other people that you don't have to deal with. Try to understand where they are coming from. For instance, your spouse and your children, depending on their age, will have to assume some of your responsibilities for the family. Friends will have to tread the fine line between wanting to help and interfering, or showing concern and appearing nosy. Family members may not know whether to step in with help or wait for you to ask. If they assume you can't perform certain tasks, they may fear they will discourage or insult you.
- E-mail is a wonderful way to keep a number of people informed about your progress without the burden of dozens of phone calls.

## Close Friends

- Give them something to do to help.
- Give them clues about how much you want to talk about. Tell them up front that you may say at some point, "I really don't want to go into that just now."

## Extended Family

- Ask one family member to inform others in the family of the diagnosis and pass on updates as they are available.

## Young Children

- Assure them that you are not contagious.
- Assure them that they did not do anything to cause your illness.
- Keep their schedules as normal as possible.
- Arrange care with people they already know and trust. Tell your child who will take care of him if you are not able. Security is important at this age.
- Answer their questions honestly and with the same candor you would their questions about anything else—information that is appropriate for their age. Their imaginations will paint a much bleaker picture than reality. Also, they know when something is amiss and feel insecure if they don't understand what is wrong. Give their clear feeling of unrest a name: breast cancer.
- Be sure that caregivers (teachers, parents of friends, other adults in the child's life) are fully informed so they can be supportive in appropriate ways.
- Realize that your children will mimic your attitude. If you are positive about your outcome, so will they be. In fact, they may appear to be indifferent after a while, which merely means they are comfortable with what you have told them.
- Distinguish your cancer and treatment side effects from other common illnesses that may befall anyone.
- If you are hospitalized a few days, give the child a notebook to draw or write in for you to "read" when you return. Or give her a calendar to check off the days until you come home. A short phone call during your hospital stay can reassure the child.
- Before you go to the hospital, give the child something personal to keep until you return, such as your keys. If she knows the item is something you need every day, she will be reassured that you are coming back soon.

## Adolescents

- They may be so afraid of your dying that they don't know how to talk about your illness.
- Being different is hard for children this age, so they may act more embarrassed than sympathetic if you lose your hair or are in bed a lot when their friends come over.
- Keep their routines as normal as possible. Arrange for them to continue extracurricular activities and encourage them to visit at friends' houses. Assure them that they do not have to be home entertaining or helping you every hour they are not in school. Most children will be glad to help, but they are still children and need to distance themselves from your troubles occasionally.

- Invite them to ask questions, but don't be surprised if they don't. Answer honestly. If you don't know the answer, say so and try to find out.

- Talk honestly about your fears or your fatigue. Putting on a brave face all the time may not give them permission to express their own fears and curiosity. Answer the hard questions truthfully. "Will you die from this?" Don't give the knee-jerk, "I'll be fine." Say, "We're doing everything we know to do to stop the cancer." Maintaining trust is important for current, as well as future, relationships.

- Don't wait for the "right" time to talk: when you have all the information or when you can say things perfectly. That time won't come. Use opportunities as they arise. In Chinese, *crisis* means both danger and opportunity. Take heed.

- Inform teachers or the school counselor about your illness. Ask them to notify you of any troubling behavior in your child that might stem from your situation.

- Don't overlook the "good kid," who is around the house all the time and neglects her friends to help Mom. She may need help dealing with her emotions.

## Older or Adult Children

- If children live far away, it may be hard for them to handle the guilt of not being near to help combined with the fear of the illness itself.

- Girls especially may be afraid of what your diagnosis means for their future health.

- Children just breaking away from home for college or a first job and apartment will be torn between the natural instinct for independence and guilt at leaving home just when you need them. Try to work out arrangements so that they can continue their plans if at all possible.

However and whenever you tell people about your breast cancer, be honest in what your share, whether feelings or facts. Although the decision of whether to tell or not is a personal one, consider that if you don't tell, you deprive yourself of emotional as well as tangible support. The guise of "I'm just fine" may add more stress to your life. Although I'm a modest person, I decided early on to tell everyone about my breast cancer and how I was dealing with it. Many friends have told me how helpful that was so that they had some clue as to the feelings of another friend who had breast cancer and would not discuss it. I consider my sharing educational—and it also has brought wonderful support into my life.

# Fighting with Your Spouse:
# More Frequent? More Friendly!

Don't be surprised if you and your spouse argue more after a diagnosis. This can happen when fear collides with fatigue and anxiety. Being open will help. Voice your fears and listen to your spouse's concerns. Encourage your partner to be honest, not stoic. Be reassured that nonverbal actions speak loudly. Maybe your husband does yell more, but he continues to do the grocery shopping and occasionally buys your favorite ice cream and asks if you need a back rub. He is dealing with his own feelings. Give him space to adjust his vision of the future.

To reduce the ability of arguments to harm a relationship at such a vulnerable time, consider the following:

- Set a timer. Let each partner have the same amount of time (maybe five minutes) to vent while the other listens. Really do listen rather than spend that time planning your rebuttal.
- Practice reflective listening. Before answering your partner with your side of the issue, rephrase what you heard him say and ask if that is correct. If you understand each other's viewpoint, sometimes a resolution can be reached quickly. You may find that you mean different things by the same word or that one has misunderstood something.
- Be respectful. Avoid name-calling, yelling, and belittling. Don't interrupt the other or label the other's ideas in a negative way.
- Know when to table an argument. When information is missing or emotions are too high, agree to come back together at a set time and resume the discussion.
- Stick to the topic. Don't bring up unrelated irritants.
- Compromise. See what you agree on and then determine what you must have and what you can forfeit for resolution.
- Respect privacy. Don't air your side with a friend. Keep the issue confidential.
- Close the argument with whatever feels right to each of you: a hug, a trip to your favorite restaurant, sex. It's a way of affirming the relationship.
- Assess. When all is over, ask each other what you each could have done to make the process easier. Don't be defensive. Just listen and learn.

## Assertiveness

When your life is threatened, your survival instinct often takes over reflexively. When you face a serious disease such as breast cancer, you begin to cherish each day of wellness and may be surprised to find yourself fighting for the best care and best circumstances for you. Even women who have spent their lives deferring to others' needs often break out of their emotional shells and begin standing up for their needs.

Such assertiveness does not have to be unkind or demanding. In fact, a request or need is much more effective if stated calmly and firmly and with the expectation of being acted upon. Obviously some conditions may be impossible to arrange and compromises will always have to be made by you as well as by your family and medical team. However, it is important for your long-term health that your needs are explained so that solutions may be found when possible.

There are three levels of communication: passive, assertive, and aggressive. Passive communication is mostly one way: One person does not contribute to the exchange. She may be listening; she just does not say much. Aggressive communication by one person can be a cause of passive communication in another. Aggressiveness means fighting, hurting, belittling, yelling, and dominating.

Neither of those communication styles is helpful for maneuvering through the breast cancer journey. Cancer robs you of your feeling of control, but it should not discourage you from being very involved in decisions regarding your care and your life. So being a passive communicator is not best for you now. If you choose to be aggressive and take out your fears and frustrations on those around you, you will drive off (maybe not physically, but emotionally) your support team, whom you need greatly now.

Assertive communication is in the middle. It's clear and kind. It reflects that you value yourself as well as others. It says, "I have something to say and I'd like you to listen." You may want to tell someone how you felt in response to something she did or said (maybe you felt hurt when a friend discounted your fatigue). You may need a particular action to be taken (you need a copy of a medical report by Friday). In either case, an assertive person will state the message without judgment or anger and will politely persist until a request is granted.

Assertive communication is:

- **Clear.** Know what you want the outcome of the conversation to be. Do you want to tell someone how you feel or do you want something to happen? Identify any feelings you want to express. Give them a name: "I felt sad/hurt/left out/patronized...." Compare them to some experience your listener can identify with: "I felt like you must have felt when...." If you are making a request, give the details: "I need my test results before my doctor's appointment on the 10th. Whom shall I speak to about this?"

- **Personal—to you.** Make "I" statements. Say, "I felt discounted when you said...." "I" statements do not erect barriers to communication the way "you" statements ("You always put me down.") do.

- **Positive.** Begin with a positive message. The first few sentences of a conversation affect how the listener "hears" what you are saying. Try saying, "I really appreciate your rearranging your schedule to take me to the doctor today. Do you think next week we could leave 10 minutes earlier?"

- **Specific.** Instead of yelling at your child, "I need some help around here!" say, "Sarah, will you please chop the carrots, and, Tom, will you set the table?"

- **Thorough.** We communicate with our whole body, so be conscious of bringing nonverbal messages in sync with your words. Arms crossed over your chest show resistance. Having your eyes focused anywhere except upon the other person's eyes can show disinterest or inattention.

- **Kind.** Forego name-calling, accusations, a raised voice, a sarcastic tone, judgments, and hostility. If you want results and good relationships, put away these communication blockers.

- **Timely.** Be sensitive to the other person's agenda. Give your husband time to unwind after he gets home before approaching a heavy subject. Don't interrupt a favorite TV show or call your friend when you know she is fixing dinner.

- **Persistent.** When dealing with medical facilities and offices, you may have to employ the "broken record" technique. No matter what excuse you get, just keep stating your request clearly and politely ("I understand that the office is shorthanded and I still need my report by noon. Whom shall I talk to about this?"). Sometimes the person you are talking with does not have the authority to grant your request. When that becomes obvious, switch to the "move up the ladder" technique. Say, "I understand that you do not have the authority to help me, so whom should I talk to?" Often that person will have to "call you back." An assertive response might be, "Is there someone who is available now to help me?" or "What time should I expect a call?"

Assertiveness means you have something clear and positive to say, either you need to share a feeling rather than stuff it inside you to fester or you have a problem that needs a solution. Some women shy away from assertiveness as not being "ladylike." I think they confuse assertiveness and aggression. To keep them distinct, I think of the g's in *aggression* as growls and the s's in *assertiveness* as smiles. You can be pleasant and persistent at the same time.

## Resilience

Many women are surprised, and pleased, to find that they cope very well with breast cancer, a terrible challenge that none wanted. The way you respond to your diagnosis has been termed *resilience*.[1] What do you do to cope?

Some women begin taking care of themselves for the first time in their life through exercising, eating more healthy meals, refusing to get stressed about much, and savoring the moment. They learn that they are not in control, and they learn to stare death in the face and move beyond their fear. Some have to "forgive" themselves for developing cancer (as though it were their fault). Getting involved in treatment decisions and seeking support are other good ways to cope.

What have you done that is out of character for your prediagnosis self? Many women I know have become assertive and feel empowered to be who they are, not who someone wants them to be. They value friendships more, are bothered by fewer things, and squeeze as much out of every hour as they can—and usually that involves relationships and enjoyment rather than career steps.

Assess how you have coped and feel good about the steps you have taken.

## Attitude

"Mind over matter." "Be positive." "Look on the bright side."

You've heard them all—and, if you're like me, you've wanted to reply with a hardy scream.

As in most aspects of life, moderation is the key to maneuvering through breast cancer. If you are angry and sulking all the time, your caregivers will wear out quickly and not want to come around. If you deny your fears and act as if you have no care in the world, you are only adding another burden to your stress quotient, according to a recent study from Australia.

All you really have control over—with or without cancer—is your attitude. The healthy approach is to acknowledge your true feelings, work through them (with professional help, if necessary), and choose how to respond to this crisis in your life. Responding rather than reacting is the key to staying in control of your attitude.

Some people find that prayer gives them the emotional balance they need. Others have a best friend who will listen nonjudgmentally. Others journal, draw, or write songs. Choose a way to identify and express your deepest feelings, the ones you really don't want to admit even to yourself. Then you must work through those emotions. Admitting "I'm angry about all this" is a start, but it's not enough to resolve the anger. For women especially, just talking about emotions helps untangle them, put them in perspective, and work out a plan to deal with them.

Your attitude does reflect on your physical well-being. When you're in a bad mood, your muscles tense. If you can't reason yourself out of a bad mood, step into a warm shower or try one of the techniques described under "Relaxation" (page 241) or "Stress" (page 231)—and your mood will no doubt improve also.

## Self-Image

Breast cancer can be a blow to self-image. Men with breast cancer feel less masculine and women feel less feminine. Treatment may leave you unable to handle all former responsibilities, so you may question your self-worth.

Now is a good time to assess your value apart from how you look or what you can do each day. Make a list of what you mean to the important people in your life. Do you make your friends laugh? Do your kids enjoy having you listen to their chatter? Does your husband relish your support and affirmation? Can you throw silver linings into gloomy conversations? The inner you that is personified in your speech and attitudes is what people who love you react to, not your body shape or chores you do. At work, people may appreciate your level head, cooperative spirit, or creative solutions. Your level of activity may return. In the meantime, concentrate on who you are, not what you do, to define yourself. If this is hard and you feel worthless, this is a good time to visit a counselor.

## Control

Illness is when insignificant things become significant and significant things become insignificant. If you cannot be at the office to supervise 10 employees, you may focus on what is in your immediate environment: the way the potatoes were salted or the way your daughter folded the towels.

Control is a way of saying to ourselves, "I am valuable. I am needed." Cancer robs you of your feeling that you can handle anything. Maybe you do sail through treatment without a hesitation in your step, but the idea that something unwanted and dangerous has entered your body without your permission will probably make you stop and think, "Am I as in charge as I thought?"

Facing the fact that you are not may turn you toward taking control in whatever areas you can so you can maintain your belief, however irrational. This trying to force reality into your preferred mold is stressful and counterproductive. If you try to micromanage your caregivers, they will burn out and may even begin to resent you. Your illness has impacted their life and schedule also. A dose of gratitude has much more effect than a detailed list of instructions.

It's better to admit, "Okay, I see that I cannot control my entire destiny. I'll do the best in what I *can* influence." One healthy form of control you can adopt is to learn all you can about the cancer, treatment options, and lifestyle influences on your disease. Knowledge may reduce feelings of powerlessness as you feel confident to make decisions about future treatment and recovery plans.

## *Limitations*

Although breast cancer can set limits on our dreams and goals, we can choose to reshape those instead of forfeiting them. For instance, if you can no longer play baseball with a grandchild, you can still be head cheerleader at his games. If your body lets you down, be creative in looking for other ways to enjoy an activity.

Often our self-image is tied to what we can do. If that gets curtailed, our self-esteem can plunge. Many people find prayer an antidote to this situation. By allowing God to offer a perspective, they begin to see themselves through God's eyes and often find value they had missed.

Hopefully you will be able to break into the world again once treatment is completed. Realize, though, that you may have less energy and fewer resources than you had when you stepped out of the world. Ask your medical team about realistic expectations for regaining your energy and modify your daily schedule accordingly. Fearlessness is as much a deterrent to recovery as withdrawal. If you refuse to admit any limitation from your treatment, you may overdo and delay your recovery. If you just give up, you won't provide your body with tools it can use.

Permanent limitations are harder to accept. Try to rethink who you are and what people love about you. Grieve the losses; then grasp your new reality. I have found much comfort in a saying by Ted Geisel (Dr. Seuss): "Don't cry because it's over. Smile because it happened."

No, I can no longer weed my flowerbeds, or lift my granddaughter, or work a full day, but I can spend more time at my computer encouraging friends, have my granddaughter over to play, and be productive a few hours each day. I enjoyed having nonstop energy before cancer, but now I am thankful I have more than I did during chemotherapy. Put in that perspective, my current level is more acceptable.

Set aside perfectionism. Learn to accept "good enough." Be content with what you can do instead of regretting what you are missing. Keep your expectations realistic and you won't be so disappointed.

## *Denial*

Denial can be healthy or unhealthy, depending on how you allow it to influence you. Many women go through the first few weeks or months of their diagnosis thinking, "This is not really happening. It's just a bad dream and I'll wake up in a few minutes."

Just that thin boundary between yourself and the awful diagnosis can ward off fears that are too overwhelming to handle at the same time you are choosing doctors, beginning treatments, delegating responsibilities, and trying to keep up a brave "front." In such cases, denial is probably a useful emotion.

It becomes unwise, however, if a woman denies that she has a disease and refuses to seek medical help. Though a few weeks delay in treatment usually makes no difference in the long-term outcome of breast cancer, indefinitely postponing any treatment can seriously undermine your chances of controlling the disease.

James W. Pennebaker, Ph.D., professor of psychology at the University of Texas at Austin, writes in *Opening Up: The Healing Power of Expressing Emotions*:

> Over time, the work of inhibition [keeping thoughts and feelings hidden] gradually undermines the body's defenses. Like other stressors, inhibition can affect immune function, the action of the heart and vascular systems, and even the biochemical workings of the brain and nervous systems. In short, excessive holding back of thoughts, feelings, and behaviors can place people at risk for both major and minor diseases.[2]

Some people try to cope with unpleasant emotions by burying themselves in work, staying busy so they can't think, getting angry, crying, clamming up, joking about the situation and never taking it seriously, or doing anything else so they don't have to face their emotions. If facing your fears and the stresses of rearranging your life are overwhelming, seek professional help so you don't undermine your healing.

## *Guilt*

Some people feel guilty when they are diagnosed with breast cancer. "I must have done something to cause or deserve it," they think. No one knows what causes cancer. It probably develops from a combination of factors. None of us has eaten the optimal diet, exercised every day, avoided stress and anger, or done the dozens of things that make for a healthier life. We do better some weeks and worse others.

And no one deserves cancer. We are imperfect people living in an imperfect world where disease is an unfortunate part of life. Do not blame yourself for the cancer. Instead, educate yourself about healthier ways to live and incorporate as many as you can into your routine, but don't look back. You can't change the way you were. All you can do is change some things about the future and hope for the best.

## Irritability

When things are not going the way you want, it is normal to be irritated. If the situation continues for very long, however, irritability can become a habit. If you notice you are irritable, talk to your caregivers and ask what they suggest. Realize that there are some parts of your situation that no one can change, so you all may as well make the best of it. Some parts are temporary and maybe together you can come up with a solution. Try to identify what is behind the irritability—fear, lack of control, pain, feelings of worthlessness, fatigue—and seek remedies.

## Grief

Everyone with breast cancer has suffered a loss. If it's not a part of her body, it's the loss of security about the future and perhaps disappointments about friends who disappeared after the diagnosis.

Identify what you have lost as a result of your breast cancer diagnosis or treatment. Spend time remembering what was lost and appreciating its role in your life. Let the tears flow. Gradually you will recognize replacements for the lost parts or beliefs. You may realize that your breast did not define your self-worth, that you still have plenty of wisdom and love to offer. You may acknowledge that the future is more uncertain than you had once thought and yet feel confident to meet whatever it brings because of new strengths you have identified during your breast cancer battle.

By all means grieve your losses. Then take comfort from the fact that you are still alive with lots more life to live.

## Holidays: Happy or Heartache?

Major holidays can be hard for breast cancer patients. A recent diagnosis may keep you from feeling like celebrating. You may be so consumed with treatment decisions that you do not have time for the niceties of the holidays. If you are undergoing treatment, you may not have the energy to participate in holiday events as you would like. Even with a good prognosis, holidays intensify your emotions and your fears about the future.

Talk to your family about your preferences and plan ahead. What do you enjoy most about the holiday? Save your energy for that. Delegate responsibilities. Send a form letter instead of individual cards. Buy gift certificates instead of carefully selected gifts. Modify your celebration so you can enjoy the most important parts.

## Anxiety

Anxiety can be that vague feeling that something is amiss and you are powerless to do anything about it. Studies have found that up to 64 percent of breast cancer survivors feel anxiety.[3] You may find anxiety to be a regular companion during treatment. There are so many unknowns, and you probably had no previous training in cancer management. Even the routines of everyday life take on new dimensions and you are constantly facing another change you have to incorporate into your lifestyle. When will it all plateau?

The best antidotes to anxiety are knowledge and planning. Ask questions and learn about your disease. If you are too tired or overwhelmed to research, ask a friend who wants to help to find answers for you. If you are anxious about finances, helping your children cope, or telling your boss about your cancer, read tips in this book and make a plan. Write out what you can do to manage each situation. Seeing that solutions exist may dissipate the anxiety, and acting on those solutions almost certainly will drive it away. There may be times when medications can be effective in managing anxiety. If you have always been an anxious person (a "worrier"), you will probably continue to be with cancer. Your basic personality will not likely change.

Anxiety can have a variety of causes: medications, unrelieved pain, anemia, low oxygenation, infection, abnormal electrolytes, or delirium. The treatment depends on the cause.

## Fear

Fear is usually heightened by the unknown. Therefore, learn as much as you can about whatever you are afraid of and you will be surprised how your fear will recede. For instance, if you are afraid of chemotherapy or radiation, visit the place where you will receive treatment before your first treatment. Ask whatever questions you have about the equipment, who will administer the treatment, or how long it will take. You should save questions about side effects and results for your doctor, but just seeing the treatment facility and the other patients there will allay some of your fears.

If the disease itself is the basis of your fears, request information on your particular type of breast cancer from a national cancer organization (see Resources) and learn all you can about it. Be sure that you keep statistics in the proper perspective. Percentages are two-sided. Someone has to be in the "lucky" numbers; it might as well be you. There are no guarantees that treatment will cure the breast cancer and prevent its coming back. Likewise, there are no guarantees that you will die from the cancer. Because no one yet knows who will be the long-term survivors, decide to act as though you are in that elite and growing group. Just telling yourself that you are a survivor will produce health benefits in the form of endorphins that boost immune activity.

And don't panic if you fall back into fear occasionally. That is a normal response to a cancer diagnosis. This fear is often triggered by things such as follow-up visits with doctors, birthdays, anniversaries of events in your cancer journey, illness of a family member, symptoms similar to ones you had around your diagnosis, or the death of someone from breast cancer.

Another way to deal with fear is to identify what you are afraid of, look at the worst possible scenario, and sculpt a plan of action. For instance, are you afraid of dying? Of being in pain? Of leaving children without your guidance? Of losing your self-image or your job?

Write a sentence or two that pinpoints your exact fear(s):

"I am afraid of _____

_____

_____

_____."

Follow that fear through to its logical (and scariest) conclusion. Then brainstorm until you have several options for whatever is the worst you can imagine happening if your fear came true. Choose which option would best solve the problem. You may even find that your fear will mysteriously have evaporated by the time you decide what action can be taken.

For example, maybe you are afraid of pain after surgery. Ask your doctor or nurse about the level of pain her patients normally experience, what is available to alleviate the pain, how long it usually lasts, and how likely it is that your particular surgery could result in pain. Once your fear takes the form of knowledge, it might diminish.

If you have trouble seeing options on your own, ask a trusted friend or family member to help you think through situations. Another good choice is to visit with a pastor, counselor, or social worker and see what new options you might identify. Studies show that talking out your fears is the only way to get rid of them. Don't be embarrassed about being afraid. It is normal. If dealt with, fears can give you a sense of control. If not dealt with, they can lead to depression.

## *Depression*

As if a cancer diagnosis were not enough to cause depression, other parts of treatment can cause or trigger brain chemical changes, and, therefore, blue moods, in many people—medications, fatigue, hormonal imbalance, and altered self-esteem. Whatever the cause of depression, there is a solution.

Depression is a medical condition that affects behavior, mood, thinking, and physical health. The most common obstacle to relieving depression is the mistaken notion that depression is a sign of weakness or that it is a result of some shameful action or inaction. Depression is chemically based and has many forms of treatment. Depression is not a choice. Who would choose to feel depressed? Nice people, religious people, charming people, healthy people, and educated people all can be affected by depression at some time in their life *through no fault of their own.* Just as you sought treatment for the cancer, seek treatment for depression if it occurs.

Depression is not the same as clinical depression, which some people mistakenly relate to mental illness. Clinical depression lasts longer, goes deeper than circumstances warrant, and is not due to physical illness or normal bereavement. The depression you may experience is transitory, and any counselor you consult will see you as struggling with a particular circumstance and not as someone who is mentally ill.

Depression colors your entire world and can paralyze you so that you cannot function. Depressed people are tired, irritable, unhappy, irrational, and unpleasant to be around. Please do not needlessly suffer this burdensome affliction or subject your family and friends to your difficult behavior.

Depression can occur at any phase of breast cancer treatment. Some women are surprised to find themselves depressed shortly after treatment has ended. Although this seems incongruous at first glance, it begins to make sense upon further study. During treatment you are surrounded by medical professionals who are fighting the battle for you and supporting you on a regular basis. Suddenly all those allies are withdrawn. Unconsciously you may wonder if the battle against your disease is continuing, you may feel abandoned now that you don't meet your medical team as often, and you may feel panic as you face the unknowns: Will the cancer recur? Will I ever feel rested again? Will there ever be a day I don't think about breast cancer? Will I ever get back on my feet financially?

Know the signs of depression and seek help when you notice the first sign. Remember that depression is partly chemical, so just "toughing it out" may not work. Get help early and you can get on with your life sooner.

## Common Signs of Depression

Unfortunately, a depressed person often does not have the ability or interest in seeking help. As soon as you notice a sudden change in your attitude or any of the following, mention them to your family or doctor so intervention can begin right away:

- Feeling hopeless, worthless, unusually irritable, guilty, or suicidal.
- Feeling blue for extended periods of time.
- Losing interest in routine activities; losing zest for life, work, hobbies, relationships, or sex.
- Chest pain, heart rhythm irregularities, fatigue, headache, bowel irregularities, loss of libido (these can have many other causes, but depression is sometimes the culprit).
- Unusual sleep disorders: insomnia or wanting to sleep all the time.
- Major gain or loss of weight.
- Pronounced fatigue.
- Prolonged crying spells.
- Inability to concentrate, think clearly, or make decisions.

## Medications for Depression

SSRIs (selective serotonin reuptake inhibitors) regulate the release of serotonin in the brain. Serotonin contributes to our sense of well-being. Common SSRIs used for depression are Prozac, Lexapro, and Zoloft. Side effects can include nausea, loss of appetite or libido, headache, nervousness, anxiety, insomnia, or sexual dysfunction. These may lessen after a few weeks.

Another class of prescription drugs used for depression, tricyclic antidepressants, include Tofranil, Pamelor, and Elavil. Possible side effects may include drowsiness, dizziness, dry mouth, heart-rate irregularities, and blurred vision.

Not all antidepressants affect all patients the same. The drugs can steady your emotions until you can benefit from counseling or emotional support or the physical cause of the depression is identified and removed. Antidepressants are nonaddicting, so do not hesitate to ask your doctor about their temporary use. Once you have started them, do not stop taking them abruptly. You need to taper off most antidepressants and take them for at least six months after the depression is under control.

Many herbs and supplements are advertised as mood lifters. Ginkgo biloba and inositol may be safe herbal alternatives to antidepressants. Discuss these or others with your doctor to eliminate any dangerous interactions. For instance, do not take ginkgo biloba if you are taking blood thinners such as

Coumadin[4] or have liver problems. Do not take St. John's wort with conventional antidepressants or if you plan to spend time in the sun. Although controversy exists about the effectiveness and safety of this herb, some studies show its effectiveness for mild depression. St. John's wort may have fewer side effects than prescription antidepressants, but it can cause dizziness, tiredness, stomach irritation, and dry mouth, and it may reduce the effectiveness of some cancer medications. Supplements made from this herb are classed as prescription drugs in Germany and other European countries, so you should not self-medicate with this potentially powerful substance.

Check with your doctor about any herbs or over-the-counter medicines that might interfere with antidepressants.

## Lifestyle Aids for Depression

Although medications can be tremendously helpful, they can't accomplish the goal of emotional stability on their own. Here are some things you can do to help beat the blues.

### Diet

No one food or beverage can prevent or cure depression; however, a balanced diet can provide many nutrients that contribute to mood and energy.

- Include protein sources such as lean animal products, beans, nuts, and nut butters. They contain the basic amino acids that help form mood-elevating serotonin and dopamine.
- Increase your B vitamins, especially B6 and B12, through liver, seafood, legumes, whole grains, fortified cereals, and dark green vegetables. Depression could be a sign of insufficient thiamin. A three-ounce pork chop will satisfy your requirement for a day. Beans can also provide B vitamins.
- Be sure you have enough omega-3 fatty acid in your diet (see page 315).
- Selenium in beef, seafood, mushrooms, whole wheat, sea vegetables, Brazil nuts, and poultry can boost your mood.
- Get a boost from the serotonin and norepinephrine in bananas.[5]
- A dip in blood sugar can make you feel down or depressed if you are hypoglycemic. To control blood sugar levels, eat protein at breakfast and eat every two hours, keeping sugar intake low, especially in the morning.

### Activities

- Exercise. This is a known mood lifter. Start slowly, with maybe 10 minutes a day, and work up to 30 if you can.
- Get adequate rest. Avoid caffeine late in the day, keep a regular bedtime, and relax before lying down.

- Get out in the sunlight. If the weather prohibits this, investigate a full-spectrum light box.
- Just do something whether it's the optimal activity for the moment or not. Taking a small step empowers and recharges you.
- Surround yourself with upbeat music, fresh flowers, funny friends, supportive family—anything that brings personal satisfaction.
- Take a citrus bath. Mix four drops of lemon and three drops each of grapefruit and peppermint essential oils in a small glass with a teaspoon of unscented liquid soap. As the tub fills with water, add this mixture. Soak for 15 minutes and see your blue mood wash away.
- Place fragrant flowers around your house where you can enjoy the scent or burn candles in your favorite fragrance.

## Attitude

- Concentrate on short-term goals such as getting dressed, walking the dog, or going to the mailbox. These keep your mind off larger tasks that seem overwhelming when you are depressed.
- Avoid sad or intense movies or books.
- Maintain healthy personal relationships. Other people provide emotional support needed to overcome depression. Seek out a family member or friend you can talk to. Concentrate on having fun with him or her as well as sharing your deep thoughts, fears, and dreams. Avoid people who put you down or discourage you.
- Do something helpful for someone else. Volunteer or do a one-time act of kindness.

If you still are depressed after a few weeks, ask your oncologist or a psychiatrist whether you are a candidate for antidepressants. Don't let false pride stand in your way. Having antidepressants prescribed is no more a reflection of your character than having penicillin prescribed for an infection. Also consider talking with a trained counselor and airing emotional baggage.

## Loneliness

Cancer is a lonely disease in two ways. You may not feel well enough to continue social or work functions that put you around people. Also, you might feel that no one really understands what you are going through. If you go for treatment often, the support staff at the doctor's office becomes your support group. When treatment is finished, suddenly they are gone and you may feel exceptionally lonely.

You are the only one who can let others know if you feel lonely. And you may have to step out of your comfort zone to dispel that feeling. Your family probably cannot be with you all day every day. You may have to be inventive to find ways to be around other people.

If your family or friends are not physically nearby, look for a support group. Contact a cancer organization to put you in touch with someone you can visit with on the phone. If you are well enough, enroll in a class or join a religious or special interest group. Making new friends is sometimes a welcome relief from the heaviness of the cancer world. Don't take current friendships for granted. Nurture them by giving the other person a chance to talk about his life and establishing rituals that will enhance bonding (getting together once a month for bridge or a movie, or celebrating birthdays together). If you feel withdrawn from family members, talk to them about it. Say what kind of support you'd like from them and hear their concerns about the relationship also.

## Stress

Stress is a factor of life. It can be stimulating and promote creativity, but too much can be unhealthy. A breast cancer diagnosis adds to your normal stress level at a time your body is actively combating the cancer and dealing with treatments, so you should do whatever you can to de-stress.

## Some Negative Effects of Stress

Stress affects not only quality of life but physiological functioning and perhaps even how disease responds to treatment, according to Dr. Lorenzo Cohen, assistant professor in the Department of Behavioral Science at M. D. Anderson Cancer Center.[6] He says an area of research called psychoneuroimmunology, or "mind-body medicine," has found that stress suppresses cell-mediated immunity, which is a first-line defense against metastasis. Stress also changes mechanisms within the cell that affect DNA damage and repair capacity. How this happens is not understood. Part of the explanation could be cellular and part could be that people under stress often adopt poor habits such as increased smoking or alcohol consumption, decreased physical activity, and poor eating and sleeping patterns.

Some physical effects of stress include:
- Increased blood pressure and heart rate.
- Increased appetite.
- Fluctuating blood sugar levels.
- Depressed immune system.

- Increased cortisol levels, which can lead to weight gain.
- Accelerated bone and muscle loss.[7]
- Increased inflammation.

# Ways to Reduce Stress

In general, you can reduce stress by breathing deeply, relaxing the body, and quieting the mind. Getting enough sleep is also a proven stress reducer.

## With food or herbs

- Eat as healthy as you can.
- Savor a piece of good-quality dark chocolate. Cocoa contains phenylethylamine, a compound that boosts production of mood-elevating brain chemicals dopamine and adrenaline.[8]
- Stay hydrated with six to eight 8-ounce glasses of water a day.
- Drink up to 2 cups of passionflower tea after dinner. Steep 1 teaspoon of dried passionflower in 1 cup of water for 10 minutes. Strain and drink. The herb relieves stress and anxiety and promotes sound sleep.[9]
- Sip tea made from chamomile or lemon balm if your oncologist gives permission. Steep one tea bag or 1 teaspoon fresh or dried tea in a cup of water for five minutes and drink. You can add more herbs if you want a stronger flavor.
- Anxiety is sometimes associated with a deficiency in selenium. Brazil nuts abound in this mineral.
- A few of the herbs that can alleviate anxiety are ashwagandha, magnolia bark, and passionflower. Theanine, an extract of green tea, can relax you. Pills give you the benefits without the caffeine in the tea.[10] Ask your doctor before you use any herb. A mineral supplement such as BlueBonnet Multimineral and Boron can help you sleep. GAIA's Melissa Supreme is good to combat anxiety, stress, and mental clouding.

## With activities

- Make time for yourself. Set aside just 15 minutes each day to do what you like: read, journal, sit on the porch, wander around the backyard, play solitaire. A 1998 study of 400 Japanese women with breast cancer reported that gardeners, painters, and others with hobbies outlived those without hobbies and had less stress.[11]
- Reserve the fifth Monday (or some other day) in a month for doing what you enjoy. If you work, reserve it for tasks you enjoy most.
- Make a regular date, weekly or monthly, for an evening with your spouse or special friends.

- Stick with routines—for sleeping, socializing with your support team (family, friends), or exercising. Our body functions at its highest level when we do something the same time every day. Don't stress over breaking your routines, but do aim for regularity and habit.[12]
- Breathe deeply. Inhale through your nose, expanding your abdomen; then exhale through your mouth with a quiet "ahhhhh."
- Try something new: a new hobby, friend, food, leisure class, route to work, weekend spot. Even little changes get the mental energy flowing, which reduces stress.
- Do something creative. Go to an art museum or crafts fair, paint, dance, take a class in origami or pottery, play an instrument, anything that can awaken your "inner artist."
- Pinch the bottom of one earlobe between your thumb and index finger. Hold for two minutes while you breathe deeply. Repeat with the other ear.[13]
- Press your thumb just below the ball of your foot (under your big toe). Hold for one minute and repeat on your other foot.
- Meditate, pray, or practice t'ai chi, qi gong, or yoga.

## With exercise
- For covert stress reduction at the office, place hands on your desk and push down for a few seconds. Now place them under the desk and push up. Turn your head slowly to the left as far as it will go and hold for three seconds; repeat to the right. Flex your feet so your heels touch the floor and your toes point upward; hold for three seconds. Reverse.
- Take a brisk five- to 10-minute walk, which can dissolve tension for an hour.
- Exercise a little each day.

## With environment
- Place wind chimes on your patio or porch for a calming sound. Play a CD of nature sounds or baroque music such as Mozart in your office or home.
- Take a sensory walk. For the first few minutes concentrate on your sense of sight. Appreciate colors, textures, movement, beauty. Then switch to each other sense: hearing, touch, taste, smell. Be aware of the sense in the present moment as well as how it has brought you pleasure in the past.
- Take a news break. The violence and urgency in the daily news can create anxiety. Go a few days without the media. Spend that time focusing on the moment.

## With attitude

- Be grateful and express it. If you don't feel gratitude, express it and soon you will feel it.

- Celebrate three things every day: a stunning sunrise, a visit with good friends, a juicy piece of fresh fruit, the fragrance of a flower, the smell of fresh air, your grandmother's picture that reminds you of how she loved you.

- Write down everything you are afraid of or worry about. Crumple the paper and throw it away. The symbolism may actually calm you down.

- Take charge. Write down what stresses you. Rank the stressors. Choose the most bothersome. Brainstorm as many solutions as you can think of. Write down every idea; it does not have to be feasible. Now rank the possibility of each idea actually diminishing the stress. Choose one or two ideas to implement and a time period. At the end of the period, choose another. Action is a potent weapon against stress. Sometimes all you need is to identify the problem very specifically and decide you can do something about it.

- For 10 minutes, fantasize about a dream vacation. Close your eyes and "see" every detail: what you'll be wearing when you arrive, who will be beside you, what you will see and eat.

- Let perfection go! Emotional stress lowers your mood-lifting neurotransmitters and the glucose levels in the brain, interfering with your brain's functioning. Stressing about being perfect may actually interfere with achieving that goal.

- Examine your priorities. Decide what's most important to you, what really mattered on the days you felt your worst, what flashed through your mind when you got your diagnosis and thought your days might be numbered on this earth. Work on maximizing those things in your life and let the others go. Don't let the rude driver or overbearing boss color your day. Flash him a big smile, confuse him with kindness, and save your anger for a life-threatening situation. Once you have decided what you value, the rest of life shrinks back into proportion.

- Mend relationships as far as you are able. Forgive or ask forgiveness. Decide to let go of anger or resentment whether or not the other person deserves a reprieve. The anger you hold on to hurts only you. Forgiving does not mean the other person never wronged you; it means you refuse to injure yourself emotionally any longer by holding on to the anger. If you are the one who erred, tell the other person you are truly sorry, make amends if possible, and ask forgiveness. Even if the other person refuses to forgive, you can be free of the weight of that incident and the toll it takes on your mind and body.

- Enjoy life! Play, move, laugh. Even on sick days you can find some incongruity to laugh about. Laughter is good medicine.

## Worry

Worry is a waste of time and energy, but how do you avoid worrying in the face of something as serious as breast cancer?

The main key is to distinguish between worry and concern. Worry seldom leads to action, makes you feel powerless, distorts the problem, makes you vulnerable to depression, distracts you from thinking about other things, and results in tension and stress, which interfere with sleep and relaxation. Worry is akin to a rocking horse: it gives you something to do but does not get you anywhere.

Concern, on the other hand, is productive. It leads you to analyze areas of your life and seek solutions for difficulties. It identifies potential problems and motivates you to take preventative or corrective measures. Whereas worry is like racing your car in neutral, concern is shifting into first gear and moving ahead.

To reduce the effect of worries on you, list them, consider what you can do to change the situation, and determine if the problem is yours or someone else's. Worry drags you down, whereas confronting challenges and concerns can energize you.

One popular "worry topic" among cancer patients is whether they made a wrong decision—about the timing of treatment, choice of doctor, and so on. Our choices change every day as new options become available and our information quotient enlarges. Be an aware patient. Learn as much as you can about the decisions you are making. Ask for more time if you aren't prepared to make a decision. Use good education, reliable research, sound medical advice, and your family's blessings to make your choice. Once you decide, don't look back. If you make the best decision with the information you have at the time, that's the right decision. "I wish I had..." or "I should have..." just adds stress that you don't need. Nothing can change by thinking those thoughts, so give them up and concentrate on the next decision you'll be called upon to make.

## Mood Swings

Closely related to depression, mood swings can trip you up at unexpected moments. You may be having a good day and suddenly your husband says something that makes you want to deck him. You *know* he didn't mean anything unkind by it, and you normally would not react to such a statement, but right now you are convinced he hates you and always has. Often your mind will be tussling for which assessment will win out: what you *know* to be true or what you *feel* is true.

Welcome to the strange world of mood swings. One moment you are yourself. The next you know the world is against you. Everyone. Gloom surrounds you. There is no hope. At the same moment your mind is telling you, "What you are feeling is untrue. What's the matter with you?"

What may be the matter with you is hormone imbalance. How you deal with mood swings is similar to how you deal with depression. First, check your lifestyle for healthy practices you can implement such as daily exercise, balanced nutrition, or reduction of stress, alcohol, and caffeine. Locate a support group where you can vent your feelings. Practice visualization, relaxation, meditation, prayer, affirmation, or yoga.

Visit an herbalist or homeopath for recommendations or ask your doctor about an antidepressant. One study at St. Luke's-Roosevelt Hospital Center in New York City found that 1,200 mg of calcium carbonate daily, specifically Tums for Life PMS (now called Tums E-X), relieved mood swings along with other symptoms of PMS.

In the meantime, hang on to any positive thoughts you can dredge up. If you feel suicidal, tell someone so you can get help. Try to get out in nature or around animals or children. Rent a funny movie. Fill your house with fresh flowers and your days with joyful activities, even if you do not share the joy. One unexpected moment you will.

## Hopelessness

Although hopelessness is a very sad condition, it is important to recognize it as a valid and acceptable emotion. When reports continue to show progressing disease and you continue feeling poorly, it is normal to lose hope, at least some of the time. In the midst of what you have lost, try to enjoy things you can still do and be grateful for them, no matter how limited. Applaud any progress and take hope from it.

If the hopelessness persists, mention it to your doctor or family so they may have you evaluated for depression. Hopelessness is a lonely place, so get help to escape from it.

## Hope

Hope is an elixir. With it, most things are bearable. Without it, life is difficult and stressful.

How do you clutch onto hope? Some find hope in their beliefs of life after death and in a God who loves them now. Some are hopeful that new treatments are surfacing almost monthly. Some look for the proverbial silver lining. They see their cancer experience as an opportunity for personal growth, for closer relationships, for healing old conflicts, for redefining the meaning of life.

Sometimes you find hope by stopping looking for it. Immerse yourself in helping others or in new hobbies or interests and you will suddenly find your attitude is more hopeful. Growth stimulates more growth and hope for the future.

Setting a goal can bring hope. What do you want to do when you regain your strength and have completed therapy? Travel to Europe? Keep the grandkids for a weekend? Learn gourmet cooking? Start your own business? Pick a goal and spend time researching, planning, and dreaming about it. When the future looms large and exciting, hope can't stay away.

## Meaning

Some women are comforted by looking for meaning in their cancer experience. They look for constructive ways to understand what happened to them. They may talk to their religious leader about the meaning of life and about faith issues. They may consider the diagnosis a wake-up call to reevaluate the way they spend their time and the relationships and values they have focused on. Many breast cancer patients end up making big changes: leaving a destructive relationship, rearranging schedules to accommodate healthy relationships, placing value (and time) on different priorities, turning their focus to helping others instead of concentrating on themselves.

Some others don't bother with finding the big "meaning of life." Instead, they look for little moments that feel meaningful. What are such moments for you: sewing a special outfit for your child, playing with your pet, fishing off the pier at dawn, reconnecting with old friends? Find what is meaningful to you and do it!

Illness is not a punishment. Life is not over, even if your former life has vanished. Find new possibilities for a meaningful life.

## Mind/Body Connections

"Mind over matter" is not just a cliché. Scientific studies are showing that what you think and concentrate on can produce physical effects in your body. Researchers have discovered links between the immune system, endocrine system, and messenger molecules such as neuropeptides. In other words, the brain and the body do influence each other.

One Stanford study of metastatic breast cancer patients[14] showed, for instance, that patients who attended weekly group therapy sessions along with their medical care survived twice as long as those who received only standard medical care. The Institute for Cancer Prevention is currently studying whether prayer has physiological effects on breast cancer patients.

Larry Dossey, author on medicine and prayer, tells us to view our bodies as music rather than as a machine. We are a work in progress, not a static set of parts. All aspects of ourselves (mind, body, spirit, emotions) are interconnected. Though there are limitations to our mind's power, it can play a part in our healing and quality of life.

Some mind/body techniques include:

- **Self-hypnosis.** Forget crystal balls and swinging pendulums. Self-hypnosis simply involves willingness, a state of intense attention, and readiness to accept an idea. You have total control over your mind and body during this technique. As you learn to achieve a state of concentration somewhere between waking and sleeping, you are more open to suggestion and can block out unpleasant thoughts or physical symptoms. Some people have the capacity to enter a hypnotic state easily, although about one in four does not. Once people learn how to enter into a deeply relaxed state, they can use the technique as anxieties or problems arise. Basically, hypnosis helps people look at an old problem in a new way and opens their mind to new behaviors. Hypnotic messages are usually couched in positive terms ("Smoking is a poison" rather than "I won't smoke"). Hypnosis is attentive, focused concentration, which makes it easier for the patient to relax and control her mind and body. What happens during hypnosis depends entirely upon the patient, not the hypnotist. Ultimately, all hypnosis is self-hypnosis.

- **Progressive muscle relaxation (PMR).** Used effectively with such diverse conditions as nausea, pain, depression, nervousness, and anger, this technique involves progressively tensing and relaxing various muscle groups. Find a quiet place where you will not likely be disturbed by the phone or another person. Lie down with your arms at your side and close your eyes. Begin by concentrating on your head. Squeeze your eyes, hold for three seconds, then relax them. Clinch your jaw, hold, and relax. Tense your neck muscles, hold, and relax. Continue to your toes, tensing, holding, then relaxing each muscle group. By the time you reach your toes, you will be calmer.

- **Systematic desensitization.** This technique takes advantage of the truth that practice makes perfect. A person imagines an anxiety-producing situation and in her imagination reduces the anxiety. The mind apparently "learns" from the imagination and enables the person then to experience the real-world situation with less anxiety.

- **Distraction.** Just as it sounds, distraction is anything that takes your mind off your pain or fear. You can apply internal techniques such as singing, praying, meditating, affirming yourself, or counting. Or you can use external techniques such as reading, listening to radio, tapes or CDs; watching TV; watching children play; doing crafts; or visiting with friends. If the distraction is too energetic, however, you may feel more tired and irritable afterward.

- **Mindfulness.** This technique involves focusing on the present moment without judgment or expectation. Have you driven to a store and suddenly realized that you don't remember a moment of your journey? Mindfulness aims to capture all that is contained in an experience. It teaches you to look at the details: textures, colors, and shapes. Instead of glancing over the lawn, you would focus on the individual blades of grass and notice their unique shapes, lengths, and shades of green. Mindfulness can reduce effects of stress and identify reactive ways that you handle stress so you can change for the better. The practice can also improve adaptation to change, enhance appreciation for life in the face of difficulties, and increase self-esteem.

- **Focusing.** Focusing is a technique that helps you tap into your subconscious to find "gut" answers to problems. Practitioners talk about a "felt shift," a moment of knowing, almost as if the analytical left brain has suddenly given a name to a nebulous feeling that has existed in the creative right brain. In a simple series of steps people can approach old problems and often find answers from deep within themselves.

Eastern societies have practiced mind/body connections for thousands of years. There are many formalized styles of "moving meditation." Try several and see which you enjoy. They all can stretch and massage every organ in your body to create energy and peace.

## *Intuition*

Listening to their inner voice is a trait many females are aware of but may not pay much attention to. Many breast cancer patients have learned the wisdom available from their instincts, their gut feeling, their "knowing." Call it what you will, your unconscious can often gently prompt you in the right direction. If you just "know" that a doctor is right for you or if some part of your plan just "doesn't feel right," speak up. Don't wait for this phenomenon to be explained by science. Take advantage of it now.

## *Play*

Do you want time to stand still and have joy fill your heart? Do you wish you could abandon your worries the way a 2-year-old playing with a watering can and a flower pot can? Adults have forgotten the healing power of play. Many of us "play" sports, but that is different from spontaneous child's play. Sports means we have to perform, usually we engage in competition, and most often we are trying to win. There is nothing wrong with those motivations. They are just different from healing play.

Play has no agenda, no rules, no desired outcome. We are simply totally absorbed in enjoying the moment. Watch a child and see how this works. To recharge your play batteries, play with a child—on his level. Let him determine what you are to do. If he says you are a monster one moment and a tree the next, go along with him. Throw logic out the window because, if you don't, spontaneity will jump out on its own and you will become frustrated trying to organize the wind. Play catch not to hone your grandson's skills, but because it's fun. Make up stories and don't try to keep the child on a particular theme. That may be appropriate for reading class, but play is different.

If you are not around children, you can still play with your adult friends—or some of them. After years of refusing to have anything to do with a game that did not require intense strategy, my husband has agreed to play board games with me that use a tiny bit of strategy and a great deal of luck. It's a way of connecting and relaxing at the end of busy days. We are still competing, but it's a haphazard contest. We know we both win because we spend time teasing and touching.

Real play will give your smile muscles a workout, your worries a vacation, and your immune system a little prod.

## *Laughter*

It's no joke that laughter can extend your life. Research studies show that laughter has measurable health benefits. It is a mild cardiovascular workout. It relaxes muscles and relieves pain from tense muscles. It enhances the immune system and produces endorphins, which counteract stress hormones.

To increase your laughter quotient:

- Watch funny movies.
- Keep a joke book handy.
- Cultivate a friend with a well-developed sense of humor.
- Look for oddities or absurdities in your present moment. Carry small inconveniences to an absurd degree in your mind. The results can be hilarious.
- When you're in a stressful situation, shout out a positive statement that contradicts the situation so much it's funny. I remember my great-grandmother sighing deeply whenever something bad happened and saying, "Oh, joy!"
- Laugh for no particular reason several times a day. Laughter is contagious. Soon you'll have others laughing and enjoying a hilarious ripple effect.

## Pets

Rover may be guarding more than your home. He may be guarding your health. Studies have shown that surgical patients returning home to loving pets fare much better than those returning to judgmental spouses. Convalescent homes often invite volunteers to bring pets for patients to play with because a cuddly kitten or playful pup can bring a smile to a depressed soul.

If you live alone, you may benefit from having a pet around to give you attention. Just watching a baby animal's antics brings laughter, and many pets keep their playful ways for years. However, be sure to assess the responsibilities of pet ownership and your ability to meet them.

## Relaxation

Some people shun relaxation as if it were a disease. They associate it with sloth, laziness, and boredom. On the contrary, it is a vital tool for keeping healthy. Our bodies need time to regroup, regenerate, and restore. Even God rested on the seventh day.

You may enjoy learning a specific relaxation or mind/body technique such as meditation, t'ai chi, or yoga, or you may design your own agenda. Either way, arrange for a few minutes of relaxation each day—even if you have to lock yourself in the bathroom to do so.

When the anxiety level rises, try one of the following to calm your nerves.

## Activities

- Fill a bathtub with hot water. Add mineral salt or an herbal bath blend. (Fill a clean sock, stocking, or cheesecloth with 1 ounce each of thyme, lavender, and sage herbs, dried or fresh, or bring 2 ounces of lemon balm leaves or chamomile to a boil in a quart of water. Simmer for 15 minutes, strain, and pour into your bath water.[15]) Rosewood, rosemary, pine, peppermint, and eucalyptus are also soothing. You may want to start with a single herb and add others later. Lean back on an inflatable pillow and close your eyes.

- Chill a gel eye mask in the refrigerator or freezer and place on your eyes to cool and soothe your eyes as well as your soul.

- Tap tension away. Taking slow deep breaths, lightly tap your knuckles against your scalp for 10 seconds. This yoga trick increases energy and relaxes tense muscles in your neck and head.[16]

- Drape a U-shaped pillow filled with herbs or grain around your neck. The weight relieves muscle tension.

## Foods

- Brew a cup of caffeine-free tea such as hibiscus, lemongrass, passionflower, or chamomile. For a calming treat, steep a chamomile tea bag in 1/2 cup boiling water for 10 minutes. Add 1/2 cup warm almond milk. Do not drink herbal teas without your doctor's permission if you are pregnant.
- Steep three fresh basil leaves or 1/4 teaspoon dry leaves in a cup of hot water for 10 minutes. Inhale the aroma; then sip the tea. Basil is very calming, but long-term use might not be safe.
- Add extra calcium, which is also calming to the nervous system, to your diet.

## Environment

- To facilitate a tranquil mood, light an aromatherapy candle, particularly sandalwood.
- Meditate on a pleasant, calming scene in your mind's eye.
- Add nature sounds or classical music to any activity for a refreshing feeling.
- Relax in your own tub by adding one cup sea salts or Epsom salt (magnesium sulfate) to your bath water, as minerals in seawater can relieve tense or sore muscles.

## Rest

If you suffer from fatigue, just had surgery, or are undergoing chemotherapy or radiation, you need more rest than you normally got so your body can heal. You don't have to sleep; just quiet your mind and relax your body.

Here are some tips on getting that rest:

- Plan regular rest breaks. Schedule them on your calendar as you would any other important appointment.
- Rest before you are exhausted.
- Lie down for optimal rest.
- Adjust light, temperature, noise level, and distractions. Turn off the phone. (Get an answering machine or voice-mail service.) Your health is top priority right now. Everything else, even possible emergencies, can wait a few minutes.

(Also see "Insomnia," page 132, for tips on sleeping better at night.)

## When Treatment Is Completed

Expect the unexpected once you have completed treatment. Your emotions are raw, you are probably fatigued and stressed, and you are still living with fear and unknowns. Anyone who says you should snap back to normal is uninformed. You will spend the next few months trying to define "normal," much less determine how to get to that state.

The top 10 symptoms reported by breast cancer survivors between one and five years after treatment were identified by Patricia Ganz, M.D., and colleagues at UCLA. They were:[17]

- 70 percent: general aches and pains.
- 69 percent: unhappiness with body appearance.
- 64 percent: stiff muscles.
- 64 percent: forgetfulness.
- 62 percent: joint pain.
- 59 percent: headaches.
- 55 percent: hot flashes.
- 53 percent: short temper.
- 52 percent: waking up early.
- 51 percent: sensitive breasts.

Physical and emotional recovery from these and other issues takes time. You can't rush either. Go easy on yourself. Give yourself time to reconsider priorities, energy levels, and interests. Don't accept any new committee assignments for a few months. Ease back into work responsibilities.

To protect your health, avoid stressful situations and people. Identify a few people you can unload your feelings on and do that when necessary. Listen to them also or they may burn out quickly. Consider taking a few days off for a special outing or vacation as a marker to separate treatment from "the rest of your life." If you can't get away, indulge yourself with flowers, a special dinner out, a new piece of furniture, or a pet. Try to avoid major decisions for several months. You will still be recuperating for a long time.

## Recurrence

If your cancer recurs or spreads, you may have a more difficult time emotionally than with your first diagnosis. In addition to the predictable fears of a cancer diagnosis is the realization that your first treatment failed. This leads to additional stress and anxiety and possibly feelings of hopelessness or guilt: "Did I eat French fries too often?" "I should have made myself exercise every day."

Rest assured that you did not do anything or fail to do anything that caused the cancer to come back. Because the disease is microscopic, there is no way to know if treatment has left any cells untouched.

Treatment may affect you differently this time. Although some patients with metastasis or recurrence are put on hormonal medicines, others end up taking chemotherapy. The effects of chemo on red blood cells are cumulative through treatment and, if you had chemotherapy before, you may experience a quicker drop in red blood cell count. This may translate into more severe fatigue than before.

You face more irritating delays and more unknowns. You may feel lonely if you don't have a support group of other breast cancer patients who have had recurrence or metastasis. Your feelings of loss of hope or loss of your image as a healthy person may intensify. You may be angry ("I did all that and now this?!"). You may worry more about your family ("What will they do without me?" "Will our support network be able to take up the slack once more?"), your finances ("Will our resources last through this?" "Can I continue working?"), or any pain or dysfunction that may lie ahead.

Your instinct may be to focus on the worst outcome, and your awareness of your mortality may heighten.

You can turn this chaos into a positive. Decide to do the things in your life you have always wanted to do. Get your estate in order. Designate a legal guardian for your minor children. Work on your legacy: Finally organize and label the family photos. Record memories of family members that will be lost when you are gone.

Squeeze the meaning and pleasure out of every day. If you wonder about the meaning of the recurrence, you may end up on a fascinating spiritual journey that ultimately brings peace and hope. People who have faced death seem to find each day more vital and important than those who have not. Perhaps you can instill this sense of enjoying the moment in your friends and family as they watch you enriched by little things they are too busy to notice.

Almost certainly you will experience random acts of love and concern, sometimes from people you would least expect.

Your dealing with the reactions of others may be the most frustrating part of recurrence. Some will be in complete denial; others will write you off as gone already. Usually this is from their own discomfort with disease and mortality, not from anything you have done. Tell them you are managing just fine and let them off the hook. Others will stay in contact although they are scared. Give them something tangible to do to help. It allows them to take their focus off your disease and the possibility of their ending up in the same situation someday.

Try to maintain balance in your life. Add pleasures in abundant proportions to your schedule. Plan for fun just as you do for treatment. Also plan time alone for reflection. Recurrence or metastasis can make you disassociate with your body. Try gentle exercises, massage, or breathing techniques to connect back. Seek out movies, books, music, or spiritual experiences to help identify your feelings and nurture your soul.

Keep your doctors informed on how you feel so they may help where they can. Know that, as soon as you have figured out what you want to do or can do, the situation may have changed, so be as spontaneous and flexible as possible. Take advantage of every opportunity for expressing your love for others and having fun. You'll have no regrets over time spent in positive activities.

## Survival

What I've learned about survival is that living is not the same as experiencing life. Now that my days are uncertain, I concentrate on enjoying everything I can and giving as much pleasure as I can. I am conscious of the years I lived in a fog, unaware of people close to me and not totally conscious of all the blessings I enjoyed. Since diagnosis, my senses of wonder and gratitude have erupted, and I wonder how I missed so much of the beauty and love around me.

Survival instincts may motivate you to change parts of your lifestyle, express your appreciation and love more, or reevaluate how you spend your time. They may open your eyes to see the reality of your environment and motivate you to make changes. They may prod you to take care of unfinished business with family members or friends or to mend relationships. Hopefully they will also buoy you with hope and strengthen you to comply with treatment requirements.

You will experience a range of emotions during your cancer journey. They will not be the same mix as the next person. Whatever you feel, know that any feeling is valid. It's what you do with it that matters. If you face any feelings you cannot resolve, please seek professional help. The relief good counseling can provide is invaluable and the reduction of stress might even help your healing.

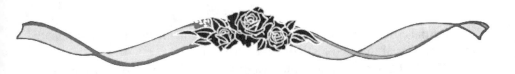

*Chapter 6*

# *Money Matters: Financial Concerns, Insurance, and Workplace Issues*

Cancer not only takes a physical and emotional toll. It can land a crushing financial blow on families. Even if you are covered by insurance, co-pays, deductibles, and uncovered costs can mount up quickly. Your health may require you to pay for services you normally perform and it may mean you have to stop or curtail your employment, at least temporarily.

## *Paying for Care: National Resources*

Fortunately, our society offers options to people whose savings accounts or support network cannot cover the full extent of cancer costs including food and rent. Check for eligibility requirements for Social Security Disability Insurance and Supplemental Security Income (Social Security Administration, *www.ssa.gov*, 1–800–772–1213), Medicare and Medicaid (Centers for Medicare & Medicaid Services, *www.cms.hhs.gov*), and food stamps (Department of Agriculture, *www.usda.gov*, or a local welfare office). Do not automatically assume you do not qualify. Definitions of eligibility change with new legislation, so at least investigate if you have no, or reduced, income. Check for other federal assistance programs at *www.GovBenefits.gov* or *www.FirstGov.gov*.

Don't overlook the Veterans Administration (*www.va.gov/vbs/health* or 1–877–222–VETS) if you or your spouse served in the military.

Hospitals that receive federal funds for construction through the Hill-Burton program are required to provide some free services to those who meet certain financial guidelines. You may apply even after you receive a bill for services. Contact *www.hrsa.gov/osp/dfcr/obtain/consfaq.htm* or 1–800–638–0742 for details. You will find a listing of participating facilities at *www.hrsa.gov/osp/dfcr/obtain/hbstates.htm*. Inquire about eligibility at the facility's admissions, business, or patient accounts office.

Partial costs of treatment may be covered if you are willing to participate in a clinical trial through a major cancer center.

The AVONCares Program for Medically Underserved Women provides some financial assistance to low-income and under- and uninsured women receiving treatment for breast cancer (see *www.cancercare.org*).

## *Paying for Care: Community Resources*

Most communities have some agencies to help people with disabilities or low income. To locate local sources of help, contact:

- American Cancer Society and other cancer organizations for local chapters.
- National Cancer Institute.
- Your doctor's office, hospital, clinic, or medical center.
- Librarians at public libraries or patient libraries at hospitals.
- Local human services or social services agencies. Ask about programs for the type of help you need: rent, food, medication, and so forth.
- Local bus systems, which may provide free or low-cost rides for people with disabilities. Some Red Cross chapters may provide transportation to doctors' appointments. (See Resources for organizations that provide free airfare to medical centers.)
- Local utility companies, which may have programs for people with low incomes.
- Meals on Wheels.
- United Way, Catholic Charities, Salvation Army, Lutheran Social Services, Jewish Social Services, Lions Clubs, and similar organizations.
- Local bar associations, most of which offer discounted or pro bono legal work in some cases.

Also consider hospitals operated by your local or state government that might have payment plans or discounted rates. Local cancer organizations and health departments may be able to provide limited financial assistance. It's worth a phone call to find out.

## *Paying for Care: Personal Resources*

If your assets are too great to qualify for government assistance, check into these possibilities. (Consult a tax advisor about tax implications before proceeding.)

- Payment plans. Most medical facilities will work with you on a payment plan of even a few dollars a month.

- Cash value of life insurance policy. If you own a whole life or universal life insurance policy, it may have accumulated cash value that you can borrow against.

- Reverse mortgage. This option is available only to homeowners older than 62. Basically it is a loan against your home that does not have to be paid off as long as you live there. It may affect your eligibility for other assistance programs.

- Home equity loan. Some states permit using your home as equity for a loan.

- Borrowing against a retirement plan. Some plans allow holders to borrow from them for "hardship" situations. Although there may be no penalties, the income may be taxed and affect your eligibility for government programs.

- Withdrawal from an IRA. Consult with the IRS about penalties.

- Viatical settlements. This is the sale of your life insurance policy for a percentage of its value, which is less than the death benefit and more than the cash value. Typical settlements are between 35 and 85 percent of the face value of the policy.[1] See the Viatical and Life Settlement Association at *www.viatical.org* or call 1–407–894–3797 for more information.

- An accelerated benefits program. Ask whether your insurance company offers one.

- Flexible spending account. Some employers offer a way of reducing taxable income through a flexible spending account (or arrangement). The employee chooses an amount to be withheld from each paycheck. This money is reimbursed to you for qualified medical expenses. The advantage of this plan is that you save taxes on the amount withheld. The disadvantage is that any money not spent is usually not refundable. Contact the IRS or your human resources department for more information.

- Tax deductions. Consult the IRS or your tax advisor about deducting expenses that are not covered by insurance: co-payments, transportation to appointments, supplies, medicine, and so on. In some cases a taxpayer can deduct medical expenses that are greater than 7.5 percent of her income.

## Ways to Trim Drug Costs

The cost of medications can be enormous and ongoing. Here are ways to chip away at the cost:

- Shop around. The cost of a medication at two stores can vary tremendously. Compare the cost of the same quantity of your drug at several places. Don't overlook large wholesalers such as Sam's Club or Costco. Weigh cost against such factors as distance from your home, hours of operation, services such as delivery or drive-through windows, and ease of shopping in that store.

- Mail-order services are often less expensive than brick-and-mortar pharmacies. However, if you need the medication in hours rather than days, this is not a good option.
- Ask about mail-order services you might qualify for through your insurance plan. Often you can fill a prescription for 90 days at one time for less than if you filled it three times for 30 days each. Be sure this is a medication you will be taking for a long time. Your doctor may have to write a special prescription to cover the extended time.
- Ask your doctor about generic substitutes for the medication, which are cheaper. Many work just as well as the patented variety. However, your doctor may have a reason she does not want you taking the generic.

## When You Can't Afford Medicine

Not all medical insurance plans pay for prescription medicine, and some pay only for the least expensive, generic drugs. Fortunately options exist.

If paying for medicine is a problem, talk with your doctor's office or hospital. They may have samples to give you or work with your insurance company to get a particular medication approved. Most major pharmaceutical companies have drug assistance programs for those with limited income or insurance. Each program differs in qualifications although most require that patients have no third-party prescription coverage. Some will work with your insurance company and some will discount their medication or give it at no cost. The nonprofit Cost Containment Research Institute offers a booklet of 1,100 brand-name drugs available from the manufacturers at a substantial discount for those who qualify (*www.institutedc.org*). The Pharmaceutical Research and Manufacturers of America (*www.phrma.org*; 1–800–762–4636) describes patient assistance programs for which you might qualify. (Also see Resources.)

Another possibility is to participate in a clinical trial. Ask your doctor about any trials that might be appropriate for you.

Many drug companies, retail pharmacy chains, groups of doctors, and nonprofit organizations offer prescription drug discount cards (sometimes called point-of-sale cards or consumer cards). Plans vary by enrollment fee, monthly fee, co-payments, drugs covered, and other provisions, so read the fine print before joining such a plan. The Harvard Medical School Website (*www.health.harvard.edu/health*) lists some cards.

### Other Financial Concerns

One area that trips up some cancer patients is splurging. Whether conscious or not, they think, "Well, if I'm going to die, I may as well enjoy life now!" or they declare, "I deserve this because of what I'm going through."

A little of that attitude is appropriate. Just be aware that you could be overspending for emotional reasons and creating more stress if spending gets out of hand.

## *Insurance*

One of the first questions you will need to answer after your diagnosis is: "What does my insurance cover?" If you are insured through an HMO (health maintenance organization), PPO (preferred provider organization), POS (point-of-service system), IPA (independent practice association), or Medicare/Medicaid, you may be restricted in your choice of doctors, facilities, and even tests or procedures.

Although most insurance companies will pay for a second opinion, some women feel they need a third opinion to "break the tie" of treatment options or to continue searching for a physician they feel comfortable with to be their coordinating doctor. If you end up paying for a second or third opinion, you can reduce the cost by having any required tests at a facility covered by your insurance.

Carefully monitor your hospital bills and explanations of benefits from insurance companies. Equifax, a national credit reporting agency, has estimated that 90 percent of medical bills contain errors.[2] Insist on itemized hospital bills. Ask what codes mean if you don't know. Keep close tabs on your deductible. Keep bills to prove your numbers.

## What's Covered?

Call either the insurance company or your employer's benefits department and ask someone to guide you through your payment responsibilities and any limitations on your choices of medical treatment. If you are not clear about anything or think a benefit has not been explained properly, do not hesitate to ask for a copy of the part of the policy in question. Also record the name of the person you talked to, the time and date of the call, and the information given. This will be useful in case you have to appeal for a denial of a claim.

Be aware that terms may mean something different to the insurance company than they do to you. I was told, for instance, by an insurance company representative that my compression sleeve was "covered 100 percent," so I expected to owe nothing. The sleeve retailed for $54 and the store asked me for $9. That's when I learned that the representative meant the company pays 100 percent of their allowable. In other words, they pay up to a certain amount (in this case, $45) and anything beyond that is my responsibility. Why the rep couldn't explain that, I don't know. So ask for clarification in dollar amounts: "So you mean that whatever the cost is, the company will pay it all?"

A phone call with a silly question might save you money. One patient was able to save sales tax on a treadmill by having her doctor write a prescription for it.

Some large insurance companies have special assistance for cancer patients, but they might not tell you about it unless you ask. For example, they may assign you an oncology caseworker to coordinate your claims, advise you of cancer benefits, and guide you through the paperwork maze.

## I Don't Have Insurance!

If you do not have insurance, there are often community resources to help you. Begin with the American Cancer Society office nearest you or a financial or account representative at the hospital where you would like to be treated. Sometimes they will work out a payment plan or suggest another facility that provides treatment in circumstances such as yours. You can also call your state board of insurance or local, state, and federal health agencies and inquire about subsidized healthcare or health insurance or companies that sell insurance to high-risk or uninsurable people.

When buying individual health plans, your health status may be used to deny you coverage. This is not true for many group plans. Your eligibility for individual policies is sometimes determined by your recent history of health insurance coverage, so avoid a lapse of coverage of any length of time.

If you are having trouble finding health insurance, check with professional, trade, or college groups that might offer insurance plans. Some states have high-risk pools that offer insurance to those who find it difficult to buy insurance. An insurance broker can provide information on several plans or contact the National Insurance Consumer Help Line at *www.iii.org* or 1–800–942–4242 with your questions.

Some women choose to go back to college and qualify for student health insurance. Check the restrictions for the school you are considering. You may have to take more hours than you want or fulfill other requirements.

Medicare rules keep changing, so check with that agency for current coverage.

## Preexisting Conditions

The Health Insurance Portability and Accountability Act of 1996 prohibits employer-sponsored group health plans, insurance companies offering group plans, and HMOs from discriminating against employees or their family members based on their health status. It also limits exclusions for preexisting conditions.

If you had a medical condition in the past and have not received treatment, advice, diagnosis, or medical care (including follow-up or check-up visits) concerning it in the past six months and meet certain insurance coverage requirements, that condition may not be excluded from your health insurance coverage. This period may be shortened under state law in certain circumstances. For details in your state, contact your state insurance commissioner's office. In general, the identification of a gene mutation in BRCA1 or 2 genes should not qualify as a preexisting condition because it is not a medical condition.

## What if the Insurer Denies a Claim or Treatment?

Every insurance company has an appeals process. If coverage is denied for a treatment your doctor recommends, call the insurance company and find out the appeals procedure. Usually it will entail writing a letter or filling out a form explaining why the denial should be overturned.

Sometimes your doctor's office will assist you in filling out the form or at least explain the reasons for the treatment so you can write them into a letter.

It is important to remember a few pointers about an appeals letter:

- Begin your letter with the action you want the company to take. Don't make them wade through three single-spaced pages to discover the problem.
- Stick to the facts. Include as many applicable statistics and medical reasons as you can.
- Be as brief as possible, but do give all the information (dates, names, and so forth).
- If appropriate, attach copies of test results or reports from doctors or procedures.
- If you feel there is an urgency to receiving an answer, ask that they respond in seven to 10 days, or sooner if necessary. Often the appeals process takes 30 days, but some conditions cannot wait that long. If this is the case, explain why you are asking them to expedite your request.
- Do not threaten a lawsuit.
- Maintain a pleasant tone.
- If you feel your policy includes coverage for the denied cost, include a copy of that portion of the policy with the section highlighted.
- End your letter thanking them for their "consideration" of your request.
- Many insurance companies have a doctor or a group of doctors who review appeals letters for the medical necessity of the procedure. Sometimes explaining why a treatment is necessary in your situation is enough to reverse a denial.
- Don't placidly accept a "no" the first time around. Occasionally someone has convinced a company to pay for a procedure in an unusual case that is routinely denied.

## Appealing an Insurance Decision

- Be sure the forms are filled out completely and accurately.

- To prove a charge is "reasonable and customary" (meaning comparable to what other providers charge in your area), check medical libraries, medical societies, or medical schools for a book that shows the charge for every medical procedure in every zip code.

- Keep scrupulous notes on all conversations with the insurance company. Record the date, time, person talked to, ID number (if any), and what was said.

- Engage a medical claims advocate if necessary. (Look in the Yellow Pages under "Insurance Claims Processing" or ask your doctor or hospital for names. Ask how long the company has been in business and how they charge.)

## External Review of Claims

Your insurance company does not necessarily have the final say about a claim. If you feel a procedure has been denied unfairly, you can contact your state's department of insurance and inquire about the external review process. Most states have an independent review board that reviews claims. Recent figures show that about half the claims were upheld. You may not be eligible for this service if your company is self-insured. Try to work with your human resources department. If that fails, your options include filing a grievance against the company or suing. Weigh carefully the pros and cons of such extreme measures: cost, time, energy, and outcome. If you lose—or even win— will you feel comfortable at work?

For a detailed guide to appealing an insurance decision, see the Kaiser Family Foundation Website at *www.kff.org/consumerguide*.

For guidelines state by state on keeping health insurance, visit *www.healthinsuranceinfo.net*.

# Disability and Life Insurance

Disability and life insurance might be hard to get once you have been diagnosed with cancer. If you switch jobs and your new employer offers them as benefits to all employees, you will qualify automatically. It is only as an individual purchaser that you can encounter difficulty.

If you have either coverage already, be diligent about paying bills on time so your policy does not lapse. If you do find a company to insure you, expect to pay premiums much higher than average. If either insurance is through your work and you leave your job, ask about converting the policy to an individual policy that does not require a medical exam.

## Workplace Issues

Many cancer patients find a supportive team in their coworkers and employer. In fact, some companies allow a sick bank, through which employees can donate hours of sick time or vacation time to fellow employees who have crises such as cancer.

However, some experience discrimination in promotions and job assignments. Such discrimination may be illegal as long as you have the necessary skills and can perform the essential duties of the job.

## Myths You May Face

Unfortunately, uninformed people can make your work situation more difficult than it has to be. When choosing whom to tell about your cancer, keep in mind some common myths people react with:

- Cancer is a death sentence. (Why should I train/promote this person if she's going to die?)
- This person is contagious.
- Cancer survivors are an unproductive drain on the economy. (Truth: They schedule chemo so they can be sick on the weekends.)

## Searching for a Job

Many people fear that a history of cancer or being in cancer treatment will prohibit them from finding a job. As long as you are qualified to do the work, this should not happen. Generally, you control the information. Though you must always be honest, you may not have to reveal your diagnosis, so do not volunteer information about the cancer if you are not asked for it.

So you don't tip your hand, do not ask about medical benefits in your first interview. Instead, when a job is offered and benefits are being discussed, get in writing how long it will be before you are covered under the new employer's plan.

Look for a larger company (15 or more) so you may be covered by some federal laws that help protect your rights in the workplace.

Apply only for jobs you can handle and for which you are trained.

### Interviewing

Interviewers can ask only job-related questions; you don't have to tell about cancer if you can perform the job requirements. If a job application asks about your illnesses, the question is likely illegal and you don't have to answer it. If you do answer the question, emphasize your current state of health and your ability to do the job. Of course, do not lie, whatever you do.

After extending a job offer to you, a new employer is permitted to ask about your medical history and to conduct medical examinations. When you are asked for a medical history by a new employer or an insurance agent, it is very important that you answer honestly. Cancer will not affect premiums for a group policy although it may mean higher premiums for an individual policy. Medical facilities and insurance companies have access to the Medical Information Bureau (MIB), which stores medical information that you have given to doctors, hospitals, insurance companies, and so on. They may check what you have submitted for accuracy. If you have not been truthful, they can use that as a reason to deny insurance or terminate you. Mistakes can be made, so you might want to contact MIB (1–781–329–4500) and request a copy of your medical profile.

If you have a visible disability (such as a lymphedema sleeve) and the interviewer could reasonably believe it could affect your ability to perform the job, questions about your ability to perform the work are legal. Also, gaps in your employment history could prompt some legitimate questions. To avoid these questions, arrange your resume by skills, not by date. Otherwise detailed questions about your health can be asked only after you have been offered a job. Do not volunteer your cancer history unless it directly impacts your ability to do the job. Focus on your current abilities.

## Sharing the News with Your Boss

It is not necessary to tell anyone at your workplace about the cancer if your diagnosis and treatment will not interfere with your work duties. The decision depends on many factors including your role at the company and your relationship with your coworkers. One attitude that should help you in the long run is keeping in mind the needs of your employer as well as your own. Usually the time from diagnosis to beginning of treatment is just a few weeks. That's not much time to prepare for your absence. Give your employer as much notice as you can and you may experience exceptional support.

Many federal and state laws require an employer to provide "reasonable accommodations" to help a disabled person do her job. However, an employer is not required to incur any "undue hardship" to accommodate you. This could include any change that is costly, extensive, or disruptive to the business. Many courts have ruled that cancer is not a disability under the Americans with Disabilities Act but more like a temporary illness. Many employers are willing to accommodate cancer patients but may not be required by law to do so.

If an employer asks for documentation of your diagnosis, it's not from mistrust but for protection on his end. Your cooperation should benefit you in the long run.

## Sharing the News with Coworkers

You may decide to wait until you have a treatment plan before you share your diagnosis with coworkers. In addition to concern for you, they will naturally wonder how your illness will affect their work situation. Assure them you will leave detailed instructions about your responsibilities and be available to answer any questions that arise during your absence. Let them know whether you do or do not want to talk about the cancer.

## Ideas for Workplace Changes

- Switch to part-time or flextime.
- Switch to another position with different hours.
- Find a place to nap during the day.
- Do some work at home.
- Arrange your office so items you use frequently are in easy reach.
- Schedule work appointments at the time you are at your best.
- Resist the "they can't do it without me" syndrome. Delegate responsibilities.
- Designate a point person for interaction with the office. Ask others to go through her to reach you. Explain your organizational system thoroughly to this person so information can be found most of the time without contacting you. Decide how mail and e-mail will be handled in your absence.

## Document, Document, Document

Even if you can't imagine encountering difficulty with job promotions or job retention, it is safest to keep records from the day of your diagnosis. Keep a daily log and a file of printed evidence of accolades as well as incidents/remarks that are suspicious regarding your ability to perform your job because of your diagnosis. Record who was present during a conversation and exactly what was said. Also record your requests for special consideration (schedule, equipment, and so forth) and the results. Write down what happens to your responsibilities while you are gone. Keep a log of times and days worked.

If you do have a dispute about the termination or downgrading of your position, keep these factors in mind:

- Stay cool. Don't get angry with your boss or HR department.
- Consider how awkward it would be to work with someone you have sued and whether that would peg you as a troublemaker. Are the stress and legal costs worth the ultimate outcome?
- Do you need a job at this particular company (nearness to home, only one in town, longevity there)?
- Minimize confrontation and maximize mediation.

## Resolving Differences

Sometimes a letter from your healthcare team stating your ability to work will help an employer decide to accommodate your needs.

Investigate your employer's policies for resolving employee disputes and try that avenue. Be very careful what you say because it might be used against you if the case does end up in court. Be aware of filing deadlines under federal and state law so you don't lose your ability to file a complaint. Generally, you have 180 days to file a complaint with the EEOC (Equal Employment Opportunity Commission) or with a state agency. If you work for the federal government, you may have only 45 days.

Is a lawsuit worth it? Determine first what outcome you want: your former job, certain benefits or accommodations, or something else. Lawsuits can mean stress over several years, legal expenses, hostility between you and those you work with—plus there is no guarantee of success. Only you can decide if the results would be worth the cost.

If you are eligible to file complaints with more than one agency, you may file with them all or choose the one with the best potential outcome, the quickest resolution time, and the closest office.

## Returning to Work

You may have mixed feelings about returning to your job. You may be afraid you'll be treated differently or that you can't manage the physical or mental strain. Consider returning slowly, half days for a while. Find out if your company has a formal return-to-work program or other requirements you must meet.

If you feel you are facing discrimination because of your illness, talk with your supervisor. If the situation continues, contact the EEOC to learn about your rights and your choices to have them upheld.

## Not Returning to Work

If you will not return to your former company, you may gain confidence by taking refresher courses in some of your skills. Be aware that you also might have to repay some health insurance costs.

## Laws That May Offer Some Protection

When cancer interferes with your job performance, federal and state laws may offer some relief. Depending on the number of employees your company has and other criteria, you may be eligible for flextime or other considerations to meet your treatment needs.

To learn about your rights as an employee with cancer, ask your human resources department, a social worker at your doctor's office or hospital, your state department of labor, or your state or congressional representative.

You should expect reasonable flexibility from your employer. If you try to ease the burden your illness will place on the company, hopefully your supervisors will reciprocate. If that does not happen, you may find protection in some federal laws that deal with health issues.

## ADA (Americans With Disabilities Act)

This law applies to employers with 15 or more employees and prevents discrimination against individuals with disabilities or chronic illnesses who meet certain requirements: physical or mental impairment that limits major life activities such as walking, working, or breathing; having a record of such impairment; or being treated as if you have an impairment. The employer is limited in the decisions he makes based upon your disability.

An employee or job applicant with a disability is protected under ADA if she can, with or without reasonable accommodations, perform the essential functions of the job. "Reasonable accommodations" may include job restructuring, modifying work schedules, or reassignment to a vacant position. The employer is not required to make such accommodations if it will place an "undue hardship" on the business nor is he required to lower production or quality standards.

Complaints under ADA are handled through the EEOC. You must go to the EEOC within 180 days of the adverse action about which you want to complain.

## FMLA (Family Medical Leave Act)

This law applies to employers with 50 or more employees within a 75-mile radius and only to employees who have worked 1,250 hours during the previous 12 months. If a company has offices in two locations and one has 60 employees and the other has 20, only the larger office is covered under this law. The FMLA grants 12 weeks of unpaid leave with continuing health insurance every 12 months to a person with a qualifying serious health condition or whose spouse, parent, or child has such a condition. During your leave, your healthcare benefits must remain intact.

Qualifying health conditions include any illness or physical condition that involves inpatient, resident medical care, or hospital care; evaluation of a condition; and continuing treatment by a healthcare provider. Chemotherapy and radiation are considered continuing treatment.

You can use your 12-week total intermittently, taking the leave in blocks of time for various qualifying treatments. For instance, you can reduce the hours you work each day or take off two hours each day for radiation or be off three days every three weeks for chemotherapy. The employer can transfer you to another position with equivalent pay and benefits and can't make you take more leave than necessary. When you return to work, the employer must place you in the same or equivalent position with the same pay, responsibilities, skill requirements, status, and privileges if you are able to do the job. If you are unable to perform at your former level, you don't have a right under this law to another position.

Planning runs both directions with this law. You must give notice of leave within 30 days or as soon as possible. Together you need to work out a schedule that accommodates your employer's needs as well as yours. Your employer has a right to ask you periodically if you intend to return to work. If you do not return to work, your employer can charge you for healthcare premiums the company paid during your leave. Also, you can use your paid and accrued vacation and sick time as part of the 12 weeks, in which case you would receive wages for that time.

Complaints under the FMLA are handled by the Wage and Hour Division of the U.S. Department of Labor. Call the referral line (1–866–487–9243) for the number of your local office. Find more information on the FMLA Website at *www.dol.gov/esa/fact-sheets-index.htm.*

## HIPAA (Health Insurance Portability and Accountability Act)

Also known as the Kennedy-Kassebaum bill of 1996, this law enables you to move from one job to another without fear of penalty for preexisting health conditions if you have had medical coverage for 18 months, have not been without health insurance for more than 62 days, and have already met a preexisting condition exclusion period under a previous plan. The law sets no limits on premiums that can be charged, although group plans are required to charge the same amount for everyone in certain demographic groups (such as age or employment longevity). Such requirements apply only to group insurance plans bought through an insurance company, not to employers who are self-insured. It is a complicated law, and you will probably need a benefits representative from your company or a claims advisor to help you understand the benefits of the law.

## Federal Rehabilitation Act

This law, as does the ADA, prohibits employers from discriminating against employees because they have a disability. This act, however, applies only to employees of the federal government and federal contractors. Disability is defined the same as for ADA. For more details, contact the Access Unit, Civil Rights Division, Department of Justice (P.O. Box 66118, Washington, D.C. 20035).

## ERISA (Employee Retirement Income Security Act)

Among many other provisions, this federal law prohibits an employer from terminating an employee in order to interrupt or suspend her health benefits.

# Is Breast Cancer a "Disability"?

A "disability" usually refers to a major health condition that substantially limits your ability to do everyday activities, such as drive a car or climb stairs. In some cases, a past disability qualifies you as disabled. Courts have ruled both ways regarding cancer, and state laws differ considerably. Consult your state human rights or civil rights commission. To find the appropriate agency, look under state agencies in your phone book or visit *www.eeoc.gov* online. Different agencies define "disability" differently, so check with each one to see if you qualify for assistance.

# State laws

Every state's laws on disability and employment are different. Check with your state's attorney general's office, department of labor, or division of human rights office. The federal Equal Employment Opportunity Commission (*www.eeoc.gov*) may be able to answer questions also.

# Other Laws to Protect You during Treatment

Several federal laws exist to protect your employment rights during cancer treatment. However, very small companies (less than 15 for the ADA) and very large companies may not be subject to them. Large companies may be self-insured and not required to comply with federal or state guidelines. Some states have similar laws that apply to small employers. Check with your state insurance commissioner's office. You are entitled to the same health insurance coverage as anyone else in your company.

If you resign from your job, be sure to obtain a certificate of creditable coverage from your employer's HR department. It will be the proof you need to be covered under HIPAA's limitation of preexisting conditions.

## COBRA (Consolidated Omnibus Budget Reconciliation Act)

The Consolidated Omnibus Budget Reconciliation Act (COBRA) is a federal law that protects your group medical insurance benefits when you retire, resign, are terminated, or change jobs or if you divorce and had insurance through your ex-spouse's employment. Companies with 20 or more employees must offer an extension of benefits for up to 18 months after a job termination. You will pay the full cost (including what the employer paid before) and must select the option within 60 days of being informed of your leaving. It will be less expensive to pay the full group premium than to pay individual insurance rates.

Before you drop COBRA coverage, be sure you have fulfilled any waiting period for new insurance and that the new plan covers preexisting conditions. If you should let your insurance lapse, you may find it virtually impossible to locate a company that will cover you. A lapse of 63 days of coverage is enough for even your next employer to be able to deny insuring you.

Several government agencies are responsible for administering COBRA. See *www.cms.hhs.gov/hipaa/hipaa1/cobra/fedrole.asp* for which department handles your issue. Departments of Labor and Treasury have jurisdiction over private-sector group health plans. The Department of Health and Human Services has jurisdiction over public sector (state and local government) health plans. For general information, contact the Department of Labor's Office of Pension and Welfare Benefits Administration (1–800–998–7542) for the office nearest you.

Cancer-related money matters can create stress. If they get out of hand, locate an agency that might help and learn your options. Don't assume anything. Laws and requirements are constantly changing. Perhaps you qualify for just the program that will fill in the gap in your financial structure.

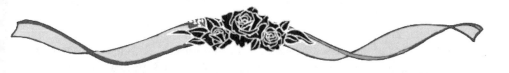

*Chapter 7*

# *Concerns of Special Populations*

## *Male Breast Cancer*

Among newly diagnosed breast cancer patients each year are approximately 1,400 men, and approximately 400 men die each year from breast cancer. This comes as a shock to most people. Because men do not have routine screenings for breast cancer, their disease is often found at a later state. However, survival rates are about the same as for women at the same stages.

The rate of male breast cancer began to increase sharply in 1991. The reason is not known. Because approximately 85 percent of male breast cancer is estrogen-receptor–positive, some researchers are looking at the possible role of estrogen in this population.

### Signs That Should Be Investigated

Most breast cancer in men is discovered when they notice something unusual on their chest. Some symptoms that might mean breast cancer in men are:
- Lump or swelling in breast area.
- Inverted nipple.
- Skin dimpling or puckering.
- Scaling or redness of nipple or breast area.
- Bloody or other discharge from nipple.

### Risk Factors

Men with a family history of breast cancer (in females or males) should ask their doctor about routine screenings. Men with the BRCA2 gene are at increased risk for cancer of the breast, colon, and prostate. One strong risk factor is Kleinfelter's Syndrome, which indicates a man has an extra sex chromosome. However, only 4 to 6 percent of diagnosed males have this condition.[1]

Many adolescent boys develop gynecomastia, or female-like breasts. Up to 40 percent of diagnosed males have this condition. Radiation to the chest, high estrogen levels, liver disease, and being African-American or Jewish are other risk factors. Most male breast cancer is detected in men between 60 and 70.

## Treatment

Staging and diagnosis procedures are similar for men and women. The most common type of breast cancer in men is infiltrating (or invasive) ductal carcinoma. Because of the small size of the male breast, a modified radical mastectomy is the normal procedure. Chemotherapy or hormonal therapy may follow, depending on the same factors as in women's breast cancer treatment. Tamoxifen is the most common drug used.

Surgical removal of the testicles used to be the standard treatment for male breast cancer because the testicles produce androgens that may be converted to estrogen by other body tissues. However, with the development of hormonal therapies, this operation is seldom done.

## Side Effects

Men undergoing treatment for breast cancer can experience the same range of side effects as women: hot flashes, mood swings, weight gain, and loss of sexual desire. In addition, they may lose the ability to have an erection.

Even without side effects, the diagnosis of breast cancer can be devastating to a man. He may feel isolated or embarrassed and think the disease reflects on his masculinity.

## *Young Women and Breast Cancer*

Breast cancer is not common in young women. In 1991 approximately 4,200 women in their 20s and 30s were diagnosed with breast cancer. In 2000 that number had grown to 5,500.[2] Doctors sometimes miss symptoms because there are so many benign explanations for them. The women themselves may not be familiar with symptoms to look for or think they are too young to have to look for them. Also, they may not have good insurance and neglect their annual checkups. Any lump that changes in size after two menstrual periods should be evaluated. Women with the mutated BRCA1 or BRCA2 gene tend to develop breast cancer at a younger age than the general population and should monitor symptoms carefully.

A cancer diagnosis can leave young women feeling isolated from their peers who are focused on career, dating and marriage prospects, and raising families. Mortality looms large for the cancer patient, whereas her friends probably have not given it a thought. In addition to the normal concerns about treatment, young women need answers about fertility, safety of pregnancy, telling someone in a long-term relationship about the disease, or dealing with young children while undergoing treatment.

Women in their 30s may regain reproductive capability after breast cancer treatment. The younger you are upon diagnosis, the less likely you are to go into menopause. Even if you go into menopause after chemotherapy, it can be temporary, and periods may resume after even two years, so take proper precautions against pregnancy unless you and your doctor have agreed a pregnancy is not a problem in your situation.[3]

## Pregnancy

A major issue for many younger women with breast cancer is pregnancy: "What if I'm pregnant when my breast cancer is detected?" "Can I become pregnant after treatment?" "Is it safe for me and the baby?" There are numerous factors, both emotional and physical, that enter into this issue. Is your prognosis good enough that you can reasonably expect to care for a child? Do you want to leave a legacy, knowing that your extended family can step in if you cannot continue caring for the child? No one can tell you and your spouse what to decide.

Because breast cancer treatment targets hormones among other factors, getting pregnant during treatment is not advisable. If you have intercourse, be sure you are on some form of birth control other than birth control pills *because you can get pregnant during breast cancer treatment*. The hormones in birth control pills might disrupt your treatment and vice versa, and some chemotherapy drugs can cause birth defects. Ask your doctor about condoms, spermicidal agents, diaphragms, or other contraceptive options. Chemotherapy drugs differ also in their effect upon the ovaries. Cytoxan may be one of the most damaging.

If you are already pregnant when you are diagnosed, be sure your doctor is informed so your treatments can be delayed or modified as necessary. The National Cancer Institute states that "ending the pregnancy does not seem to improve the mother's chance of survival and is not usually a treatment option."[4] Between 2.8 and 7.3 percent of breast cancer cases are diagnosed in pregnant or breastfeeding women. Radiation can increase the risk of birth defects; however, breast biopsies and even modified radical mastectomies are considered safe for the mother and baby. The American Cancer Society reports that recent studies show that chemotherapy may not increase risk of birth defects, stillbirths, prematurity, or low birth weight in the second and third trimesters. Radiation or chemotherapy treatment during the first trimester is generally not recommended.

Becoming pregnant after breast cancer treatment is another story. Some treatments cause early menopause, in which case pregnancy is not possible. More than half of women who develop breast cancer in their 30s, however, regain their reproductive capability.[5] There is no way to determine when you will go into menopause, with or without the cancer, so you might factor that into your plans. All women begin menarche with a finite number of eggs, and if some were damaged during chemotherapy, for instance, you could conceivably stop your periods sooner than you would have otherwise. Because recurrence of invasive breast cancer usually occurs within two years after treatment, some doctors suggest waiting until that time has passed to get pregnant. It is recommended that you wait one year after radiation before you get pregnant. The effects of certain cancer treatments on later pregnancies have not been studied, although it does appear that breast cancer itself does not harm the developing baby.

A confusing area is tamoxifen. Generally, oncologists don't want a woman getting pregnant while on tamoxifen, although the drug is sometimes used as a fertility drug. Apparently because of this, there is no recommended waiting period after completing tamoxifen before becoming pregnant.

Pregnancy does not cause recurrence, and a relapse due to stimulation of hormones during pregnancy is rare. In fact one recent study concluded that mortality in young women was *less* in those who got pregnant after breast cancer than in those who did not.[6] Pregnancy is generally not recommended for a woman on hormone therapy or one with metastatic disease because pregnancy could interfere with her treatment.

If you want to get pregnant after treatment and you had a small tumor, you might be able to avoid chemotherapy, which in effect poisons the ovaries. However, look at all risks of that decision before you make it. If chemotherapy is necessary, consider using LHRH (luteinizing hormone-releasing hormone) agonist or LHRH antagonist drugs, which suppress ovulation and may protect unripe eggs from damage from chemotherapy. (Zoladex is one drug to ask about.) Ask your doctor which drugs have the least effect on fertility. Blood tests done about six months after chemo can predict future fertility fairly accurately, although blood tests done during chemo cannot. If you have periods during most of chemotherapy, you will probably retain your fertility afterwards.

Studies of women who became pregnant after breast cancer treatment show that pregnancy did not seem to affect recurrence, new cancers, metastasis, or death rates.[7] A myth has long circulated that women whose breast cancer was diagnosed during pregnancy had a worse outcome. This is not scientifically accurate. However, some women may have later detection of a cancer because their breasts are enlarged and doctors are not usually looking for breast cancer in women young enough to be pregnant.

Consult an infertility specialist about harvesting and storing your eggs or fertilized embryos for later implantation. You will probably have to have your oncologist call on your behalf to get an appointment within a few days. Unfortunately, the rate of success for unfertilized eggs is small. Fertilized eggs have a better track record, but the process could delay your chemotherapy for several weeks and might be risky from a hormone standpoint. Chances are 20 percent or less of having a child through in vitro fertilization.[8] Because of the increase of hormones involved in the fertilization process, the safest time for this procedure may be the six weeks or so a woman is waiting between surgery and the start of chemotherapy. She will be waiting anyway so this procedure will not delay her treatment further. The older you are, the less likely it is that the procedure will be successful because of the fewer eggs you have available for harvest. Of course each case is different; talk with your doctor.

The safety of fertility drugs for women with breast cancer has not been studied. Are they safe for one cycle to produce more eggs to store? Answers are not readily available.

Some women have had a small portion of ovarian tissue removed during surgery and frozen on the theory that, if it were replanted in the body, it could possibly restore ovarian function. This has not been proven, and no known pregnancies have resulted from it. Another possibility is taking a GnRH agonist (such as Zoladex, Lupron, or Trelstar) during chemotherapy to protect ovarian function. CMF (cyclophosphamide, methotrexate, and 5-fluorouracil) has a much higher rate of chemotherapy-induced menopause than AC (Adriamycin and Cytoxan) followed by a taxane (Taxol or Taxotere), according to Dr. Hope Rugo, associate clinical professor of medicine in the Division of Hematology and Oncology at the University of California San Francisco Comprehensive Cancer Center.[9]

Other options are donated eggs, surrogate implantation or adoption. A team of specialists is best to advise you on this difficult issue. You also need to consider cost because many insurance plans do not cover fertility treatments. Also consider ethical questions of the ultimate disposition of frozen eggs, sperm donation if your husband's sperm count is insufficient to fertilize a frozen egg, and so forth.

# Breastfeeding

Breastfeeding after breast cancer might be possible if surgery or radiation did not prevent milk from traveling to the nipple. However, you need to consider some other issues as well:

- Stop breastfeeding if surgery is planned to reduce blood flow to the breasts and reduce their size.

- An infection in the breast during breastfeeding (known as mastitis) could be harder to treat.
- You can breastfeed from only one breast (not the treated one) if you don't mind the difference in the size of your breasts. A radiated breast will produce very little, if any, milk. One breast can feed a baby. However, it will get considerably larger than the other one—and may stay somewhat larger after weaning.
- A lactating breast is harder to examine via mammogram, so your follow-up schedule could be compromised. It can take six months to two years for a lactating breast to return to its normal state after pregnancy and breastfeeding.
- Do not breastfeed during or possibly after chemotherapy, as the drugs may appear in high levels in the milk and could harm the baby.
- If you cannot breastfeed, ask about a breastfeeding simulator, a reservoir that holds milk and attaches to your nipple through a tiny tube. The baby sucks your nipple and the end of the tube at the same time.

## Abortion and Miscarriage

In February 2003 more than 100 of the world's leading experts on pregnancy and breast cancer risk met at the invitation of the National Cancer Institute to review population-based, clinical, and animal studies on pregnancy and breast cancer, including induced and spontaneous abortions (miscarriages). This prestigious group concluded that neither induced abortion nor miscarriage increases a woman's risk of developing breast cancer. They felt that some earlier studies that showed the opposite were flawed in such a way as to lead to unreliable results.

### Older Women and Breast Cancer

Women older than 65 with breast cancer face different issues than middle-age or younger women. Often doctors are reluctant to treat them as aggressively. Certainly quality of life needs to be considered. However, if a patient is in good health otherwise, there is no reason to deny her the same treatment, such as adjuvant chemotherapy, as women of other ages. Recent studies show the same survival benefits for many treatments for women of all ages.

Of course elderly women are more likely to have other complicating medical conditions that might sway a doctor to recommend a particular treatment. Just be sure to ask the reasons for his recommendations and inquire about other alternatives he has not mentioned.

Older women are likely to be concerned with enjoying their remaining years. This may lead to their refusing treatment because of side effects. Ask thorough questions so you are making a decision based on fact instead of rumor. For instance, if you need assistance walking, you will need to know possible side effects from radiation or chemotherapy.

Self-image may be even more important to older women than healthcare professionals realize. Already they are dealing with sagging breasts, weak muscles, and lined faces. The loss of a breast may just intensify their feelings of worthlessness.

Women in the older generation should take a close friend or family member to appointments where treatment options are discussed because they tend to treat doctors as the final word and may not think to question a recommendation. Some even see no need for a second opinion: If the doctor said it, it's the plan.

Finances can also be a concern for older women on retirement or fixed incomes, as Medicare and insurance probably will not cover all expenses. Check *www.seniors.gov* for eligibility for federal assistance programs. Women living far from family may worry about the availability of caregivers during treatment.

Many communities have resources available. Groups you belong to, such as religious organizations, may also be a support network. Online or phone support groups are very helpful for emotional issues although they cannot address physical needs.

## *Ethnic Groups*

Women of all ethnic groups develop breast cancer. However, some groups have better outcomes than others. For example, non-Hispanic white, Hawaiian, and black women have the highest levels of breast cancer whereas other Asian/Pacific Islanders and Hispanic women have lower levels. Korean and Vietnamese women have the lowest levels of risk. The reasons are unknown, although some studies are investigating this issue.

Breast cancer is the most common cancer among African-American women and the second most common among Caucasian. The five-year survival rate among African-American women with breast cancer is 72 percent and 87 percent among Caucasian women.[10]

| Ethnicity | Incidence/100,000 women[11] | Deaths/100,000 women |
|---|---|---|
| Caucasian | 115.5 | 24.3 |
| African-American | 101.5 | 31.0 |
| Asian/Pacific Islander | 78.1 | 11.0 |
| Hispanics | 68.5 | 14.8 |
| Native Americans | 50.5[12] | 12.4 |

About one-quarter of all women who get breast cancer are younger than 50; however, about one-third of African-American women who get breast cancer are younger than 50. Also, lower income African-Americans who get breast cancer are three times more likely to have an advanced disease than African-Americans in higher income brackets.

Differences in ethnic statistics may depend on a variety of factors. No one is sure yet whether they reflect differences in attitude toward disease, education about cancer, availability of healthcare, or other factors. Regardless, here are some disturbing statistics from 1999:

|  | % Caucasian | % African-American |
|---|---|---|
| Cancer found when still confined to breast | 62 | 50 |
| Cancer found when spread to lymph nodes under arms | 29 | 35 |
| Cancer found when has metastasized | 6 | 9 |
| 5-year survival for localized cancer | 98 | 89 |
| 5-year survival for metastatic disease | 23 | 14 |

One study showed that foreign-born people, particularly Hispanics, Asian-Americans, and Pacific Islanders, were less likely to have cancer screening than people of the same ethnicity born in the United States. Researchers do not know if that is due to unavailability of healthcare in their home countries, different beliefs about healthcare or use of conventional medical practices, or some other factors.

## *Lesbians*

Lesbian women have a greater risk of breast cancer than other women—not because of their sexual practices but because of not bearing children. Most women connect with the healthcare system for reproductive issues, which can lead to detection of other conditions. Because fewer lesbians have children, they may not have routine health checkups as frequently as other women. Of course, checkups do not prevent breast cancer. They may, however, facilitate detection at earlier stages, in which treatment has more favorable results.

To have your unique concerns addressed, be open with your doctor. Ask questions freely and contact cancer organizations for more information about your particular area of concern.

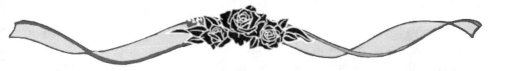

## Chapter 8

# Looking Good

How you look affects how you feel about yourself. Breast cancer treatments can have a major impact on your looks. Not only may you lose a breast, you can lose the hair on your head as well as *all* your body hair, experience dry skin, and not have the energy to apply makeup.

## Appearance

The aspects of appearance you deal with will evolve as you move through your cancer experience.

The goal of grooming during treatment is to make you look as though it's any other day of your life! If you look good, you will feel good about yourself—and that attitude affects your mental, emotional, and physical states as well as the attitudes of those around you.

Two aspects of your appearance that are lost temporarily during treatment are contrast and movement. Your hair contrasts with your skin tone. Your eyebrows contrast with your face. Once your hair is gone, you can add contrasts through innovative and colorful headwear. Texture can also add to the illusion. Pick something sexy such as crepe or suede for evening affairs (maybe in a glittery, shimmering material) and something soft and colorful for casual occasions.

Movement can be mimicked with long, dangling earrings, wigs and hairpieces, and the wavy ends of scarves.

## Bathing

Chemotherapy dries your skin, so choose bath products that add moisture. Choose unscented products, which are less likely to cause allergic reactions or skin irritations or to contain alcohol. Baby skin products such as baby oil are good during chemotherapy because they are so mild.

Try to bathe every day. If necessary, bathe only essential areas such as under arms, feet, and your genital area. If you are too fatigued, attempt a sponge bath while seated on a stool near the bathroom basin. Smelling and feeling fresh will give you a lift.

When undergoing radiation treatment, it is essential that you not wash off any marks your radiotherapist or doctor has made on your skin. They will fade eventually. In the areas being irradiated, use clear, warm water instead of soap or creams. Pat dry gently.

## *Posture*

Whether it's a physically or psychologically motivated act, many women who have had a mastectomy tend to hump their shoulders forward. This posture not only tends to shorten and therefore tighten the pectoral (chest) muscles but also strains the back muscles.

Regaining full range of motion with your arms depends in part on stretching the pectorals, so after surgery be aware of your posture and consciously pull your shoulders back so they are just under your ears. (See "Frozen Shoulder," page 120.)

## *Skin Care*

Because your body's defense mechanism has been compromised by the cancer and by treatments, choose products that are as natural as possible. Any ingredients in skincare products are absorbed through your skin, so try to minimize the chemicals in the products you use. Avoid products with alcohol (any ingredient that ends in "-ol"), which is drying.

If you develop acne from chemotherapy, do not use astringents that contain alcohol. Wash your face with warm water and mild soap.

## Cosmetics

Use unscented cosmetics whenever possible to minimize chemical absorption. Because of concern about the prevalence of estrogen-mimicking chemicals in our environment, some women switch to natural makeup in their new quest for health, seeking brands with no chemicals and only natural substances.

## Moisturizing

Cracked, dry skin is an invitation to infection, and your body does not need to deal with anything else during treatment. Wash with mild soap, creams, or cleansing lotions and lukewarm (not hot) water. Avoid all types of hormone creams (such as those containing hydrocortisone)[1] unless your doctor has approved them.

Keep all your skin well moisturized—from your face to your heels. Apply moisturizers while your skin is still damp to seal in more moisture. Try to avoid activities that make you perspire because you lose moisture through perspiration. If you do perspire, use moisturizer often.

Good options for body moisturizers are:

- Olive oil.
- Soap with moisturizers such as Dove or Cetaphil.
- Creams or moisturizers with aloe vera or vitamin E.
- Eucerin cream/lotion, which has no fragrance.
- Vaseline with vitamin E.
- Aloe skin creams, Nivea cream, cornstarch, Keri soap, or Shower to Shower (for dry, itchy skin).
- Dry oil spritzers to get moisture to hard-to-reach places, such as your back.

### Facial moisturizers

- Mix two to three drops of an essential oil (lilac, lavender, rose, or your favorite scent) in a spray bottle filled with 1 cup of filtered water. Chill overnight. This makes a refreshing spritz for moisture and fragrance.
- Mash meat of an avocado into a bowl and add one egg white as a binder. After washing your face, spread the paste on your face. After 10 to 15 minutes, rinse with cool water.

## Sunscreen

Some chemotherapy drugs and radiation can heighten your skin's sensitivity to sunlight. If so, avoid direct sun as much as possible. If you will be outdoors for any prolonged period during chemotherapy, use sunscreen of at least 15 SPF. An SPF of 30 or a sunblock that does not allow any rays to touch the skin is even better. Choose one that has no PABA, alcohol, or fragrance that could irritate sensitive skin.

During radiation treatment, avoid exposing your treated area to the sun. Do not use sunscreens during treatment unless your doctor agrees.

## Hands/Feet

If you had lymph nodes removed during surgery, you are at risk of developing lymphedema. This condition, which involves swelling, can occur in your hands as well as your arms. Preventing trauma and infection is essential. (See "Lymphedema," page 137.)

To keep your hands and feet soft, lather them well with moisturizer or Vaseline just before bedtime (Bag Balm from feed stores works as well on human hands as on cow udders!). Wear a pair of soft, cotton gloves or socks to bed. In the morning your skin will be as soft as a baby's. This technique is also helpful under gloves when you wash dishes.

Wear gloves when you wash dishes so your hands don't dry out. Use a thimble when you sew. Always use protective gloves when you garden, work with chemicals, or do any other task that could injure your skin.

## Stains

Use lemon slices or lemon juice to remove many stains from your skin so you can avoid harsh chemicals. If that doesn't remove the stain entirely, try a thick paste of water or lemon juice and baking soda. It's magic!

## Scalp

Your scalp may itch or tingle as your hair falls out. For relief try baby powder or Sea Breeze, a soothing astringent. (Refrigerate it for an especially calming effect.)

## Discoloration

Although rare, radiation may cause blotches on the skin in places that were not treated. These may fade or disappear in time. In irradiated areas "spider veins" may appear. If these show and you are bothered by them, use a thick foundation to cover them.

## Makeup

The most important factor in applying makeup during cancer treatment is cleanliness because your immune system is already weak and overtaxed. To minimize the risk of infection, wash your hands before applying cosmetics. Apply makeup with clean cotton swabs, cotton balls, or makeup sponges. Apply powdered cosmetics with brushes or sponge-tipped applicators that you wash frequently. Avoid sharing cosmetics.

Keep makeup containers tightly closed and replace on the manufacturer's schedule to help prevent infection. When shopping for cosmetics, apply test samples to your hands or wrist rather than to your face.

## Basic Makeup

Choose a foundation with a minimum SPF of 15. Not all foundations have this added feature, so shop carefully.

Choose a foundation color that best matches your normal skin tone to even out your complexion. Choose a moisturizing foundation if your skin is dry. Set the foundation with a light application of translucent powder.

Temporary weight gain or loss due to chemotherapy is especially visible in your face. Blush is the best and easiest way to produce a vibrant, healthy glow. Brush a light coating of blush over your cheekbones and out toward your ears. Brown-tone powder can hide puffiness due to weight gain; light-colored concealer cream can make thin facial areas appear fuller.

## Eyebrows

If your eyebrows have fallen out, re-create them using the following steps and two shades of eye pencil. The goal is to duplicate your natural eyebrow arch. Short feathery strokes will give the most natural look. To understand what you are trying to achieve, look at a close-up photograph of yourself taken before treatment.

- Hold an eye pencil straight up along your nose, parallel to the inside corner of your eye, and place a dot just above the brow bone. This is where the eyebrow should begin.

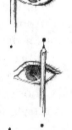

- Hold the pencil so that it's in line with the outer edge of your iris (the colored part of your eye) and the middle of your brow. Put a dot here to locate the highest point of the eyebrow.

- Hold the pencil at an angle from the outside corner of your nose to the outside corner of your eye, and place another dot on the bottom of your brow bone. Be sure the outer edge of the brow is not lower than the inside edge.

- Using an eye pencil (or eye shadow with an angled brush) the color of your natural eyebrows and another one to two shades lighter, connect the dots with short feathery strokes. Most brown eye shadows look darker on your skin than they do in their case. Make the brow fuller at the inner corner and thinner at the outer corner.

## Eyelids

Eye shadow can brighten your eyes and thus add sparkle to your entire face. Try using three complementary colors for a stunning effect. Apply the lightest shade just below the arch of the brow. Apply the primary accent color across the entire lid. Add a deeper shade in the crease for emphasis. Soften by blending the colors where they meet.

Occasionally chemotherapy drugs can cause allergic reactions to the eyes. If this happens, do not use eye shadow or eyeliner. No law says you have to use blush only on your cheeks. Powdered blush can serve as a good base on your eyelids too. One light stroke of the blush brush across your forehead, when you've finished your cheeks, will give your face a warm glow.

Eyeliner can help re-create the look of full lashes. Use liquid or pencil. Draw thin lines along the upper and lower lids.

Cetaphil makes a good eye-makeup remover. It won't sting your eyes and does not leave any oil behind.

Dark colors make a feature recede. Lighter colors bring it out. Brown or grey eyeliner gives a softer effect than black. For a still softer look, stop the liner at the corner of the eye.

To make close-set eyes appear farther apart, thicken your eyeliner at the outer corners of your eyes.

False eyelashes that have been trimmed and thinned are another solution to losing your own lashes. As your eyelashes thin, apply mascara to the top and underside of your lashes for a fuller look. Mascara wands can be breeding grounds for bacteria so change yours about every six weeks to avoid infection.

## Lips

Your lips may dry out along with other parts of your body during treatment. Apply lip moisturizer frequently during the day. If you are outdoors for longer than 15 minutes, apply sunscreen to your lips.

Outline your lips with a soft lip liner in a color that complements your lipstick to prevent your lipstick color from "bleeding" or spreading unevenly.

Choose a lipstick from the same color family as your blush. Use a creamy, moisturizing formula.

## Scars

Scars take a long time to disappear, if they ever do. In the meantime you can minimize their appearance by:

- Using scar cover-up makeup sold at better department stores. One brand is Covermark. Check with your doctor before using this type of product.
- Moisturizing and massaging the area with the oil from a vitamin E capsule or aloe vera gel.
- Applying an aromatherapy mixture for three months. Do not use this until your surgeon declares the surgical area healed. Mix 10 drops of frankincense essential oil (to rejuvenate skin) and 10 drops of lavender essential oil (to stimulate cell turnover) with 1 ounce of jojoba oil (to aid absorption) in a small glass bottle. Shake well before use. Coat the scar area twice a day with the mixture and gently massage it into the skin. Store in a cool, dry place for up to six months.
- Applying Mederma, a natural over-the-counter gel made from onions. Massage onto scar two to three times a day for two months.[2]

## Nails

Nails are another body part that can be affected by chemotherapy. They can become brittle, grooved, or discolored; become more sensitive; crack easily; or even fall off. Take care of them, not only for their appearance but because they offer protection for your fingertips and toes. Toenails are rarely a problem because they are less exposed to the environment than fingernails.

During chemotherapy:

- Notify your doctor if you notice redness or other sign of infection around the cuticles or if a nail falls off. It may take six months to grow back.
- Avoid fake nails. The adhesive may worsen your nails' condition.
- You can use nail polish to keep nails strong; however the remover can make the nails more brittle. Use an oily remover.
- Keep nails clean, dry, and trimmed to avoid snagging them on something and tearing them.
- Moisturize the nail bed daily with a cream.
- Protect nails with gloves during all tasks involving chemicals or risks of infection.
- If you get a manicure, inform your manicurist of your need for extreme sanitation and avoidance of injury to the nails or cuticles.

## Hair Loss

To many women, the loss of their hair is more profoundly depressing than treatments for breast cancer. Perhaps it is because the loss is so visible. The loss of a breast is hidden by clothing most of the time, but our hair frames our face and to some extent expresses who we are. (See "Hair Loss," page 123.)

## Headwear

Yes, it's emotionally difficult to lose your hair during chemotherapy. For a few days it may even be devastating. But cheer up! There are some colorful, stylish replacements for your hair until it grows back—and it will almost every time (except when the head area has been irradiated).

You can choose turbans, wigs, scarves, or hats—and have fun mixing them for various occasions. One motto for appropriate headwear is "cool, comfortable, covers." Be sure it is cool and comfortable to wear and that it covers your scalp. A bare scalp in the winter chills the rest of your body, and a sunburned scalp in the summer is very inconvenient, to say nothing of painful.

## Where to Find Headwear

Shop for headwear in specialty shops, in catalogs, and on the Internet (see Resources). You also can find soft and inexpensive hats or turbans at department stores.

## Turbans/Head Wraps

Turbans are a quick, easy head cover for days you don't feel well or don't want to bother with a wig. You can also purchase special soft sleep caps, made without a back seam, to keep your head warm on cold nights.

Natural fabrics such as cotton knits are the best for head wraps because they breathe and are washable. Have at least two so you can wash one and wear the other to remove perspiration from your head. Remember that, even in fashion, cleanliness is paramount during cancer treatment.

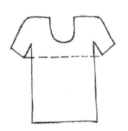

One of the tricks of the Look Good...Feel Better program of the American Cancer Society is the T-shirt turban. Cut off a T-shirt (get outrageous with the colors!) at the armpits. Use the bottom tube. Place the hemmed edge on your forehead and over your head. With both hands pull the T-shirt back on both sides. Make a figure eight with your hands in the back and pull the T-shirt up over your head. Voila! An instant turban.

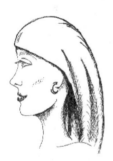
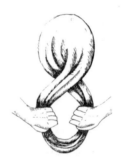
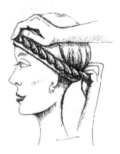

You can also tie a 38-inch scarf or bandanna around your head for a quick wrap.

Dress up any turban with a scarf fashioned into a band, rope coil, bow, or rosette.

## Headliners

Many women's health boutiques carry a turban-style scarf called a head-liner that covers the head and has slots for front and back hairpieces. You can use this combination in place of a wig.

## Wearing tips[3]

- Wear a head wrap 1 inch below your natural hairline. Wearing it too far down your face ages you.
- To avoid the flat head look, slide a soft shoulder pad under your cap.
- To make a head wrap cooler in the summer, stuff it with soft tissue to absorb perspiration.
- To add a sense of movement and the illusion of hair, wear dangling earrings with your head wrap.
- Create interest by layering your headwear with scarves or hats.
- Distract from your head wrap by wearing a scarf that matches or complements your outfit.
- Choose bright colors, which brighten your face.
- To make a head wrap smaller, fold a cuff around the ends.
- Avoid very tight turbans. Your scalp needs to breathe to prevent irritating the tender skin.

### Basic turban look

Make your own turban by folding a scarf in half to form a triangle. Now slide the fold up about a third of the way, giving you a shorter triangle overlapping a longer triangle. Tie around your head.

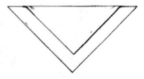

## Hats

You can go as casual or as formal as you like with hats. Choose a jaunty yachting cap or a relaxed baseball cap or a high-fashion felt or suede fedora. In the summertime straw or denim hats are fashionable, and you'll have others wanting to copy your stylish looks.

You can find some hats in specialty stores with hairpieces such as bangs, a ponytail, or a bob permanently attached.

### Wearing tips

- If a hat is too large, glue a band of foam inside for a closer fit.
- To dress up a plain hat, wrap a scarf around the band. Either tie it into a bow or let the scarf hang loose to simulate hair.

## Scarves

Scarves are an easy and colorful alternative or complement to wigs and turbans. Although any size and shape can be used, a 36- to 40-inch square is best. Rayon is the best fabric. It drapes nicely, clings to your head, and is washable. There are different types of rayon, some of which are not comfortable to wear. Rub the fabric against your wrist. If it feels soft there, it will feel good against your scalp. If it feels rough, don't buy it.

Wool challis has the same advantages although it may be scratchy. Cotton is another good choice, especially in hot weather. Silk won't stay on your head or hold knots tightly, but it makes a fashionable second layer. Polyester and other synthetics are slippery and may not stay on your head. Also they are hot in warm weather.

### Basic scarf techniques

- Lay a square scarf (36- to 40-inch square) with the wrong side facing you. Fold into a triangle and place the fold on your forehead about an inch below your natural hairline. Cuff the front an inch if you like. Tie the ends over the triangle point and in a square knot (right over left, left over right, and pull) in back. Pull any excess scarf from under the knot to give an illusion of fullness at the back of your head. Wear the scarf with the ends loose or tie in a classy bow.

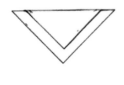 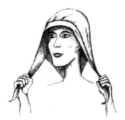 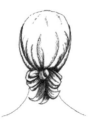

- For a different look, pull the scarf point over the knot and tuck securely in the back of the knot to resemble a bun. Take one end of the scarf at a time and coil and wrap around the bun knot. Tuck the ends of each tie securely through the center of the rosette you have created.

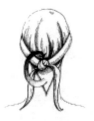 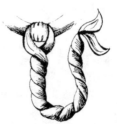 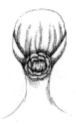

## Wearing tips

- Place the edge of the scarf approximately two finger widths above your eyebrow.
- Cut the tag or label off the scarf so you don't have to fuss with hiding it.
- After you have tied the scarf ends into a knot, tuck in the little ends for a smoother, finished look.
- Choose a color that blends with your outfit. An exact match is not necessary. Two patterns in the same color scheme can be attractive.
- Wear a scarf under a hat for a classy look.

## Fashion tricks with scarves

- Scarves with fringe feel good against your cheeks and neck and give the impression of hair.
- Fasten a long scarf into your turban. Twist each end into a rope. Wrap one end into a bun at the back of your neck. Wrap the other end around the first. Tuck the ends into the folds to hide them. You can move the bun to one side of your head or to your forehead and slip a visor under it.

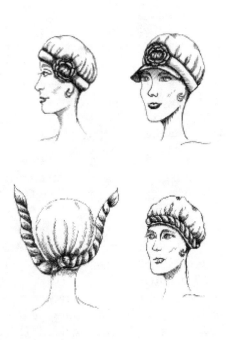

- Slip a long scarf (or one you have folded into a long rectangle) through the turban or knot at the back of your head. Twist each end of the scarf into a rope. Bring both ends to the top of your head. Depending on the length of the scarf, tie a knot there or cross the ends and take them back down to your neck and tie them there. In either case tuck the loose ends under the folds to hide them.
- Dress scarves up with pins, a man's tie, ribbons, artificial flowers, a fabric belt, or a hat.
- Sew several bandanas together to have a scarf big enough to work with.
- Buy pretty fabric at fabric stores and either hem the ends or just tuck them under.

# Wigs

If you will need a wig, buy it before you begin chemotherapy. A stylist can more easily match your style and color before your hair begins to fall out (although this is a chance to experiment on a new color or style—or several!). Also, you are more likely to feel well enough to get out and shop before treatment begins.

## Insurance issues

Some insurance companies will pay for a wig, although they may have a limit on what they pay. You will need a doctor's prescription for a "cranial prosthesis" (no kidding!).

Ask if you must purchase your wig from certain stores or providers. If not, ask your doctor or nurse for names of suppliers (or see Resources).

Any out-of-pocket cost not covered by insurance may be tax-deductible (depending on your tax status).

## Free wigs

If insurance does not cover a wig and you cannot afford one, check with your doctor's nurse or social work department at your hospital about services that provide free wigs in your community. Some major cancer centers and some chapters of the American Cancer Society (ACS) provide free wigs.

Also, some support groups have access to free wigs. When you have finished treatment and want to dump your wigs and headwear, consider donating them to a support group or your ACS chapter to continue the cycle.

## Types of wigs

The most important characteristics you want in a wig are a natural look, a proper fit, and a comfortable feel. After that you may consider price and care.

Nowadays most synthetic wigs look very much like human hair. The synthetics are available in a wider range of colors and styles. Most wigs can be adjusted to fit most head sizes. Comfort, then, becomes the biggest variable in a wig purchase.

The feel of a wig is largely determined by the material used in the base and the method of attaching the hair to that base. Handmade wigs usually have fibers hand sewn into a cap. These wigs are easily styled and lightweight. Machine-made wigs have fibers sewn into a cap in a process that may make the wig stiff and uncomfortable. Some wigs substitute a mesh lace or "artificial skin" for the cap. These are usually lightweight and flexible.

Another type of wig is called monofilament. This type gives the appearance of real hair as each filament is tied into a fine mesh base. This design offers ventilation and comfort and makes the hair look as if it is growing out of your scalp. The wig is easily styled and parted in any direction. This type is available in both synthetic and human hair wigs. A monofilament remy human hair wig is at the top of the line for comfort, flexibility of styling, and natural appearance.

| Types of Wigs | | |
|---|---|---|
| **Type** | **Advantages** | **Disadvantages** |
| Machine-made synthetic | • Washes out and dries overnight as hose do. <br>• Holds up under adverse weather conditions. <br>• Often cooler and lighter in weight. <br>• Less expensive ($50–150). | • Style cannot change except to have it cut or taken in to fit better. <br>• The fibers can melt if they get too close to heat (such as an oven). <br>• Can look artificial. <br>• Can be warm to wear. May not fit well. |
| Hand-tied custom synthetic | • Custom-fitted. <br>• Natural look. <br>• Lighter weight and cooler. | • More expensive ($600–900). <br>• Limited sources. |
| Grade B human hair (made from Asian hair) | • Can be customized by color and texture. <br>• Looks and feels like real hair. <br>• Blends well (through attachments, bangs, etc.) with any hair you still have. <br>• Available in wide variety of styles and colors. <br>• Can be styled many ways. <br>• Can be styled by yourself or a professional. | • If machine-made, is perhaps less comfortable. <br>• Not amenable to dying or perming. <br>• Can be more expensive ($100–600). <br>• Must be restyled after every washing, as human hair does. |
| Grade A human hair (European HH) | • Can be customized by color and texture. <br>• Often looks more natural. <br>• Style can be changed. <br>• Hand-tied onto lightweight mesh base so is cooler. <br>• May be dyed or permed. | • More expensive ($500–3,000). <br>• Fragile due to hand-tied hair and lightweight. <br>• Must be styled by a professional after each washing. |

## Wig measurement

You will be happier with your wig if you try it on before you buy it. However, if you order online or from a catalog, compare three measurements to the company's sizing chart:

- Around your head. Starting at your forehead, wrap a tape measure around your natural hairline to just above your ear, around the back along the bend of your neck, just above the other ear, then to the place where you began.
- Front to back. Measure from your natural hairline in front, over the crown of your head to where your head meets the top of your neck.
- Ear to ear. Measure from in front of one ear where the hairline ends, over the crown, and to the front of the other ear.

## Wig styling and sizing

- Besides full-cap wigs, you can purchase partial fill-ins, bang fringes, and attachments.
- If a wig is too full or too long, a hair dresser can thin or shorten it. Have the cutting done while the wig is on your head. Do not leave the wig with a stylist to be adjusted solo.
- Some wigs have open ear tabs to facilitate wearing glasses.
- Some wigs have permanent lift or tease, meaning they are specially made for lasting volume.
- Some wigs have Velcro bands for adjusting the circumference up to 1 inch.
- Some wigs have a comfort band around the front rim for softness next to your skin.
- Use a wire brush for straight styles and a pick for curly styles. Standard brushes can damage the fragile wig filaments.

## Wig accessories

- **Wig cap.** You can buy a wig cap to make your wig fit snugly or make your own using a queen-size knee-high stocking. Knot the end and place it on your head. Don't worry about the knot on top; it will add some fullness under your scarf, turban, or wig. It may also reduce irritation from the wig base.
- **Wig stand or head form.** This keeps your wig styled while you are not wearing it.
- **Wig grip.** This soft band that fits around the perimeter of your wig keeps it from touching your head where it binds. It's nice for sensitive skin.
- **Wig shampoo, conditioner, and hair spray.** Use brands especially made for wig fibers.

- **Wig pins or chin strap.** These hold the wig onto the styling stand so you have both hands to work with.
- **Wig carrying case.** This is nice for traveling when you won't be wearing your wig all the time and want to preserve the style. However, you can just as easily place the wig in a plastic bag in a suitcase.

## Wig care

These common-sense precautions will extend the life of your wig:

- Take your wig to your hairstylist or the store where it was purchased for styling. Be sure the stylist has experience with wigs. A mistake in cutting will not grow out!
- Wash your wig after six to eight wearings in warm weather and 12 to 15 in cool weather. If you are very active, wash it once a week to remove perspiration.
- Before washing your wig, brush it gently or use a pick to remove tangles and teasing. Wash in cool or lukewarm water (see your manufacturer's recommendation). Use a special wig shampoo and conditioner. Wigs can dry out if washed too often.
- Add a capful of wig shampoo to a basin of water. Saturate the wig and gently dip it up and down. Do not rub or soak for more than two to three minutes.
- For shine and softness, apply wig conditioner for five minutes.
- Rinse in clear water and gently squeeze out excess water. Hang and gently blot with a towel. Air dry. For curly styles, gently squeeze curls while hair is damp. When dry, gently shake the wig and brush back into its original style. Synthetic wigs will naturally return to their original shape.
- Do not brush synthetic wigs while wet unless you are completely restyling them. Do not use a hair dryer or curling iron or dry in direct sunlight. Do not stand in front of an open oven door or the wig may frizz. This may also happen over a steaming pot of food on your stove or any similar heat source.

# Be Bold: Go Bald

Whereas some women won't even go to the kitchen without tissue stuffed in their bra, others would rather stay in their room than appear in anyone's presence without a wig or head wrap. What you decide is up to you.

It is not unusual to see women these days wearing closely shaved hairstyles. If you choose to leave your shiny scalp showing, do it with flair. Consider wearing big, bold, colorful earrings for contrast with your skin. You might don a hat occasionally for a change of pace. Have fun with your new look.

At the same time, realize that those around you may not be as cavalier about a woman's bald head as you are. You'll have to decide what to do. The people in the grocery store have no emotional ties to you, so you don't have to consider their feelings. Those who see you a lot will soon get used to your smile beneath the bald; however, your professional life may demand a more classic look.

If someone you care about has not heard that bald is beautiful, you must decide whether or not to cover up when you are around her. Yes, the cancer is your crisis, but everyone who knows you is affected by it. If your bald head makes someone very uncomfortable, consider your options:

1. Covering it when she is around.
2. Trying to humor her into accepting your new look.
3. Ignoring her discomfort because it's your "right" to dress as you please.

Only you know the relationship you have with that person and how this decision will affect it.

Although you may look different on the outside, remember that you are the same, and maybe even wiser, on the inside than before your cancer diagnosis. There are lots of tricks to take attention off those areas that have changed or don't look the way you want them to.

Looks are not the defining criteria for who you are and what people enjoy about you. Hold your head high, and people will look into your eyes and see courage and hope. You'll begin to see it also in your reflection in the mirror, right above a genuine smile.

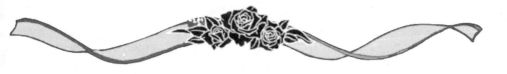

*Chapter 9*

# Getting Back in "Shape"

Once treatment is over or manageable, many women are ready to "get back to normal." Of course, the "new" normal is different from the "old" normal, but the longing for normalcy is valid and healthy.

There are many products available today to help you look the way you did before surgery, and every day research is identifying lifestyle options that can support your desire to be healthier.

## Clothing
### Breast Forms

Breast forms, or breast prostheses, are a viable alternative to reconstruction. Made from materials that approximate natural tissue in weight, feel, and movement, forms are available in a wide variety of materials, weight, shapes, colors, and sizes. Most forms are made from silicone or polyurethane, a few have rubber or polyester pellets, and others are mostly fiberfill to accommodate tenderness. Some forms have side extensions that gently taper the area between your breast and your underarm. You can even buy nipples separately and attach them to the forms or your skin, although most forms have nipples as part of their design.

Take someone with you to the fitting who will tell you honestly whether a particular size or shape matches your remaining breast under your clothing or whether the form complements your overall size and posture. My friend Bonnie did this for me, and I referred to her as my Bosom Buddy thereafter. Have your friend check for centering, placement, and matching the shape of both breasts. You might have fun and buy swim forms of one size and another size for everyday wear.

When you shop for forms, wear a shape-revealing garment, perhaps a sweater, so you can know exactly what your shape might be. Wear the bra in which you plan to wear the forms. Comparison shop (unless insurance limits your choice of stores) because not all stores carry all brands. The price of the form has little to do with how it suits you.

## Considerations for choosing breast prostheses

- To match darker complexions, ask for colored prostheses and foam covers or dye yours using strong coffee or tea or fabric dye such as Rit in brown shades.
- A fabric backing on a form generally makes it cooler to wear in hot weather.
- A seamless backing prevents irritation to your skin.
- If you have had a lumpectomy, look for fillers or enhancers to fill out your profile. Shells can compensate for breasts of unequal size. Most fitting shops can produce custom enhancers to correct any problem.
- Some forms have a back pocket that can be filled with fiberfill for a flexible amount of fullness.
- For even balance and posture, choose a prosthesis that approximates the weight of your real breast.

## Types of breast forms

Basically there are two types of forms: those that adhere to your chest and those that slip into a special pocket in a bra.

| Pros and Cons of Each Type | |
|---|---|
| **Attachable Prosthesis** | **Non-Attachable Prosthesis** |
| Moves with you | Don't have ongoing cost of patches |
| Weight is shared by shoulder and skin | Weight carried by shoulder only |
| Can be worn with any bra and with most formal wear; works well under lingerie | Large prostheses cannot detach with normal wear or in water |
| Warm in hot weather | Not warm in hot weather; does not affect sensitive skin; can be worn swimming |

Prostheses that adhere to your body are held to the skin with gel adhesives. They should be fluid in back to hug the unlevel chest wall and soft in front. You do not need a special bra with these forms. Though these breast forms give you the option of going braless, they can be hot and uncomfortable in the summer. Some of these attach by surgical tape or by Velcro to a soft adhesive-backed cloth patch. These patches last about five to14 days.

Breast forms that slide into special bra pockets are made from foam, fiberfill, or silicone gel. The lightweight foam or fiberfill is ideal for postsurgical weeks when you may be tender in that area and for swimming. If possible, try one on before you buy. The unweighted ones may tend to ride up as you move your arms.

Silicone prostheses are almost impossible to distinguish from the real thing under clothing. You can also pay (handsomely!) for a custom-made breast form, cast to fit your chest wall and to match your remaining breast. Some insurance companies do not pay for these.

## Care of breast prostheses

To make your breast prosthesis last:

- Wash as needed in warm water and mild soap. Do not use perfumed or deodorant soaps. Gently pat it dry immediately afterward. Buildup from perspiration, body acids, oils, perfume, bath powders, and so forth, over an extended time, could deteriorate the form's skin and reduce its life. Attachable prostheses need water to reactivate the stickiness.

- Remove jewelry from your hands before washing your prosthesis. The edges of rings and stones could damage the form.

- Do not drop or crush your breast form. It might break open. However, do not be afraid to hug while wearing it!

- To maintain its shape, store your prosthesis in its shaped box when you are not wearing it.

- Avoid getting close to heat for long periods.

- If you wear a name tag or jewelry on your bodice that fastens with a pin, place it on your clothing before you put the garment on. A tiny pin prick can weaken the prosthesis and cause it to split over time.

- Be careful playing with pets. A kitten's claws could puncture the form through your clothing.

- Salt water, hot tubs, and swimming pool water can damage silicone prostheses over time. Buy an inexpensive set for swimming or the beach.

To get your forms to fit naturally in your bra, after you fasten your bra, lean forward slightly, grab the bra at the bottom just below and at the outside of each cup, and gently jiggle the bra. The forms will settle into the center of the pockets at just the right angle.

Heavy prostheses may require a bra shoulder pad under the bra straps for comfort. Weighted postsurgical forms are available for large-breasted women.

### Make your own forms

If you prefer to create your own prosthesis, you can make a cup to fit your bra cup (order American Cancer Society's free *Mastectomy: A Patient Guide*, publication 97-75M-No. 4600-CC) and fill it with Dacron or polyester fill from a crafts or sewing store. Cotton quilt batting will be more comfortable in hot weather. Use drapery weights or fishing sinkers to give weight so it will not ride up as you move. Be aware that the weights could set off metal detectors at airports.

Lightweight forms could result in the bra strap pulling toward the middle of your chest. To prevent that, pin the strap to the shoulder seam of your garment.

## Lingerie

After breast cancer surgery, many women struggle with feeling feminine. Whether you choose reconstruction or not, do pamper yourself with feminine lingerie to enhance a feeling of wholeness and femininity. Lacy mastectomy bras are harder to find, but they are worth the extra trouble. Many women are surprised at the emotional lift they get from knowing they are wearing lace, even if no one can see it.

Special garments are made to accommodate breast prostheses, including bras with side pockets, camisoles (some have the forms already inserted and others have a pocket), and nightgowns. Breast forms slide into the side pockets of the garment and do not touch your skin. Some department store lingerie departments carry a soft bra, sometimes called a leisure or night bra, that some women like to wear under a gown. It is more comfortable for sleeping than a regular bra.

### Tips for proper mastectomy bra fit

- A properly weighted form will anchor your bra and prevent it from riding up.
- A properly fitted bra should not bind the chest too tightly. Your bra should feel as one did before surgery.

- A higher price does not necessarily mean a better bra.
- If your chest is tender after surgery, a bra extender can ease the pressure on that area.
- Some department stores will help fit you with a bra and even sew in a pocket to hold the prosthesis.
- Check with your doctor about wearing an underwire bra. You do not want the wire to rub the area near surgery.

## Special Bras

Leisure bras and lightweight breast forms are available for wear right after surgery when your chest is too tender for a normal bra. Mary Jane surgical bras are prescribed by many plastic surgeons following reconstruction. Another option for postreconstruction is Frederick's Mammary Support by Jobst, which claims to reduce the need for surgical dressings and helps minimize scar tissue formation and postoperative swelling. It also holds surgical implants firmly in place and eliminates the danger of adhesive tape burn. The adjustable Velcro closures at the shoulders support the implants. Both of these bras are available in surgical shops.

## Swimwear

Of course you can swim after breast cancer surgery! You can purchase special mastectomy swimsuits with higher-cut necks and arms and lightweight breast forms that will give you a nice silhouette and will not ride up in the water.

You can also sew a pocket for your own swimsuit and fill it with old nylon stockings or fish tank filter for an aquarium. Be cautious of using sleep forms in swimsuits. They can ride up or even float out of the pocket!

## Insurance Tips

Check with your insurance company before you shop for breast forms and mastectomy bras. Have your doctor write a prescription for both. Many plans pay for two mastectomy bras every year and prostheses every two years.

Your part of the cost of breast forms and mastectomy bras may be tax-deductible. Check with your tax advisor about the deductibility of related expenses, such as having bras altered to fit a prosthesis. When you purchase either a bra or form, have invoices and any check you write marked "surgical" to facilitate income tax deductions.

Medicare and Medicaid cover some of the expense for bras and prostheses for eligible women.

## Exercise

The "conveniences" of modern life have robbed many of us of opportunities for physical activity. Think of indoor plumbing vs. hauling buckets of water inside, scrubbing boards and hanging clothing on line to dry (230 calories burned per hour) vs. washing machines and hanging clothes to dry (140 calories per hour) vs. automatic washer and dryer (120 calories per hour), or beating rugs and scrubbing floors (325 calories per hour) vs. using a vacuum cleaner (150 calories per hour) vs. hiring a cleaning service (0 calories).[1] Yet physical activity has been linked to lower risks for breast cancer.

This could be because exercise turns body fat into lean tissue. Fat produces estrogen and other hormones. After menopause, conversion of some hormones into estrogen happens mostly in fat tissue. Women who gain 20 or more pounds in their adult years have a 50–100 percent increased risk for developing breast cancer than those who have carried excess weight since childhood.[2] The American Cancer Society released findings from a large study of breast cancer and weight in the spring of 2004. The study showed that women who gained 20–30 pounds after high-school graduation were 40 percent more likely to develop breast cancer than those who maintained a stable weight.

Exercise forces the body to burn excess fat and its accompanying hormones.[3] The optimum range for cancer prevention is from 10 percent below ideal body weight to 10 percent above. A study from the University of Southern California showed that only four hours of physical exercise a week could reduce a young woman's risk of breast cancer by 50 percent.[4] This could be because aerobic exercise can alter menstrual patterns and thus modify the production of hormones by the ovaries. Overexposure to ovarian hormones is being researched as a risk factor in breast cancer.

A small study from the University of Alberta tested participants' immune functions before and after a 15-week program involving 35 minutes of exercise three times a week. Natural killer cell activity was elevated. Insulin-like growth factor (IGF1), which can cause cells to grow and divide, was reduced in the exercising groups and not in the control group. The study points to the need for more research into whether exercise can affect molecular factors of tumor growth.[5]

Although physical activity may be the last thing you feel like doing, it may be one of the best things to get you back to your normal routine. With a condition such as breast cancer, there is a fine line between pushing yourself and listening to your body's limits. If you are fatigued, more strenuous activity will only make you feel worse, but some exercise will increase your energy.

Be aware of the many benefits of even mild exercise and begin incorporating short walks or other activities into your day as soon as you can. The Center for Disease Control emphasizes that it's never too late to begin exercise and reap its benefits. Some benefits of exercise are:

- It stimulates the appetite.
- It gets you in the fresh air, which has a soothing effect.
- It enhances well-being by stimulating chemicals in the brain that assist in the healing process. It also promotes a healthy immune system.
- It helps with weight loss.
- It lowers blood pressure and cholesterol and improves circulation.
- It reduces stress.
- It lifts depression.
- Aerobic exercise (swimming, biking, brisk walking) can modify the amount of hormones the ovaries produce.
- It helps you sleep more soundly.
- It helps you concentrate more fully.
- It can improve your sex life and your social life.
- It helps move the bowels.
- It strengthens the bones.
- It reduces your risk of many diseases including some cancers, cardiovascular disease, obesity, diabetes, osteoporosis, and arthritis.
- It gives you a sense of accomplishment.

After getting approval from your doctor, do some mild exercise every day. Start slow and gradually increase your time and intensity. A good first goal is 10 minutes of stretching, muscle strengthening, or cardiovascular exercise. Rotate these three kinds of exercise. Ralph S. Paffenbarger Jr., M.D., a Stanford University scientist, says, "You don't have to be a marathon runner. However, there is a need to be up on your feet, moving about and using the large muscles every day."[6]

Studies have shown that regular exercise, even if for short periods (10 to 20 minutes), was more beneficial than lengthy exercise less often. Also, those who exercise regularly have lower incidences of cancer and other diseases than those who don't. Fitness experts are suggesting that three 10-minute sessions of exercise four days a week will give significant health benefits. The National Institute on Aging reports that after just two weeks some of the effects of endurance or muscle-building exercise begin to deteriorate if you cut back substantially.[7]

## What Is Exercise?

Is all exercise puffing and sweating? Not necessarily. Exercise is moving your muscles and body. This can be walking from the bedroom to the kitchen or skiing down the black slopes.

**Mild exercise** can include gardening, housework, leisurely cycling, and walking.

**Moderate exercise** can include dancing, water aerobics, brisk walking, washing a car, pushing a stroller, jumping rope, volleyball, basketball, or shoveling snow.

**Strenuous exercise** can include biking, participant sports, running/jogging, or swimming.

Obviously how you participate in these activities determines the level of exercise you do. If you cut roses and stoop to pull a weed or two, that is mild exercise. If you trim the hedges, mow the lawn, and spread fertilizer, that is strenuous exercise.

A study published in *Medicine & Science in Sports & Exercise* in September 2001 concluded that being physically active reduces the risk of breast cancer. The study reported that the frequency and duration of physical activity were more important than intensity. The greatest reduction in risk of developing breast cancer came from moderate intensity occupational or household activity, such as doing laundry or gardening.[8]

Remember that some types of exercise may put you at risk for lymphedema. Weight lifting, repetitive pulling on a rowing machine, and some resistance exercises (such as gardening) may not be recommended. Any increase in your level of exercise should be attempted very slowly. Check with your surgeon, oncologist, or a physical therapist or personal trainer who is familiar with lymphedema.

## When Not to Exercise

If you have any of the following symptoms, do not exercise until you have consulted with your doctor:

- Irregular pulse or resting pulse higher than 100 beats per minute.
- Leg pain or cramps.
- Chest pain.
- Fever.
- Anemia.
- Shortness of breath.
- Unusual fatigue, faintness, or weakness.
- Mental confusion/disorientation.

- Blurred vision.
- Dizziness.
- Recent bone, back, or neck pain.

# I Don't Have Time to Exercise!

That's a common complaint (or excuse?). The three to four hours a week that is recommended is less than 2 percent of your week. The benefits are worth finding the time. You can add bits of exercise into your day in ways you won't even recognize after a while. Try these tips:

- Park farther from the door of the store. If the store is a few blocks away, walk instead of driving.
- Take the long route to the water cooler, restroom, or the building cafeteria.
- Get off the bus one stop early and walk that extra distance.
- Use stairs instead of the elevator.
- Take a walk on your lunch break.
- Enter a charity walk with a friend.
- When you go outside to pick up the newspaper, walk around the block first.
- Decide to walk 10 minutes; then see if you can stretch that to 15 or 20.

Some people have found a pedometer to be an easy way to monitor their exercise. The Centers for Disease Control and Prevention recommends walking 10,000 steps a day, or roughly five miles.[9] Strap a pedometer onto your waist and see what your typical day entails. Then think of creative ways to increase that amount.

# Ways to Work Exercise into Your Lifestyle

- Choose something you enjoy—whether gardening, biking, hiking, dancing, swimming, water aerobics, walking, skiing, tennis, and so on.
- Find a companion to exercise with. Having someone else depending on you is a great motivator. You might even assign family members a day of the week to take a walk with you. Not only will this get you moving, it will give you special time with that person.
- Sign up for a class. When you have put money on the table, you are more likely to work the activity into your schedule. The closer you are to your gym, the more likely you are to go on a regular basis.
- If cost is a factor in your exercise choices, walk, use community resources, buy used equipment, join a YWCA instead of a gym, rent exercise videos from the public library, or buy used videos at garage sales or on the Internet.

- For a quick workout at home, use a 1-pound can of food for weights or turn on your favorite music and dance or move for 10 minutes.
- If you travel a lot, stay at hotel chains that have fitness rooms or swimming pools, take a walk during breaks in meetings, do floor exercises in your room, or take a resistance band or travel weights that fill with water. While you wait for your flight, walk around the airport instead of sitting. Find out if the hotel has VCRs in the room and, if so, take an exercise tape.

## Types of Exercise

Exercises can be categorized different ways. Mainly there are three types of exercise you should work in every week: strength training, cardiovascular (aerobic) workout, and stretching. With a mixture of all these you will be on your way to improving the five components of fitness for women vulnerable to bone loss: posture, flexibility, balance, strength, and endurance.

**Strength training** does not give you Popeye arms. It does protect and strengthen your bones. The *Journal of the American Medical Association* reported that strength training is the only exercise that can reverse loss of lean body mass or bone density.[10] Strength training also fortifies muscle fibers. Muscles burn five to 10 times more calories per pound than fat, regardless of the type of exercise.

As with any exercise program, start slow with light weights and work up gradually. Choose a weight that offers slight resistance and do eight to 12 repetitions. If you can't do that many, reduce the weight. Do exercises that focus on upper and lower body and alternate strength training with another form of exercise on consecutive days.

**Aerobic exercise** not only strengthens your lungs and heart, but it helps regulate mood swings, reduces stress, and promotes general well-being. A good goal is 15 to 40 minutes four times a week. Exercises such as jogging, cycling, walking, stair climbing, and aerobic dance fall in this category.

**Stretching** can be done in as little as five minutes a day. Its benefits include extending your range of motion, improving flexibility, and reducing stress. Unless you have a tape to follow, you can simply stretch each set of muscles and hold for 20 seconds. Stop the stretch if you reach a point of pain.

## Walking

Walking is the most popular exercise because it can be done in any setting (urban or rural), at almost any time, and without the constraints of cost, finding classes, obtaining equipment, and so forth. All you need is well-fitting, sturdy shoes. Begin by just doing it!

After you have walked a few days, you can hone your program with the following tips:

- Schedule the times on your calendar. Aim for 30 minutes three times a week. You can break the time into two 15-minute or three 10-minute sessions with the same effect.
- Have a plan for inclement weather: a nearby mall, a route in your house, and so on.
- Pick a safe place with level ground and clean air if possible. Choose a place that is well lit. Carry a cell phone or whistle. Be careful wearing headphones because you cannot hear someone approaching from behind. A street is easier to maneuver than a field with clods of dirt. A path along a country lane or through a neighborhood will have less pollution to breathe than a highway feeder road.

While walking, observe these guidelines:

- If you walk in the dark, wear light-colored clothing and know where to go for help if necessary.
- Keep your head up, looking 10 feet ahead.
- Swing your arms naturally or make walking a total body activity by keeping your elbows bent at a 90-degree angle and swinging them from the shoulder.
- Gradually pick up your pace as you walk. Walk as briskly as you can without getting out of breath. If you can't talk while you walk, slow down.
- Be aware of your surroundings as you walk—for pleasure as well as for safety.
- Vary your route so you don't get bored.
- Add a book in a backpack for weight to help build bone. After a few weeks add a second book.[11]

The exact type of exercise does not matter. Choose something you enjoy and will stick with. The benefits have been proven. Michelle Holmes of Brigham and Women's Hospital in Boston released a study in 2004 that was taken from the Nurses Health Study. The researchers looked at the 2,167 women in that larger study who developed breast cancer. They measured their activity level two years after their diagnosis and for the following 16 years. Those who walked one to three hours a week at a leisurely 3 miles per hour lowered their risk of dying from breast cancer by one-quarter compared to the most sedentary women. Those who walked three to eight hours a week slashed their risk by half.[12] Sounds to me as though walking (or other exercise) is a step in the right direction.

Prostheses will enhance your shape artificially, whereas exercise can improve your physical body shape as well as the physiological shape of your body functions and sense of well-being. Move as often as you can with as many muscle groups as you can, and reap all the benefits.

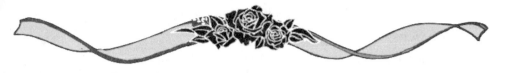

*Chapter 10*

# *Starting Over Again*

After breast cancer treatment, your perspective may have changed on many issues, your body is different, and you may know more about yourself than you did at your diagnosis. In other words, you don't really "start over." You start again. The rule of thumb is that it takes about as long for you to feel good again physically as the length of time from your diagnosis to the end of treatment (not including hormone therapy). Emotional recovery can take much longer.

Though the cause(s) of breast cancer are not completely understood, studies are showing some factors within your everyday control that may influence your body's ability to retard or stop cancer cell growth. Three factors you can do something about today are nutrition, exercise, and stress.

Sound like one of your mother's favorite lectures? Well, there was truth in her warnings to "eat your spinach," "turn off the tube and go outside to play," and "chill!" It may make you feel better to know that she probably didn't understand why these were important warnings to heed.

In 2003 the American Cancer Society published a report that weighed the evidence concerning the benefit for cancer survivors for various interventions. Although the evidence was not compelling enough to obtain the best ranking (*convincing*) for any intervention studied, there was enough evidence for ACS to declare *probable* benefit (next best ranking) for the following: Striving for healthy weight after treatment has benefit for recurrence, overall survival, and quality of life; increasing physical activity during and after treatment has benefit for quality of life; limiting saturated fat has benefit for overall survival.[1]

There was even less evidence, but it still may be true that there is a *possible* benefit for: Striving for healthy weight during treatment has benefit for cancer recurrence; increasing physical activity during and after treatment has benefit for recurrence and overall survival; limiting saturated fat has benefit for quality of life; increasing vegetables and fruits has benefit for recurrence and overall survival.

## Confession Time

When I started incorporating healthier habits into my lifestyle, I had a battle with guilt. Why hadn't I eaten the veggies my mother had urged upon me? Why had I sat inside reading during high school instead of playing tennis with my friends? And on and on.

So I coined the phrase FESS UP for my new healthier way of living. I've confessed my past lack of wisdom and have changed course. This phrase reminds me of the components of my new choice:

> F: Food
>
> E: Exercise
>
> S: Sleep
>
> S: Stress (the lack thereof)
>
> UP: the direction I'm moving toward a healthy lifestyle

I hope this helps you to admit your weaknesses and overcome them. There are no guarantees, of course, that switching to healthier choices will prevent recurrence. Breast cancer takes a long time to develop, so whatever caused it in the first place probably still has influence in your body. These new habits, however, can be new tools your body can use to get strong and fight back. They will also protect you against some other health concerns.

## It's Never Too Late

Many prominent cancer research organizations are finding that vegetables and fruit contain various cancer-fighting substances, some of which are not fully understood. Studies have also shown that moderate exercise, a low-fat diet, and a lifestyle free from stress may aid in preventing breast cancer or its recurrence. Other studies are underway examining these and similar theories. These lifestyle choices have been shown to have value in preventing other medical problems, so you can't go wrong checking with your doctor to see how you can incorporate them into your "new" life.

Slow, gradual change is more likely to succeed than trying to redo yourself in a week. Choose one area to start with—taking a walk three times a week or reducing your meal portions or resigning that committee job that keeps you awake at night. When you are comfortable with that, add something else.

If you begin to feel restricted, remind yourself why you are choosing to make the changes: they may prolong your life or make you healthier. There are no guarantees, but more and more studies are showing that lifestyle factors may account for 60 to 70 percent of all cancers.[2] The National Cancer Institute reports that as many as 35 percent of cancer deaths are diet-related.

Combine those with deaths related to smoking and alcohol, and you have almost three-quarters of all cancer deaths related to lifestyle and diet.

Apparently, it is never too late to change your diet and lifestyle. What can you lose by making some changes? If you say, "My favorite foods," think again. If research shows that a high-fat diet may contribute to breast cancer, are your chicken-fried steak and French fries still as appetizing as before? Believe one who resisted eating my "three Brownie bites" of veggies growing up and now follows a vegan diet as much as possible: Healthy food can be delicious. And an occasional "forbidden" food is not deadly. Balance is the key.

Don't judge all healthy food by that one whole-wheat cookie recipe you made 20 years ago. There are hundreds of cookbooks with delicious recipes for low-fat, high-fiber, vegetarian, or any other kind of healthy food. Find recipes that use ingredients you like. If you don't know tofu from jicama, try a recipe with green beans and marinara sauce or substitute oat flour for white flour in a favorite cake recipe. Take small steps and soon you won't even recognize your own dinner plate—or trade it for your former one.

## Nutrition

Cancer has an all-or-nothing mentality. Not only does it affect our body, mind, emotions, and self-esteem, it attacks our nutritional integrity, the basis of our health. Cancer can have the following negative effects on our nutritional status:

- Treatments or medications can interfere with digestion and metabolism, reducing the efficiency of nutrient processing.
- Infection, fever, shortness of breath, increased stress on the body, or tumor cells competing for nutrients can increase our energy requirements.
- Side effects from treatment such as mouth sores, loss of appetite, constipation, diarrhea, nausea, or vomiting can decrease our energy intake (make us eat less).

As basic as food is to our health, Western medicine is slow to include it as part of physicians' training. Of 125 U.S. medical schools, only 32 required a course in nutrition, although 106 did include the subject as part of a required course and 41 offered elective courses.[3] From 1999 to 2003 only 12 of 15,015 abstracts presented at meetings of the American Society of Clinical Oncologists dealt with nutritional intervention after breast cancer diagnosis.[4]

Because of this lack of training, many doctors dismiss food as irrelevant to overcoming disease because they didn't learn about it in medical school. The American Board of Physician Nutrition Specialists will implement in 2006 a certification for physicians who complete six months of supervised clinical nutrition training and instruction. Currently, physicians must pass a board examination for this certification. About 160 physicians had qualified by 2003. In the meantime, to receive authoritative information on your nutrition needs, consult a registered dietician or clinical nutritionist.

## Different Diets for Different Stages of Treatment

Although a cancer diagnosis may spark a desire for healthier eating, gradual changes may be best during treatment. Understand what your body needs during each part of treatment and feed it those foods. For instance, if you develop nausea, you will eat one way. If you have mouth sores, you will eat other foods.

If you are not eating to manage a side effect of treatment, provide your body with plenty of protein and calories. After treatment, low hemoglobin and hematocrit are common. Iron and vitamin B12 can help your body rebuild your red blood cells. Aim for 3 to 4 ounces of lean meat (beef, chicken, or fish) for lunch and dinner. To boost iron absorption from vegetables and beans, include a source of vitamin C (bell pepper, orange juice, tangerine, melon, grapefruit, orange) at the meal. You can also gain a little iron by cooking in cast-iron cookware. It may take up to three months for red blood cell counts to return to normal. Do not take an iron supplement without your doctor's permission.

Though your ultimate aim should be to replace all "fake foods" in your diet (processed foods, chemical substitutes for natural substances, convenience and fast foods), it may not be possible to do this during your active cancer treatment. Cooking healthy takes more time, and you may not have the energy. Also, you can make only so many changes to your lifestyle at once if you hope to forge them into habits.

Begin to learn more about nutrient-dense nourishment and make changes at a pace you can stand. For example, you might set as a goal one meatless dinner a week or substitute green tea for your afternoon cola or order water with your Mega Meal. Every change moves you closer to giving your body the fuel it needs to rebuild and keep you moving.

Also avoid diet extremes that can lead to cravings. For instance, very low-fat or low-carbohydrate diets often lack nutritional balance; some may raise your cortisol level and increase appetite.

## The Calcium Question

Because chemotherapy often causes early menopause, women with breast cancer have heightened concern about osteoporosis and other conditions that naturally occur with aging. One theory about preventing osteoporosis relies on supplying your body with adequate calcium. Some women choose to take calcium supplements to try to meet this goal. If this is your choice, be aware of the following:

- Calcium carbonate contains 40 percent elemental calcium and is the most concentrated form of the mineral in supplement form. This form often causes gas or gastrointestinal distress. Tricalcium phosphate runs second at 38 percent.

- Calcium phosphate (Posture D) contains vitamin D, which is necessary to help calcium absorption. It does not usually cause stomach distress.[5]

- Calcium citrate is about 21 percent elemental calcium and is more easily absorbed.

- Take calcium with meals so your stomach will produce enough gastric acid to absorb the mineral efficiently. Taking it with food also allows it to stay in the intestines longer, which increases its absorption rate.[6]

The dairy industry likes you to think "milk" when you think "calcium." Some alternative medicine practitioners, however, are concerned that the protein in dairy products, particularly casein, is difficult to digest. You can get calcium without the fat or other possible negative effects of dairy by eating fortified cereals and juices, beans, peas, soybeans, soy nuts, sesame seeds, poppy seeds, green leafy vegetables, bok choy, raisins, blackberries, bananas, and canned sardines and salmon (with the bones).

See how much calcium you get through food:[7]

| Food | Mg of calcium |
| --- | --- |
| Yogurt, low-fat, 1 cup | 447 |
| Orange juice, calcium-fortified, 1 cup | 350 |
| Sardines, canned, 3 ounces | 325 |
| Milk, 1%, 1 cup | 300 |
| Cheese, Swiss, 1 slice | 272 |
| Spinach, cooked, 1 cup | 245 |
| Tofu, firm, 1/2 cup | 204 |
| White beans, 1 cup | 161 |
| Parmesan cheese, 2 tablespoons | 138 |
| Frozen yogurt, 1/2 cup | 103 |
| Dry cereal, calcium-fortified, 1 serving | 100 |
| English muffin | 98 |
| Broccoli, cooked, 1 cup | 72 |
| Almonds, 1 ounce | 70 |
| Green beans, 1 cup | 58 |

The World Health Organization reports that countries where calcium intake is low do not have high rates of osteoporosis.[8] Studies also show that only about 18 to 36 percent of the calcium in milk is actually absorbed into the body.[9] The president of the Physicians Committee for Responsible Medicine commented that "the amount of calcium in your bones is very carefully regulated by hormones. Increasing your calcium intake does not fool those hormones into building more bone, any more than delivering an extra load of bricks will make a construction crew build a larger building....For the vast majority of people, the answer is not boosting your calcium intake, but rather limiting calcium loss."[10]

How do you prevent calcium loss?

- Reduce animal proteins, which cause bones to release stored calcium and prevent the parathyroid from reabsorbing the mineral.
- Reduce caffeine, which negatively impacts calcium absorption.
- Reduce alcohol consumption, which interferes with calcium absorption. Beer is the least damaging in this regard.
- Get sun. Only a few minutes sunlight on your skin helps produce vitamin D, which is essential for calcium absorption.
- Get enough magnesium, which works with other chemicals to promote bone growth. Magnesium is found in molasses, seeds and nuts, figs, whole grains, wheat germ, and apples.
- Exercise. Weight-bearing exercise helps build bones.
- Include the mineral boron, which helps prevent calcium loss, in your diet. Boron is found in almonds, peanuts, hazelnuts, apples, pears, prunes, grapes, berries, dates, raisins, and tomatoes.

## To Cook or Not to Cook?

Strong opinions exist on both sides of the raw vs. cooked vegetables question. Heat destroys some enzymes in food that you need for digestive health. The question is the percentage that is destroyed. This is a concern mostly for vitamins B and C. Minerals are not affected by high heat, and cooking makes proteins more digestible. In fact, carotenoids, powerful antioxidants in red, yellow, and orange fruits and vegetables, are absorbed better from cooked, rather than raw, foods. Carrots contain more beta-carotene after being cooked. Heated tomato products deliver more bioavailable lycopene, a cancer-fighting phytochemical, than raw.[11]

Eating some of your vegetables raw or lightly cooked may provide you with additional tools for health. Try steaming vegetables instead of drowning them in water, which is thrown away carrying valuable substances that your body could benefit from.

# *Diet*

No one food is a medicine that will cure or prevent cancer. However, researchers around the world are learning that diet and nutrition have a great impact on people's ability to fight off cancer. Whatever nutrients are supplied to, or withheld from, our bodies affect what our cells have to work with.

In 1994 the American Institute for Cancer Research (AICR) and the World Cancer Research Fund (WCRF) launched the massive Diet and Cancer Project. An expert panel of leading researchers from around the world, more than a hundred scientists, and representatives from the World Health Organization (WHO), International Agency for Research on Cancer (IARC), Food and Agriculture Organization (FAO) of the United Nations, and the National Cancer Institute (NCI) reviewed more than 4,500 research projects on diet and cancer conducted over the previous decade and held a series of international review meetings with local scientists to discuss new recommendations for cancer prevention.

The resulting publication, *Food, Nutrition and the Prevention of Cancer: A Global Perspective*, is the basis for new research and policy decisions. The bottom line of the study was that the primary causes of cancer in the United States are not pesticides, pollution, genetics, or some mysterious substance. All of us probably carry some mutated genes that could, with the right conditions, become malignant. The good news is that we also carry (mostly in our heads) what we need to empower our bodies to develop their natural protective mechanisms against the cancer-causing agents we come into contact with every day.

A "significant protective role against breast cancer was suggested, especially for vegetables," in the analysis of 45 studies that examined the role of a plant-based diet (fruit, vegetables, beta-carotene, or vitamin C). Three studies showed that increased intake of beta-carotene via food was associated with a reduction in recurrence of breast cancer. It is also theorized that diet influences circulating hormones, which may impact breast cancer risk. The Women's Healthy Eating and Living (WHEL) study and the Women's Intervention Nutrition Study (WINS) are now looking at the connection between diet and recurrence.

Determining what is healthy to eat can be overwhelming. The U.S. Department of Agriculture has helped simplify the task with a nutrient database at *www.nal.usda.gov/fnic/foodcomp*. Here you can view the nutritional breakdown of more than 6,000 foods, including generic and some name-brand foods. They will be adding fast foods and information on national restaurant chains.

# The China Project

Another landmark study on diet and disease, the China Project, began in 1983. Cornell University, the Chinese Academy of Preventive Medicine, Oxford University, and scientists from the United States, Britain, France, and other countries gathered information on the diets of people in 65 counties in China, where people tend to live their entire lives in one region with the same diet. The Chinese government had data showing death rates from specific diseases, some of which varied several hundredfold from county to county. Three basic findings were:

1. Diseases occur in groups (diseases of affluence, where breast cancer falls, and diseases of poverty).
2. As blood cholesterol and urea nitrogen (what is left over from the metabolism of protein) levels rise, so do diseases of affluence.
3. Even small intakes of animal foods—meat, eggs, and milk—are associated with significant increases of chronic degenerative diseases.

A surprising finding was that, although the Chinese eat little if any dairy and low amounts of calcium, they are at a much lower risk for osteoporosis than Westerners. The study showed that high protein intake, especially protein of animal foods, results in calcium loss through the urine. Some vegetables contain substantial amounts of calcium. They also contain boron, a mineral that helps keeps calcium in the bones. Milk contains virtually no boron. Vegetables also contain antioxidants, which are basically nonexistent in meat and milk.

The China Project compared breast cancer rates to many countries' meat consumption and found that the countries with the highest rates of meat consumption have the highest rates of breast cancer. Researchers found five things associated with deaths from breast cancer:

1. High intake of dietary fat.
2. High levels of blood cholesterol.
3. Estrogen. The study found that even relatively small additions of meat, milk, and fat were associated with higher levels of estrogen and other reproductive hormones.
4. Blood testosterone. Scientists found that women who ate more fat and animal-based foods had high blood testosterone levels and a higher risk for breast cancer.
5. Early age at first menstruation. Chinese girls begin menstruation around 15 to 19 years of age, whereas Western girls start around 10 to 14 years. Researchers found that diets high in fat, calories, and animal protein hastened menstruation by accelerating growth.

Another startling finding was in experiments with animals. Tumors stopped growing when animal protein was decreased and replaced with plant protein. When the body has all the protein it needs, the excess protein feeds tumors and precancerous lesions. In China only 10 percent of protein comes from animals; in America 70 percent of our protein comes from animals. The report suggests replacing animal protein not with low-fat versions but with a wide variety of grains, fruits, and vegetables. The report also notes that the Chinese eat about three times as much fiber as Americans. High fiber can reduce cholesterol levels.

After a while recommendations from a variety of sources begin to sound the same: more plants in our diets. Of course, we must keep in mind that most studies have looked at prevention of primary tumors, not at recurrence or secondary tumors. Until more research is available, it is just an educated guess that a diet good for prevention is also good for survivors.

## Start Slow

Do not expect to change lifetime habits, such as eating, in a few days or weeks. Rather than waiting until you are brave enough to draw a line in the sand and step forever into no-meat land or low-fat territory, try easing into the anticancer benefits of a healthy diet. Try one or two meatless days a week or switch to poultry, fish, or wild game for several meals a week. Make mealtime fun by trying new recipes with ingredients you like.

A little splurging won't matter too much—as long as you limit the excess. Out of 21 meals a week, you can probably splurge on four without losing the benefits of your other healthy choices.

## Mediterranean Diet

More evidence of synergy regarding food and health benefits comes from researchers at Harvard and the University of Athens. They followed 22,043 adults in Greece for four years and found that those who most closely followed a Mediterranean diet (fruits, vegetables, nuts, grains, cereals, olive oil, fish, wine, and dairy products such as cheese and yogurt) were 33 percent less likely to die of heart disease and 24 percent less likely to die from cancer than other participants. Studied separately, none of the factors in the diet showed a protective role. However, when the elements were combined, a benefit was seen.[12]

Again, this indicates that no one food is going to offset a generally unhealthy diet.

# Common-Sense Anti–Breast Cancer Diet

Researchers continue looking into the complex interaction between food and cancer and between estrogen and breast cancer. Some studies have suggested that increased fiber and decreased fat may reduce the risk of breast cancer because of their effects on estrogen. Fat cells produce estrogen and can encourage the growth of intestinal bacteria that enable estrogen to be reabsorbed into the body.[13] Fiber eliminates estrogen from the body. In fact, studies indicate that women eating a high-fiber, low-fat diet excrete two to three times more estrogen and have half the blood levels of estrogen than women whose diets are high in dairy and animal fats.[14]

The major cancer organizations in the United States recommend moving toward a plant-based diet. The National Cancer Institute recommends consumption of five or more servings of fruits and vegetables a day. More is better.

One thing you do not want to do is go on a fast-weight-loss diet. When you restrict calories, your body burns up lean tissue, such as muscle, to get the energy it needs. To reduce its energy requirements, the body also slows down some of its automatic functions and your metabolism slows down. When you resume eating at your previous level, your body is still in slow motion and can't keep up with the demands of additional food, so it stores excess calories as fat. And the scale creeps back to its earlier level or higher. Only a variety of nutritious foods can meet your body's needs.

A nutritious diet after breast cancer could include:

**Variety.** Each food contains its own set of vitamins, minerals, and other beneficial chemical compounds. Scientists have not figured out yet what they all are or which provide specific benefits. Probably their advantage comes from the combination with other substances. Take advantage of as many as possible by eating a wide variety of foods over the course of a week. Although some foods such as cruciferous vegetables or citrus fruits are touted by the media as being powerhouses of phytochemicals, they may be just the best studied to date. More research into micronutrients is being conducted now than in recent years, so our knowledge will continue to expand in this area.

**High fiber.** Fiber is the "vessel" that takes estrogen and toxins out of the body. If the fiber is not available to absorb the hormones, they are reabsorbed and recirculated through the body. Foods high in fiber include vegetables, fruits, and whole grains (rather than processed flours). Most sources recommend 25 to 35 grams of fiber per day.

**Low fat.** High amounts of fat in the diet can promote the growth of intestinal bacteria that permit estrogen to be reabsorbed into the body. Also, fat cells produce fatty acids that may promote the growth of breast cancer cells. Recommendations for fat intake vary among groups. Though the National

Cancer Institute and the American Cancer Society recommend fat intake be no more than 30 percent of your calories, other groups feel that is still too high for maximum benefits. They suggest a prudent goal of 10 to 20 percent of your calorie intake. Much less or much more than that may be inviting other health, not necessarily just cancer, problems. Some fat intake is necessary for proper bodily functions.

**Cruciferous vegetables.** A compound (I3C, indole-3-carbinol) found in broccoli, bok choy, cabbage, cauliflower, cress, turnip, kale, kohlrabi, collard greens, Brussels sprouts, and radishes converts estrogen into a form that is not linked to cancer. Other compounds in these vegetables are sulforaphane, a powerful detoxifier; chalcones and isoflavones, to support reproductive function; and isothiocyanates, which support healthy DNA.[15] It is unclear how much of these foods must be consumed to affect DNA metabolism.

**Yellow, dark green, deep orange, or red fruits and vegetables.** Foods such as carrots, cantaloupe, pumpkin, squash, peppers, lettuce, and yams contain high amounts of vitamin A and beta-carotene, which may help protect the body against cancer.

**Organic foods.** Evidence is still not clear about the role of pesticides in cancerous growths. Some studies suggest that more research needs to be done on DDT-like pesticides and other substances that may cause the body to manufacture cancer-promoting kinds of estrogen, xenoestrogen and 16-alpha-hydroxyestrone. Until such chemicals are proven to have no effect on breast cancer, you may want to increase the amount of organic produce you consume and carefully wash conventional produce with an organic or vegetable-based solution. Organic produce can be grown with pesticides, just a kind that has not raised concern over carcinogenic effects.

**Local vs. imported produce.** The U.S. Department of Agriculture says that "all imported products are required to meet the same food safety standards as domestic goods."[16] Of course, not every container of food reaching our harbors can be sampled. The FDA keeps a list of import alerts: firms, products, or countries that have violated standards, then works with the Customs Service and extensive databases to ferret out shipments that are most likely to violate standards, and these are sampled or analyzed carefully.

**Lots of fruits and vegetables.** Research has found that people who eat more fruits and vegetables have less risk for breast cancer and, if cancer develops, they live longer.

**Soy.** What to say about soy? Study results are conflicting regarding the consumption of soy by breast cancer patients. Japan has one of the lowest per capita rates of breast cancer. Japanese women eat a low-fat diet as well as a lot of soy. Soy contains chemicals called isoflavones, which are converted into plant estrogens. One of these phytoestrogens, genistein, is significantly weaker than the estrogen produced by the ovaries, estradiol, which binds to estrogen receptors and causes new growth. This constant stimulation of breast tissue over decades may increase a woman's risk of developing breast cancer. Genistein can block the activity of estradiol by locking into estrogen receptors in the breast and other areas of the body. It may also prevent the formation of new blood vessels, which are necessary for a tumor to grow. In other words, isoflavones are thought to act similar to tamoxifen, an antiestrogen given as hormonal therapy for many breast cancer patients. Tamoxifen also attaches to estrogen receptors to block dangerous estrogens. Soy intake could interfere with that process. Soy is not a medicine; it's a type of food. Isoflavones are also found in other beans besides soybeans. In fact, yellow split peas, black beans, baby and large limas, anasazi beans, red kidney beans, and red lentils all contain more genistein than soybeans. Black-eyed peas, pinto beans, mung beans, adzuki beans, fava beans, and great northern beans contain almost as much as soybeans.[17]

Two of the big unanswered questions about soy for breast cancer patients are amount and form. Although the data from Japan are intriguing, some researchers fear that an overabundance of soy in the diet may have a harmful effect. Remember that Japanese women have been eating soy and fish and vegetables all their lives. Perhaps the foods' benefits were highest during puberty, as some researchers have suggested, or they work together to provide protection. No one knows how much soy product is safe and how much is too much. No one knows whether some forms of soy are more or less protective than others and whether isolated soy components (such as soy powder or isoflavone supplements) are as effective as the whole food. And no one knows how a combination of tamoxifen and isoflavones reacts. Some doctors therefore recommend that a woman with breast cancer limit her soy intake to a few times a month; others encourage their patients to consume soy in as many forms as desirable. Some nutritionists feel that fermented soy (which has been heated, such as natto, tempeh, miso, and tamari) is the only form that is safe. Flora must be present in the stomach to convert genistein to an active phytoestrogen. If your digestive system is not functioning optimally, this may not happen. Keep watching for the results of research studies (most so far have tested fermented soy products) and discuss this puzzling question with your doctor or dietician.

**Flaxseed** contains lignans, which can block estrogens from breast tissue,[18] so they may arrest the growth of estrogen receptor-positive cells. No clinical studies have been done on women who have estrogen receptor–positive breast cancer and who eat flaxseed, so researchers are uncomfortable with women eating more than 3 tablespoons a day.[19] The same hesitations regarding flaxseed and tamoxifen exist as for soy products: not enough evidence exists for safe recommendations on dose, form, or effect on various stages of breast cancer. If you do decide to eat more flaxseed, remember that it must be cracked open for you to derive benefit from the oil inside. Just before serving, grind the seeds in a coffee grinder that is reserved just for flax. You can also take flaxseed oil. Remember that it goes rancid quickly, so it must be refrigerated.

**Green tea** may protect against some cancers by detoxifying enzymes and stimulating antioxidants.[20] Though the majority of studies show beneficial effects of green tea consumption, a few do not. Drink tea as you like, remembering that it does contain caffeine, which can cause insomnia, heart-rate irregularities, and nervousness. Green and white tea, which have more therapeutic properties than black tea, are made from the same plant; only the method of preparation differs.

**Juicing** with raw fruits and vegetables several times a week, or even several times a day, will add nutritional reinforcements you can't get by eating the foods, simply because of the volume required. You would have to eat 200 baby carrots to receive the nutrients in 8 ounces of fresh carrot juice. Buy a juicing machine that uses low heat to extract the juice. High heat can kill some of the nutrients before you even have a chance to consume them. A food processor won't separate the bulk of the food from the juice as efficiently as a juicer. Because of the tough cellular walls of carrots, for instance, the body cannot absorb many of the nutrients from a raw carrot. Juicing makes more nutrients available.[21]

**Glucarate-rich foods** such as alfalfa and bean sprouts, apples, apricots, broccoli, Brussels sprouts, cherries, and lettuce may reduce levels of B-glucuronidase and thus help the body purge itself of excess estrogen.

**Other foods** that are good to incorporate into your treatment diet, if you can tolerate them, are parsley, dill, carrots; garlic, onion, chives, leeks; gourds (squash, cucumber, melon); nightshade (potato, tomato, eggplant); green leafy vegetables; citrus; berries, especially black raspberries; legumes; and spices such as cayenne, curcumin, and sesame.

**Fortified vs. enriched.** Choose fortified rather than enriched foods. Fortified foods have nutrients added that were not in the food to begin with (calcium added to orange juice). Enriched foods simply add back nutrients that were lost during processing.

## Foods to Limit or Avoid

**White flour.** Most of its nutrients were stripped out in processing.

**Refined sugar.** Some nutritionists believe that sugar lowers the immune system for several hours after ingestion, creates hormonal imbalance, intensifies fatigue, and causes the bones to give up B vitamins[22] and calcium to balance the acidity of the bloodstream produced by the sugar. However, a study of 7,841 Harvard graduates found that chocolate and candy eaters lived almost a year longer than those who abstained. The key is moderation. Study participants who averaged three candy bars a month lived 36 percent longer than those who ate none. An article on the study concluded, "Perhaps it is not the phenols (powerful antioxidants also present in wine) that are healthful at all. Maybe it's the regular celebration of a special treat that boosts mood and results in longer life."[23]

Sugar can hide under other names in ingredient lists: raw sugar, brown sugar, cane, confectioners sugar, corn sweetener, corn syrup, dextrin, dextrose, fructose, glucose, hexitol, honey, invert sugar, levulose, maltose, mannitol, maple syrup, molasses, saccharin, sorbitol, sucrose, turbinado sugar, or xylitol. Natural sugars are found in healthy foods such as fruits, vegetables, and dairy products. The recommendation to limit high-sugar foods reflects the high-calorie and low-nutrient content of these foods.

**Caffeine.** It may increase breast tenderness and menopausal symptoms such as hot flashes and can deplete calcium.[24] Coffee, tea (not herbal teas), many sodas, and chocolate contain caffeine.

**Alcohol.** A few recent studies have implied, but not proven, a relationship between alcohol and breast cancer, but the mechanism is not clear.[25] Alcohol should be avoided particularly during chemotherapy because it can lower liver function, dehydrate the body, and depress the immune system. Alcohol can also aggravate symptoms of menopause and interfere with the liver's ability to break down estrogen, which can then circulate freely and do damage.[26] The AICR recommends avoiding alcohol. For women who want to drink, the AICR recommends no more than one drink (1 1/2 ounces of distilled 80-proof liquor, 12 ounces of beer, or 5 ounces of wine) per day.

**Carbonated drinks.** Phosphorous in dark-colored carbonated drinks can leach calcium from bones.[27] Because women with breast cancer can have reduced calcium from premature menopause or chemotherapy, it would be wise to minimize these beverages.

**Red meat.** Most red meats have a high percentage of fat, and processed meats such as hot dogs can be loaded with fat. Evidence shows that diets high in animal protein might present a higher risk for cancer.[28] This could be because of the fat or because such diets usually include less fruits and vegetables than low animal-protein diets. The leanest cuts of red meat are pork and beef tenderloin, ground sirloin, flank steak, and round tip sirloin. Venison and elk are also good lean meats. Most vegetables provide a higher percentage of protein per calorie than animal foods. The vegetables also give you vitamins, minerals, phytochemicals, and dietary fiber. Occasional small amounts of lean red meat are not a cancer risk. Studies show no additional decrease in cancer risk between vegetarians and those who consume no more than 3 ounces of meat a day. The Nurses' Health Study involving 90,000 women found no link between breast cancer risk and red meat.[29] However, the study researchers, noting the high fat content of red meat, did suggest eating red meat in moderation. Another reason for decreasing your intake of red meat is that it may contain antibiotics, hormone residues, and other chemicals from the feed or processing.

**Grilled or smoked foods.** Charcoal grilling and smoking meat can produce known and suspected carcinogens. Cooking with high heat can cause a substance known as heterocyclic amines (HCAs). The smoke and flames that flare up to blacken meat when fat drips on the coals deposit chemicals called phoycyclic aromatic hydrocarbons (PAHs), which raise cancer risk. For this same reason, burned meat should be avoided. An occasional grilled hamburger or smoked salmon probably won't harm you. Just practice moderation. When you grill, marinate meats; trim off the fat before cooking; precook them in the oven, then grill for the flame-cooked flavor; cook in smaller portions to cook faster; turn meats frequently to help them cook faster; minimize dripping by using a spatula or tongs instead of a fork to turn pieces; and remove all charred areas before serving.

**Salt-cured and pickled foods** contain carcinogens that may increase the risk of some cancers, although no particular connection has been established with breast cancer.

**Partially hydrogenated oils** are trans fats that have been chemically altered in processing and introduce foreign substances into the body. Avoid foods made from these oils, such as margarine, cakes, cookies, crackers, or some cereals or fast foods such as French fries cooked in these oils.

**Fried foods.** The lard or shortening used to fry foods contains trans fatty acids, which are undergoing study for their potential contribution to cancer. Choose baked chips, for instance, instead of fried ones.

**Dairy products** are under suspicion as a factor in breast cancer. Some studies link substances in milk, such as prolactin and IGF-1, with cancer promotion. The European Union Scientific Committee has identified "an association between circulating IGF-1 levels and an increased relative risk of breast and prostate cancer."[30] Research at the University of Pennsylvania Medical Center showed prolactin to be an important driver in breast cancer metastasis.[31] Other research shows some of these possibly harmful substances are contained in milk protein, not milk fat, so drinking low-fat milk won't help although the low-fat versions avoid some man-made chemicals that are stored in the fat, not the protein.[32] By substituting rice or almond milk for cow's milk, you will be avoiding possible carcinogens as well as antibiotics and hormones given to cows.

## Fat

Fat is essential to the human body. It provides energy and assists in the manufacture of vitamins A, D, E, and K. However, Americans eat much more fat than people in other countries. This fact is thought to be one factor in our higher rates of heart disease and some cancers, including breast cancer. Fat has twice as many calories per unit of weight as carbohydrates and protein. For general health as well as possible cancer prevention, some health organizations recommend lowering your fat intake to 10 to 20 percent of your total calories.

Fat cells increase estrogen production. Leaner people produce less estrogen and a less potent form of estrogen, according to Rose Frisch, Ph.D., professor emerita of the Harvard School of Public Health.[33] Estrogen is thought to be a factor in breast cancer, so less may be better. The number of pounds you weigh is not the only issue; it's body fat (or ratio of fat to lean body mass). Also, where your carry your fat may make a difference: fat around the waist may pose a bigger risk for cancer than fatty thighs or hips. Go to *www.nhlbisupport.com/bmi* to have your body mass index (BMI) calculated so you can determine if you should lose a few pounds.

Studies on fat in the diet are conflicting. Some show that countries with low total fat in the diet have less breast cancer wheras others show no correlation between dietary fat intake and breast cancer in American women. Researchers believe other factors such as activity level, other nutrients, and genetic factors play a role that is not fully understood.

Fats are found in such foods as dairy products (butter, cheese, sour cream, ice cream), salad dressings, animal protein, and processed foods (cookies, cakes, chips, snacks). Always read labels. Even veggie chips can be high in fat. Choose snacks with no more than 4 grams of total fat per serving.

Unhealthy fats are saturated (animal) fats and trans (hydrogenated) fats. It is not clear whether they increase the risk of breast cancer, but they do promote heart disease. Healthy monosaturated fats are found in plant foods such as avocado, macadamia nuts, pecans, hazelnuts, almonds, olives, sesame seeds, and olive and canola oils.

Some studies have shown the incidence of cancer to be lower in countries where omega-3 fatty acids are a major part of the diet. These healthy unsaturated fats are found in some fish. The body can convert linolenic acid, which is found in canola oil, flaxseed, soybeans, walnuts, and some leafy green vegetables, into omega-3 fatty acids. Eating a moderate amount of these fatty acids several times a week may protect against heart disease and some cancers.

## To increase the omega-3 fatty acids in your diet

- Choose olive, canola, flaxseed, soybean, and walnut oils instead of other vegetable oils.
- In baked goods, substitute ground flax flour for up to 10 percent of the flour. Because flax flour has a high omega-3 fat content, reduce the fat in the recipe by one-third. Replace the lost moisture with water, fruit puree, or juice.
- Eat fish with omega-3 fatty acids two or three times a week. If you don't like fish, try white fish. It is less "fishy" tasting. Marinate it as you would chicken or in milk to modify the taste further. Best sources of omega-3s: anchovies, Atlantic bluefish, wild catfish, herring, mackerel, sablefish, wild salmon, sardines, whitefish, pampano, shark, smelt, squid, striped bass, swordfish, trout, and tuna.
- Add a sprinkle of flaxseeds, wheat germ, or nuts to baked goods such as muffins, breads, pancakes, waffles, or rolls.
- Avoid fish oil capsules unless first discussed with your doctor. Concentrated amounts of omega-3s can lead to excessive bleeding, stroke, high cholesterol, and possible dangerous drug reactions.

### How much does a little fat cost you?[34]

| Item | Amount | # fat grams |
|------|--------|-------------|
| Butter | 1 tsp. | 4 |
| Salad dressing | 1 tbsp. | 7 |
| Mayonnaise | 1 tbsp. | 11 |
| Pan-frying meat | per 3-oz. serving | 6 |
| Deep-frying meat | per 3-oz. serving | 15 |
| Gravy | per 3-oz. serving | 2 |
| Cheese sauce | 2 tbsp. | 10 |
| Marinating, stir-frying | per 1/2 cup vegetables | 4 |
| Deep-frying vegetables | per 1/2 cup vegetables | 8 |

## Snacks

So what is left to eat on the run? Some healthy snacks are pretzels, light popcorn, air-popped popcorn, nuts (but no more than 1/4 cup), dried or fresh fruit, baby carrot sticks, baked chips and salsa, whole-grain crackers, sorbet, seeds, or vegetable juice. Unfortunately, you must read labels because wording on packaging can be misleading. Make your own smoothie from a banana, one or two servings of other fruit, ice, and a little orange juice. Make healthy trail mix from dried fruits, nuts, and puffed grain cereal.

# Eating Out

Eating healthily does not mean you have to avoid parties or restaurants. You can make healthy choices and still enjoy an active social life.

## At parties

- Start at the fresh fruit/veggie trays.
- Don't overdo on rich desserts or fatty foods. Too much fat can overload your system, especially if you otherwise eat a low-fat diet, and cause nausea and diarrhea.
- Fill up on water before you arrive at the buffet table.
- Enjoy just a few bites of rich foods instead of an entire serving.

## Restaurant dining

The type of food as well as portion sizes is important to keep in mind when you eat out. Here are some tips for dining out:

- Eye the amount of food before you begin eating. Estimate the number of servings on your plate and decide how much you will eat. Ask for a take-out box and place the excess food in it early in the meal so you are not tempted to overeat.
- Order broiled, steamed, baked, or grilled instead of fried, creamed, or breaded.
- The following hint at high fat content: au beurre, au gratin, Alfredo, batter-dipped, breaded, béarnaise, creamy, crispy, carbonara, croquette, flaky, fritters, hollandaise, parmigiana, tempura.
- Ask for salad dressing or sauces served on the side so you can control the amount. Ask for light/nonfat versions.
- Mexican: Order tacos or burritos without cheese and with more tomatoes. Choose corn tortillas instead of flour (less fat). Choose black beans over refried beans. Avoid fried tortilla chips.
- Italian: Don't overdo the garlic bread. Ask for half the cheese on your pizza and more green pepper, pineapple, and so forth.
- Chinese: Go easy on the fried noodles. Choose steamed meats and vegetables.
- French: Beware the dessert cart and rich sauces.

## Vegetarianism

Because breast cancer has been implicated in diets high in animal protein (meat and dairy), you might wonder whether a vegetarian diet is best for you. There are at least three types of vegetarian diets:

1. **Lactovegetarians** exclude meat but eat dairy products (milk, cheese, yogurt) and eggs.
2. **Vegans** exclude all animal products including dairy products.
3. **Part-time vegetarians** eat white meat and fish but not red meat.

The vegan diet is the most challenging for consuming all necessary nutrients. The other types, however, must be careful not to rely too heavily on cheese or eggs for protein. Both of these foods are high in fat, which may not be prudent for a breast cancer survivor. In fact, the University of California San Diego Cancer Center reports that studies show a preventive effect for breast cancer from a vegetarian diet. The American Cancer Society reports that "vegetarian diets that include fish and dairy foods typically contain the same quantity and quality of protein provided by nonvegetarian diets.... Adults eating vegan diets can meet protein needs if they consume nuts, seeds, legumes, and cereal-grain products in sufficient quantities."[35] The report goes on to recommend a multiple vitamin/mineral supplement containing 100 percent of Daily Values and supplementing a vegan diet with vitamin B12, iron, and zinc. Check with a registered dietician for guidance in your particular circumstance.

Protein exists in foods other than meat. For example, 1 ounce of low-fat cheese or 8 ounces of low-fat milk or yogurt have 7 grams of protein. One slice of bread; a cup of rice; 1/2 cup cooked pasta; or ½ cup of peas, squash, or corn has 2 grams of protein. Even 1/2 cup fresh or 1 cup of cooked green leafy vegetables or green beans has approximately 2 grams of protein, and 8 ounces of orange juice, a medium apple or orange, 1/4 cantaloupe, or 1/2 grapefruit has 1 gram of protein.[36] One-half cup beans/lentils has eight grams of protein.

Vegetables are powerhouses of valuable nutrients. The USDA reports that three raw carrots have 2 grams of protein, 21 grams of carbohydrates, 60 mg of calcium, 1 mg of iron, 696 mg of potassium, 60,000 IUs of vitamin A in the form of beta-carotene, 19 mg of vitamin C, 30 mcg of folate, and traces of other minerals, vitamins, and enzymes.[37]

Animal products are hidden in many foods you would not suspect. For example, gelatin is protein taken from the tendons, skin, cartilage, bones, or other parts of steer, calves, or pigs. Lactose, found in baby's formulas and processed sweets, is a sugar naturally occurring in cow's milk, and carmine and cochineal found in colored pasta, ice cream, and bottled juices are red colorings derived from the body of a female cochineal beetle. Other ingredients such as "natural flavorings," emulsifiers, and clarifying agents may have animal or vegetable sources.

You may find that being a vegetarian takes more preparation time than serving processed foods. Also, your dinner plate will be more colorful. It's a tradeoff—and one you can only profit from.

## Invisible Veggies

Here are some simple ways to incorporate veggies into your lifestyle without fanfare and with possibly beneficial results:

- Heat tomato juice with 1/2 teaspoon of basil for a quick, energizing drink.
- Increase quantities of vegetables and beans in casseroles while decreasing amounts of meat.
- Pile extra veggies on your sandwich: spinach (instead of lettuce), cucumbers, tomato, mushrooms, onions.
- Use salsa for low-fat dressing, pasta sauce, or baked potato topping.
- Add a little pureed, cooked cauliflower to mashed potatoes.
- Add grated carrots to grated cheddar cheese for tacos or pasta.
- Add finely chopped broccoli or frozen chopped green pepper and onion to omelets.
- Add thawed frozen peas and celery to tuna salad.
- Add finely grated carrots, spinach, or mashed potatoes to pasta sauce.
- Substitute pureed green peas for half the avocado in dips.
- Substitute a layer of vegetables for meat in lasagna.
- Top pizza with vegetables and pineapple instead of meat.
- Stir a little canned pumpkin into your hot cereal.

## Hidden Fruits

Easy ways to add more fruit to your diet include:

- Freeze seedless grapes for a delicious treat.
- Freeze unsweetened fruit juice in ice cube trays and crush for a delicious, refreshing snack.
- Add dried fruits to pancake or muffin mix.
- Pureed frozen fruit makes a delightful substitute for ice cream. Try pureeing frozen banana (freeze in inch cubes for easier blending) with strawberries, blueberries, peaches, and so forth for a variety of flavors.

## Smart Food Tips for Starting Over

### Meal planning

- Eat only if you are hungry.
- Plan meals that are pleasing to all the senses—sight, taste, texture.

- Know that soups or beverages with a meal can fill you up and leave no room for higher-nutrient foods.
- A salad and two vegetable or pasta dishes make a complete meal. You don't need to serve five options for each meal.

## Shopping tips

- Remember that ingredients are listed in their order of prominence, so if sugar (corn syrup, dextrose, sucrose, fructose, malt, or other "-ose" ingredients) is listed near the top, pass up that food.
- For breads, pastas, tortillas, and so on, look for "whole wheat flour." "Wheat flour" and "seminola flour" are just other names for white flour.
- Avoid foods with hydrogenated or saturated (solid at room temperature, such as lard and shortening) fats.
- Frozen or canned fruits and vegetables are acceptable alternatives if fresh is not available; however, frozen or canned have often had fiber (skins) removed and sugar added. The nutrient value of fruits and vegetables is highest if they are picked at peak ripeness and eaten within about three days. Often, the produce in your local grocery store was picked weeks ago, whereas the canned or frozen products were processed immediately after being harvested.
- Labels can be confusing. The FDA defines *fresh* as any unprocessed food in its raw state that has not been frozen or subjected to any form of thermal processing or preservation. *Fresh frozen* and *frozen fresh* mean the food was frozen quickly after harvesting, even if it was blanched first. *Quickly frozen* means the food was quickly frozen after harvest by certain methods and no deterioration has taken place. The food can have FDA-approved wax coatings or have been sprayed with postharvest pesticides.
- When selecting canned fruit, choose fruit packed in its own juice rather than sweetened syrup.
- Buy shredded cheese, frozen chopped onion and green pepper, and bags of washed salad greens to save time.

## Cooking tips

- Wash fresh vegetables only when ready to use. Wet vegetables rot faster.
- Freeze leftover peppers, onions, vegetables, herbs, or berries for use in casseroles or soups.
- Add a cheesy flavor to salads, sauces, and spreads with nutritional yeast (different from baker's or brewer's yeast).
- Look for vegetarian baked beans and other staples.

## Healthy Substitutions in Recipes

| Item | Substitutions |
|---|---|
| Butter/margarine | Flaxseed oil, almond butter, unsweetened fruit preserves. |
| Buttermilk | Add 1 tablespoon of vinegar (or apple cider vinegar) per cup of soy or rice milk. |
| Cheese, cow's milk | Soy cheese. |
| Chips (corn or potato) | Pretzels, air-popped popcorn. |
| Chocolate, unsweetened baking | For frosting or sauces: 3 to 4 tablespoons cocoa powder + 1 tablespoon oil + 1 tablespoon sugar. For cakes or cookies: 1/4 cup cocoa. |
| Cooking methods | Bake, broil, steam instead of fry. |
| Cooking oil | For cooking, extra-virgin olive oil. For baking, extra-light olive oil or canola oil (preferably organic, cold-pressed[38]). |
| Cottage cheese | Crumbled tofu (if your tumor was estrogen receptor–positive, use sparingly), low-fat/nonfat cottage cheese. |
| Cream | Soy or rice milk; evaporated skim milk. For creamed soups, add nonfat dry milk or puree some of the soup ingredients, cooked rice, or a cooked potato to thicken. When you need a sweet, thick cream, whisk soft tofu with honey or malt extract for a rich topping. |
| Croissants, doughnuts, or breakfast bars | Bagels, English muffins, pita bread, corn tortillas. |
| Dips | Hummus. Puree chickpeas and add your own spices. |
| Eggs | Select depending on the texture and flavor of the food being prepared. This is the amount for one egg: • 2 egg whites. • 1 ounce (2 tablespoons) soft tofu. • 1/2 banana, mashed. • 2 tablespoons another liquid such as lemon juice or water. |

## Healthy Substitutions in Recipes

| Item | Substitutions |
|---|---|
| Eggs (cont.) | • 2 tablespoons cornstarch or arrowroot starch.<br>• 1 heaping tablespoon soy flour mixed with 2 tablespoons water.<br>• egg replacer (Ener-G, Egg Beaters).<br>• 1 tablespoon flaxseed pureed in blender with 1/4 cup water.<br>• 1/3 to 1/4 cup canned pumpkin, ground zucchini, applesauce, or tofu. |
| Eggs used to bind other ingredients such as in burgers or loaves | Mashed potatoes, quick-cooking rolled oats, cooked oatmeal or barley, fine bread crumbs, tomato paste (about 1 to 2 tablespoon per egg). |
| Flour, white | Use other flours such as oat, almond, rice, or whole wheat. Make easy oat flour by pureeing rolled oats in your food processor. |
| Frosting | Pureed fruit, dusting of confectioners sugar. |
| Gravies | Add pureed vegetables to thicken instead of butter and flour. |
| Ice cream | Sherbet, sorbet, frozen yogurt, low-fat ice cream or ice milk, pureed frozen fruit. |
| Mayonnaise | Mustard, honey mustard, Dijon mustard.<br>Nonfat yogurt for sauces and dressings.<br>For cooked dishes, use nonfat yogurt and add 1 1/2 teaspoons of flour.<br>Nasoya makes an eggless, dairyless Nayonaise. The Ojai Cook makes an all-natural, low-fat Lemonaise Light with no sugar, cholesterol, or carbohydrates. |
| Meat | Instead of processed or marbled meat, choose:<br>• Lean cuts of beef (ground sirloin or extra-lean ground beef).<br>• Fish.<br>• Skinless poultry.<br>• Lamb.<br>• Pork loin or extra lean pork chops. |

## Healthy Substitutions in Recipes

| Item | Substitutions |
|---|---|
| Meat (cont.) | In recipes such as chili, spaghetti sauce, or casseroles:<br>• Texturized vegetable protein (TVP), made from soybeans<br>• Tempeh (cultured soybeans with a chewy texture)<br>• Wheat gluten or seitan, made from wheat protein (has a meaty taste)<br>• Vegetarian burgers or hot dogs, many of which are fat-free<br>• Substitute up to one-half with rolled oats, cooked brown rice, couscous, or cooked and chopped beans.<br>• Reduced-fat tofu. Baked tofu can be sliced thin for sandwiches, shredded for salads, or added to stir-fry recipes. Freeze and thaw to give a meaty flavor. This will change the color to off-white but does no damage to the food.<br>Ask your oncologist about the wisdom or frequency of eating soy foods such as TVP, soybeans, or tofu. |
| Milk | Soy or rice milk.<br>Nonfat/skim or 1/2% or 1% milk.<br>Potato milk<br>Nut milks |
| Oil, butter, or shortening in baked goods | For all or part of ingredient:<br>• Mashed bananas.<br>• Pureed prunes.<br>• Applesauce.<br>• Cooked pumpkin.<br>• Zucchini (will not add flavor, whereas the others will).<br>• Soy margarine.<br>• Spectrum Natural Spreads makes a nonhydrogenated margarine substitute.<br>• Flaxseed meal (ground flaxseed). Use three times as much flaxseed as the recipe calls for butter, margarine, or cooking oil (for instance, 1 1/2 cup ground flaxseed if the recipe calls for 1/2 cup butter). Baked items with flaxseed meal tend to brown more quickly than those cooked with oil or butter. |

## Healthy Substitutions in Recipes

| Item | Substitutions |
|---|---|
| Oil for sautéing | Lemon or other citrus juice, olive oil, vegetable broth, cooking spray, organic butter, or Bragg's Liquid Aminos. Add minced garlic, onion, and/or herbs for flavor. Because olive oil is unstable at high temperatures, use canola oil for frying. Other healthful oils are almond, sesame, sunflower, walnut, and hemp; they require refrigeration. |
| Oil in salad dressings | Grapeseed oil is a great source of essential fatty acids and vitamin E and is cholesterol free. Try oils from extra-virgin olives, walnuts, pumpkins, safflower, hazelnuts, or macadamia nuts; canola oil. |
| Rice, white | Brown rice, bulgur, kasha, quinoa, whole wheat couscous |
| Salt | Sea salt, herbs, spices, dulce, or kelp<br>Bragg's Liquid Aminos. Use 1 tablespoon for 1 teaspoon salt. |
| Sour cream | Nonfat yogurt or cottage cheese for sauces and dressings.<br>For cooked dishes, mix nonfat yogurt with 1 1/2 teaspoons of flour per cup of yogurt. Because yogurt loses its healthy microbes at 140 degrees, cook the rest of the dish and mix in room-temperature yogurt just before serving. |
| Sugar | Substitute any of the following concentrates for 3/4 cup sugar. Reduce the liquid in the recipe by 1/4. If the recipe does not call for other liquid, add 4 tablespoons of flour for each 3/4 cup of concentrate.<br>• 1/2 cup honey.<br>• 1/4 cup molasses.<br>• 1/2 cup fruit concentrate.<br>• 2 cups apple juice.<br>• 1/2 cup maple syrup.<br>• organic cane sugar in equal amounts of sugar called for. |
| Yogurt | Use 3/4 cup soy or rice milk with 1 tablespoon of vinegar per cup in recipe. |

## What's in a Label?

In the 1990s the U.S. government passed new rules for food labels that are mandatory, whereas some of the previous guidelines were voluntary. The new Nutrition Facts label on food products has been revised again. Labels must show the percentage of certain substances, based on a 2,000-calorie diet.

Be aware of marketing blending into labeling, however. For instance you want "100% whole wheat" bread, not "wheat bread." If in doubt, check the list of ingredients, which are listed in order of quantity in the product. If "wheat flour" is listed sixth, it probably is not a major ingredient and the label of "wheat bread" is more advertising than fact.

Serving sizes are standardized, so comparison shopping is easier than it used to be. Read serving sizes carefully. One bread may seem to have a great fiber content—until you realize that the serving size is *two* slices.

Some confusing terms you may find on labels are defined by the FDA as:

| | |
|---|---|
| **Calorie-free:** | Fewer than 5 calories per serving |
| **Low-calorie:** | 40 calories or fewer per serving |
| **Reduced or fewer calories:** | At least 25 percent fewer calories than a reference food |
| **Sugar-free:** | Fewer than 0.5 grams of sugar per serving |
| **No added sugar, without added sugar, no sugar added:** | No sugars or ingredients that contain sugar are added during processing or packing |
| **Fat-free:** | Fewer than 0.5 grams of fat per serving |
| **Low-fat:** | 3 or fewer grams of fat per serving |
| **Reduced or less fat:** | At least 25 percent less fat per serving than a reference food (full-fat version) |
| **Low saturated fat:** | 1 gram or less saturated fat per serving; not more than 15 percent of calories from saturated fat |
| **Reduced or less saturated fat:** | At least 25 percent less saturated fat per serving than a high saturated fat food |

# What Is a Serving?

There is a difference between a serving and a portion. A serving is a standardized amount used as reference on food labels, government food charts, and so forth. A portion is the amount of food you choose to eat or how much is served on your plate at a restaurant. For example, a serving size of pasta is 1/2 cup, but a typical restaurant portion is 3 cups.[39]

**Vegetable serving:**
1 cup raw leafy vegetables
1/2 cup cooked or chopped vegetables
3/4 cup vegetable juice

**Fruit serving:**
1/4 cup dried fruit
1/2 cup chopped, cooked, or canned fruit
3/4 cup fruit juice
1/2 cup raw fruit (small banana, apple, orange, and so on)

**Dairy serving:**
1 cup milk or yogurt
1-inch cube (about size of last part of your thumb) or thin slice of cheese
1 1/2 ounces of natural cheese
2 ounces of processed cheese

**Fats and oils serving:**
2 to 3 teaspoons vegetable or nut oil
2 to 3 teaspoons butter
2 to 3 teaspoons mayonnaise
1 tablespoon salad dressing

**Nut serving:**
2 tablespoons nuts or nut butter
1/3 cup nuts equals 1 ounce of meat

**Poultry, fish, meat, eggs serving:**
2 to 3 ounces of cooked poultry, fish, or meat
1 egg

**Bean serving:**
1/2 cup cooked beans

**Grains, bread, cereal, rice, pasta serving:**
1 slice bread (or 2 slices diet bread)
1/2 bagel or English muffin
3 to 4 plain crackers
1/2 cup cooked cereal, rice, or pasta
1 ounce dry cereal (Read the label. The measurement varies.)

## Quick Reference for Serving Sizes

To make it easier to remember serving sizes, actually measure out the serving size of the foods you eat or serve your typical portion and measure it before you eat it to see how many servings it is. Also you can measure what your cereal bowls or serving spoons hold.

Some other easy comparisons are:

| Serving | Equivalent | Serving | Equivalent |
|---------|-----------|---------|-----------|
| 1 cup | Tennis ball, closed fist | 1 ounce | 4 dice, 2 fingers |
| 1/2 cup | 3 ice cubes | 2 tablespoons | Ping-Pong ball |
| 1/4 cup | Large egg | 1 tablespoon | From tip to joint of thumb |
| 3 ounces | Deck of cards, palm of hand | 1 teaspoon | Tip of thumb |

## Advertised Anticancer Diets?

Several "diets" have been popularized as ways of eating that will reduce cancer activity or the possibility of developing cancer. However, none of them has been proven through accepted scientific studies to have anticancer effects. Some may in fact pose a risk of inadequate nutrition or unwanted side effects such as fatigue.

Unfortunately, there is no known "anticancer diet." Scientists and researchers have identified many foods that contribute anticancer benefits. What is not known is the ratio or interaction of certain nutrients or foods. Until this information is known, you are safest concentrating on balance, moderation, and variety.

### Macrobiotics

As practiced currently, individual macrobiotic diets take into account a person's age, activity level, medical history, and other factors. In general a macrobiotic diet would consist of 50 percent grain, 25 percent vegetables (two-thirds cooked and one-third raw), and the rest soups, condiments, sea vegetables, and beans.

Possible side effects of this diet are deficient protein, vitamins, and minerals and weight loss. Monitoring of albumin, calcium, iron, zinc, vitamin B12, and ascorbic acid levels are recommended for those who follow this diet.[40] Another concern is that frail cancer patients might not consume enough calories or fat for their status.

## Other anticancer diets

Other advertised anticancer diets include Gerson therapy, Livingston-Wheeler Regimen, Kelley/Gonzalez Regimen, and wheat grass therapy. Each is based on a theory of illness that has not been tested by research. Some elements might be beneficial, but there is concern over frequent enemas or nutrient deficiencies. Be sure to include impartial sources of information if you investigate these diets.

# Going Natural

Research shows that many of the chemicals used in our everyday products for cleaning, cosmetics, pest control, and most other basic functions may be carcinogens and have or may have estrogenic properties. This means that, as they are absorbed through your skin or you breathe them into your body, they can have the effect of estrogen inside you. Because estrogen dominance or overproduction is being studied as a factor in breast cancer, some women want to minimize their use of synthetic materials and substances.

It's not possible to avoid chemicals totally because they exist in all parts of our environment. Formaldehyde, for instance, is used as a preservative on fabrics in new cars and clothing; in some cosmetics, nail polish, hair dyes, and shampoos; and in PCBs used in lubricants, adhesives, and insecticides.[41] The problem for our bodies is overload and no one can define that. So the goal for some people after breast cancer is to minimize toxic exposure in as many ways as they can. Learn how toxins interact with our food supply, our air and water, what we wear and spread on our skin, and decide what you want to change about that.

Studying environmental risks in humans is difficult because, of course, researchers cannot select control groups to receive high doses of the chemicals being tested. Instead, they must rely on studies of animals or highly exposed occupational groups. The degree of risk from pollutants varies by concentration, intensity, and duration of exposure. Risk assessment must include the cancer-causing potential of the substance, the levels in the environment, and the extent to which people are exposed to the substance.

Then there are the ironies such as pesticide residues on fruits and vegetables. Those who eat more of these foods will be exposed more, yet they have lower cancer risks than those who eat few fruits and vegetables.

Scientists calculate acceptable standards to limit the increased risk to no more than one person per million over a lifetime. Unfortunately, many substances have not been tested, so we don't really know what is safe and what is not.

Concerned that too little is being done to investigate environmental toxins and their effect on breast cancer, the Breast Cancer Fund and Breast Cancer Action compiled a comprehensive report in February 2002 that was updated the following year. The paper has been presented at several public forums, including the first International Summit on Breast Cancer and the Environment, held May 22–25, 2002, and sponsored by the U.S. Centers for Disease Control and Prevention (CDC) and the University of California Berkeley School of Public Health. More than 100 scientists, advocates, and community representatives gathered at the summit to create a new agenda for public policy as it relates to breast cancer research. The report is titled *State of the Evidence: What Is the Connection between Chemicals and Breast Cancer?*[42]

The report states that "in today's complex, constantly changing world, absolute proof linking a particular chemical to human breast cancer may never be possible."[43] It also notes that most Americans carry in their bodies 116 synthetic chemicals and metals, according to the Second National Report on Human Exposure to Environmental Chemicals, released by the CDC on January 31, 2003. This is up from 27 chemicals in the report CDC released in March 2001. Yet only 7 percent of the 85,000 synthetic chemicals registered for use today in the U.S. have complete toxicological screening data available. More than 90 percent of these chemicals have never been tested for their effects on human health.

However, when Israel outlawed the use of certain pesticides similar to DDT, their rate of breast cancer dropped by 30 percent as rates were increasing elsewhere in the world.[44] Also, a study in 1989 found that the 339 counties in America with hazardous waste sites and contaminated ground water consistently had higher mortality from breast cancer than counties without such contamination.[45]

Many chemicals accumulate in body fat and can remain in breast tissue for decades. The amount of toxins that exist in a person's body is referred to as "body burden." Even years after a chemical has been banned for agricultural or industrial use, it can remain in our bodies. Some studies of women's body burden show the presence of chemicals that have been linked to mammary tumors in animals.

Three European scientists have developed a mathematical model for studying the combined impact of several organochlorines, estrogen-like pollutants, on humans. Reported in the April 2004 issue of *Environmental Health*

*Perspectives*, a journal of the National Institute of Environmental Health Sciences, the study showed that a combination of four organochlorines (including two forms of DDT) stimulated breast cell division and proliferation of MCF-7 cells, which are a type of breast cancer cell. The researchers point out that most studies of similar substances have been conducted on individual organochlorines at high concentrations. Because these substances are present in humans at low concentrations and in combinations, they "wanted a model of what happens in the real world." They found that "these agents act together in combination and may have an impact on individuals even at very low concentrations."[46]

A variety of chemical-free products are available at healthfood stores. Home improvement stores carry boric acid, diatomaceous earth, and cedar chips for natural pesticides. Some women even enjoy making their own cleaning products and cosmetics. For more information on environmental risk factors for cancer, see the Websites of the Agency for Toxic Substances and Disease Registry (*www.atsdr.cdc.gov*), Environmental Protection Agency (*www.epa.gov*), National Institute of Environmental Health Sciences (*www.hiehs.nih.gov*), National Institute for Occupational Safety and Health (*www.osha.gov*), and World Health Organization (*www.who.int*).

## Organic vs. Conventional Produce

Though no study has been done to prove that eating organic produce and meats is healthier than eating conventional products, it makes sense to some to reduce the toxic burden on their body by consuming pesticide- or hormone-free foods as much as possible.

Organic crops use a minimum of fertilizer and no synthetic pesticides (although natural pesticides are used) and restrict irradiation. Their farming practices are not without question. Dean Cliver, Ph.D., former principal investigator at the World Health Organization Collaborating Centre for Food Virology, for instance, questions the safety and timing of "green manure" used in growing organics.

If you can raise your own food, you have more control over its quality and how it is harvested and stored, although you cannot control the quality of the soil (unless you grow it in potting soil ) and air and the amount of sun and rain, which contribute to its overall nutrient load.

The U.S. Department of Agriculture has accredited four categories of organic labeling: "100 percent organic," "organic" (contains 95 to 100 percent organic ingredients), "made with organic ingredients" (made with at least 70 percent organic ingredients), and products with less than 70 percent organic ingredients. This last group of products may not make organic claims on the front of the package but may list organic ingredients on the side.

Healthfood stores and some traditional grocery stores carry chicken, eggs, and red meat from free-ranging animals. Read the fine print carefully to be sure no antibiotics or hormones were used at any time during the life of the animal.

Organic produce may still contain pesticide residue from the soil, water, or air supply, but it will be a smaller amount than food that is sprayed directly. In fact, *organic* does not mean that no pesticides were used, only that different kinds of pesticides were used. Bruce Ames, a biochemist and cancer researcher at the University of California at Berkeley, says that Americans "consume more carcinogens in one cup of coffee than we get from the pesticide residues on all the fruits and vegetables we eat in a year."[47] Ken Cook, president of the Environmental Working Group, says, however, "If you want to reduce your exposure to pesticides, eating organic is a very good way." Again, the facts are not clear. Do your research and make the decision you are comfortable with.

Wash even organic produce because animal manure is the main fertilizer used in organic farming. Peel fruit that is not organic before eating it. Although the skin is often nutritious, it also is often sprayed with chemicals to preserve its appearance until it can get to market and then waxed so the chemicals won't wash off. Discard the outer leaves of cabbage or lettuce.

The following foods soak up more pesticides than other foods: apples, bananas, bell peppers, celery, cucumbers, grapes and raisins, spinach, and strawberries. Buy organic whenever possible.

## Wild vs. Homegrown

The Environmental Protection Agency warns that even wild game may contain pesticide residue if it resides in an area where pesticides are used and that fish caught in the open stream can contain residues if the water is contaminated. The EPA suggests:

- Watching for posted signs at fishing spots.
- Checking with game wardens and other officials about chemicals in the area.
- Trimming wild game of fat and skinning wild fish.
- Not eating berries picked from the roadside where herbicides and pesticides may be sprayed.
- Drinking distilled spring water from glass bottles. Even well water can be contaminated as pesticides soak through the soil, so have wells tested at least annually.

## Safe Seafood

Although seafood is inherently better for you than animal products (partly because of its low fat content), pollution is a concern in our waters as well as our soil. Mercury becomes highly toxic in water, so much so that the Environmental Protection Agency (*www.epa.gov*) issues Fish and Wildlife Advisories warning the public not to consume certain fish from certain contaminated areas. In 2002 there were 2,800 advisories covering 32.9 percent of lakes, 15 percent of rivers, and 70 percent of the coastline for the lower 48 states.

Larger, more predatory fish have the highest levels of mercury poisoning, so some people cut back on their consumption of tuna, marlin, shark, tilefish, walleye, mackerel, largemouth bass, and swordfish. Orange roughy and grouper also have higher toxicity than other fish. Generally, smaller fish such as cod, halibut, wild salmon, scrod, perch, flounder, catfish, and whitefish have lower contaminant levels.

Wild fish are generally a better choice than farm-raised or freshwater fish, which are subject to pesticide and insecticide runoff and are sometimes fed antibiotics or pellets of grain and animal byproducts instead of smaller fish as they would eat in the wild. Recent research found detrimental levels of PCBs in farm-raised salmon, more than 10 times that found in wild salmon.

Don't miss out on the health benefits of fish. Just try to find the least contaminated.

## Easy Changes to Make

Here are some easy changes that can't hurt and may possibly help the overall health of your family:

- Use organically grown cotton sheets and wool blankets. Consider an all-wool mattress.

- Hang clothing from the dry cleaners in a well-ventilated area or outdoors without the bag for a day or two until the odor of the solvents dissipates.

- Buy food in metal or glass containers or transfer food (especially fatty foods) from plastic containers when you get home from the store. PVC (polyvinyl chloride) found in food packaging, water bottles, plastic wrap, and toiletry containers may contribute to cancer and other health problems because some of the chemicals leach into what the bottles contain.

- Don't microwave food in plastic containers. Use glass or ceramic instead. Some chemicals in plastics, even hard plastic, can leach into the food when it is heated. Don't let plastic wrap touch foods during microwaving for the same reason.

- Install a water filter for your whole house if possible or at least for your drinking water and shower. Even some drinking water that meets EPA standards contains contaminants, some of which mimic estrogen.[48] A reverse-osmosis purifier is considered the most effective.

- Avoid creams, moisturizers, shampoos, body gels, or other personal care products that list placenta, estrogen, estriol, estradiol, natural hormones, diethenolamine (DEA), propylene glycol, or sodium laurel sulfate (SLS) as ingredients.[49]

- Use natural pesticide/insecticides such as neemoil products. Use Avon's Skin So Soft or Bite Barrier for a mosquito repellant.

- Avoid aerosol sprays for hair, cleaning, gardening, deodorants, or other purposes. The spray contains man-made chemicals.

- Wrap food in waxed paper, then in aluminum foil instead of plastic wrap.

- Use paint that contains less volatile organic chemicals (VOCs), known to leach into the air for a month after application and which can cause kidney and liver damage. Choose water-based latex, low-VOC paint (at Sherwin-Williams and Glidden), or milk paints (Old Fashioned Milk Paint Company; *www.milkpaint.com*; 1–978–448–6336).

## In food

- Reduce pesticide consumption by trimming fat from meat and skin from fish and by discarding fats and oils in broths and pan drippings. This is where pesticides collect.

- Wash skins of vegetables and fruit that will be eaten. Although pesticide residue diminishes over time, some may still be present when you consume the product.

- Avoid artificial colorings; Splenda, Aspartame, or other synthetic sugar substitutes; BHA (butylated hydroxyanisole) and BHT (butylated hydroxytoluene); nitrites and nitrates commonly found in processed meats; Olestra; and potassium bromate in bread.

## Cleaning

For all-purpose cleaning, put 3-percent hydrogen peroxide in one spray bottle and white vinegar in another. Spray the surface to be cleaned with one, then the other, and wipe with a paper towel. Do not combine in same bottle.

- For shower mold, mix 2 cups water and 2 teaspoons tea tree essential oil in a spray bottle. Shake well and spray. The oil has a strong odor, which will disappear in about 12 hours.

- For toilets, sink, and tub, mix 2 cups water, 10 drops eucalyptus or peppermint essential oil, 1/4 cup liquid Castile soap, and 1 tablespoon tea tree essential oil in a spray bottle. Spray, scrub with brush or sponge, and rinse with damp sponge.

- Detergents leave residues on your clothing that can irritate your lungs. Try natural soap flakes or "free-and-clear" detergents or make your own from 1/4 cup borax, 1/4 cup washing soda (sodium carbonate), 1/2 cup baking soda, and 1/2 cup powdered Castile soap. Mix and use about half as much as you do of your store-bought brand.

## *Emotions*

As you start over with new habits and a new look on life, you may experience higher emotional highs and lower emotional lows than in other seasons of your life. This is because breast cancer affects not only your breast; it affects your self-image, your vulnerability, your sexuality, your energy level, your priorities, and your perspective on life itself.

Be prepared for an onslaught of emotions, sometimes at the least expected moments. Many women, for instance, tell of major depression on the anniversary of their diagnosis or fear on the eve of another chemotherapy treatment. Others reexamine aspects of their life that require energy—jobs, relationships, hobbies, recreation, social groups—and ditch those that are not fulfilling and concentrate on those that are satisfying. Some women finally begin working toward a dream they have always had and have not pursued. Still others want to share their experience with others and express themselves through art, writing, or volunteer work.

Even if you stay emotionally strong during your treatment, you may find yourself crying at unexpected moments or lethargic when you normally would be bustling about. Don't be hard on yourself. You may be suffering from depression. Depression is not a sign of weakness. It is a chemical imbalance that can be treated. (See "Depression," page 227.)

## Hope

"A will to live" may not be quantified by research, but at least anecdotally those who have a reason to live and have hope for improvement in their health may live more fulfilling, if not longer, lives. This is not true in all cases, but in general a hopeful, positive attitude contributes to a better quality of life. This does not mean denial that you have a serious, life-threatening illness. It does mean that you embrace life with anticipation, you continue to plan for your future, and you continue to pursue new treatment options if the former ones have not worked.

If people treat you as if you will be gone tomorrow, ask them to help you enjoy each day as fully as possible and to accept the possibility that you might be a long-term survivor.

## So What Do You Tell Your Daughter?

The hardest part of breast cancer for some women is wondering if they have predisposed their daughters to walk the cancer journey. If we knew that cancer was only genetic, we could relieve ourselves of guilt because genes are out of our control. But genetics has been identified as a cause in only 5 to 10 percent of breast cancer cases.[50] In families with many cases of breast cancer, genetic counseling may be an appropriate course of action.

A large study of twins found that inherited factors do not explain the majority of breast cancer cases.[51] A study by T.I. Sorensen et al. in 1988 found that adopted children whose adoptive parents died of cancer were five times more likely to get the same disease than the general population. This certainly suggests factors beyond genetics in family cancers.

One possibility of cancer running in families is that lifestyle factors tend to be passed down from one generation to the next. As a kid, I loved raw cookie dough (I had never heard of the trans fat) and proudly served it to my children also. In high school and college I didn't relish much physical activity outside of PE class and so didn't encourage my daughter to play a sport. I thought a proper Southern belle endured whatever emotional baggage was dumped on her and—no, here at least I wised up in time and taught my daughter to express her emotions, tactfully but fully. But you see the pattern. What we know now as unhealthy lifestyle factors are merely traditions in some families and could be influencing generations of family members although not directly through the genes.

What I tell my daughter is what I read about factors I now know I can, and should, control: my weight, my exercise plan, my emotions, and my environment. And I tell her to teach her daughters the good habits I did not know about so they will gain the protective benefits before and during puberty, the period researchers are focusing on as very important to breast cancer prevention.

Tell your daughters and granddaughters and nieces and sisters and anyone else who will listen that they are not pawns waiting for cancer to strike them down. They can be proactive and reduce their chances of cancer outrunning their body's immune capability. They can do this through regular exercise; a healthy, mostly plant-based diet; reduction of stress; and avoidance of as many toxins as possible. Will that guarantee a cancer-free existence? Unfortunately not, but many leading cancer organizations are saying such changes might actually help—a lot.

## Follow-Up with Doctors

Once treatment is over, you will still see a lot of your oncologist or primary care physician. Usually you may see her every three months for a year or so, then every six months. Eventually you'll graduate to annual visits.

Interestingly, many breast cancer patients prefer the more frequent visits. Once their contact slips to once or twice a year, many patients feel as if they are in a free fall. They want the security that the exam gives them that they are healing and being monitored.

Also, it is very normal to feel anxiety as the day for your anniversary tests approaches. Most women are not afraid of the tests as much as they are what the tests will show. If possible, take someone with you to the tests so you'll have someone to talk to while you wait. Try to plan several fun things the few days afterwards so you also have something to look forward to and to distract you while you wait for the results.

## Follow-Up Tests

Although you probably had a mammogram, bone scan, chest X-ray, and abdominal CAT scan before treatment started, physicians differ on the types and frequency of follow-up tests once treatment is completed. Some schedules depend upon the type of treatment taken.

A surgeon may want to check you every few weeks until your incision has healed, then every three to six months for a year. A radiation oncologist and oncologist who ordered chemotherapy will likely want to examine you every three or four months for two or three years.

Oncologists will usually take a blood sample on each visit. Whether tumor markers are measured will depend on whether they are predictive for you. Sometimes doctors will do blood chemistries to check liver or kidney or other body functions.

Controversy surrounds follow-up testing. Some doctors and patients want bone scans, CAT scans, and chest X-rays every three to six months. Others are leery of the radiation exposure and cost. The American Society of Clinical Oncology does not recommend routine radiologic or laboratory testing (including tumor markers) unless they have an impact on survival.

The guidelines from the National Comprehensive Cancer Network (NCCN) call for a history and physical every four to six months for five years, then every year and a mammogram every year. For those taking tamoxifen, the NCCN recommends a pelvic exam every year because of the slightly increased risk of uterine cancer.

Mammography is still recommended annually after breast cancer. Most doctors agree that a mammogram on the remaining breast is very important because your chance of another cancer is greater than for a woman who has not had breast cancer. Also, if you had a lumpectomy, you will want to have the affected breast checked regularly, as recurrence is a possibility. If you have had reconstruction, mammography may be useful if you are at high risk for recurrence or if it is difficult to examine the area by hand. You should still do self-examinations of the area around the breast because recurrences may develop there.

Some studies have shown that finding a systemic relapse a few months earlier does not change the overall treatment or prognosis, though others point out that those studies are at least a decade old and they feel that the sooner a metastasis or recurrence is found, the better results are possible. Whatever you and your health team decide on this issue, do inform your doctor when you have a new symptom or a pain that persists for more than two weeks. Most of these are not cancer, but if they are, you may as well get a head start on treatment.

## Hormone Replacement Therapy (HRT)

Menopause decreases the amount of estrogen produced by a woman's body. That decrease is behind the symptoms some women experience after their monthly periods cease (hot flashes, vaginal dryness, loss of interest in sexual activity, osteoporosis, and so forth).

Chemotherapy sometimes causes early menopause that can be accompanied by the same irritating symptoms. About 60 percent of breast cancer patients will be given tamoxifen as part of their cancer regimen after surgery,[52] and it can introduce some of the same side effects as menopause as well as slightly increasing the risk of uterine cancer and blood clots.

Because the role in breast cancer of estrogen and other hormones is still being determined, some women and physicians are leery of continuing or initiating hormone replacement therapy after treatment for breast cancer, especially if a woman's tumor was estrogen receptor–positive. This means that the tumor used estrogen cells to its advantage. Estrogen is known to stimulate the growth of breast tissue, and how that may or may not contribute to breast cancer is still under investigation. Most of our estrogen is produced by the ovaries, but the adrenal gland and our own body fat produce a measurable amount also.

A recent study showed that hormone replacement therapy increased the risk of breast cancer for some women. Other studies agree this is true for only some groups of women, such as those who take HRT for more than 15 years.[53] Much of the research has been done on Premarin or Prempro (Premarin and Provera, a synthetic progesterone-like drug). In July 2002 the

Women's Health Initiative study was stopped three years early after data showed that women taking combined estrogen-progestin HRT had an increased risk of developing breast cancer over women taking no HRT or estrogen alone. This confirmed findings reported in the prestigious *Lancet* that reviewed 51 studies and concluded that each year of HRT use increased the risk of breast cancer and another NCI study reported in January 2000 that showed a 40-percent increase for breast cancer for women on the combined drug.[54] Some physicians are still recommending HRT because they believe HRT protects women against heart disease, osteoporosis, and menopausal symptoms. These findings are from much earlier studies that have been overridden by more recent studies.

Some physicians feel that natural progesterone or natural hormones (hormones derived from plants that are chemically identical to those produced by our bodies) are safe. Because these substances cannot be patented, they are not made or marketed by drug companies and do not receive the same promotion to doctors via free samples, literature, ads in journals, presentations at seminars, and so forth as patentable drugs do. This may be an area to research and discuss with your physician.

In the meantime, there is some light on the horizon. Tamoxifen works by "clogging up" the entrances to the cancer cells with other estrogen-like substances so the estrogen cannot enter the cell. It has also been found to have benefits for heart disease and osteoporosis. Other new drugs, known as selective estrogen receptor modulators (SERMs), are being tested to add to the arsenal of medication available to replace HRT. SERMs provide the benefits of estrogen (such as lowered risk of heart disease and osteoporosis) but not the risks (such as increased risk for breast or uterine cancer). Currently only one, Evista (raloxifene), is available. More are being researched and tested and may be on the market soon.

Some herbs that are often recommended for menopausal symptoms include black cohosh, evening primrose, gamma oryzanol, chaste tree berry (*Vitex agnus-castus*), borage oil, black currant oil, dong quai, red clover, and motherwort. Although these have been used in women's health for years, check with a qualified herbalist or nutritionist about recent studies and any relationship to breast cancer.

## Mind/Body Connection

As the folk song says, "The hip bone's connected to the thigh bone." We are a composite of parts that overlap and do not stand as isolated entities. These parts include all aspects of the body, the mind, and the spirit. Part of your treatment plan for recovering from breast cancer will need to address mental, emotional, and spiritual issues because you will probably experience changes in these areas, which will lead you to examine some beliefs and attitudes and to investigate ways of healing these areas.

A new field of study has emerged to combine psychology, neurology, and immunology. It is called psychoneuroimmunology. It is known that high periods of stress or anxiety are often related to reduced functioning of the immune system. Even mild depression may suppress the immune system. However, other studies have shown that acute stress may stimulate immune activity by increasing production of some types of white cells that fight infection.

One of the most common forms of holistic help for breast cancer patients is a strong support system. This can be family members, friends, a religious group, a social worker or psychotherapist, or a support group. A study in 1989 at Stanford University found that women with metastatic breast cancer who participated in a support group described a better quality of life and a longer life than a similar group of women who were not active in support groups. Another more recent study did not confirm these findings.

Another controversial theory of the mind/body connection has been popularized by general surgeon Bernie Siegel. He identifies a cancer-prone personality (passive, not expressing feelings, hopeless) and claims that people who take charge of their cancer diagnosis and participate fully in their treatment decisions have better outcomes than those who don't. Other researchers have criticized Siegel's theory as being too guilt-producing and inaccurate. They feel people blame themselves for developing cancer. Also, they point to many people who are active in their fight against cancer and who die from it anyway.

Probably the most accurate statement that can be made about the connection of the mind and physical illness is that we know there is a connection, but we don't know for sure the extent of the cause/effect relationship. Did a student's anxiety cause the ulcers or was it the pizza and doughnuts she lived on and the sleep she didn't get during finals?

Any technique that can calm, refresh, or relax you is worth pursuing. Your mental state is as important in this battle as your physical state. Just remember that imaging, meditation, or journaling cannot cure cancer. They should be practiced alongside conventional therapies, not in place of them.

## Preventing Recurrence

The majority of women who have had breast cancer are plagued to some degree with the fear of recurrence: Did doctors really get it all? Recurrence can happen at the sight of the original tumor (local recurrence), the lymph nodes near the breast (regional recurrence), or in another part of the body (metastatic recurrence). Twenty to 30 percent of women with localized breast cancer and 30 to 60 percent with initial lymph node involvement develop metastasis. Breast cancer in the other breast is usually a new primary tumor.

Studies have shown that women with excess body fat are at greater risk for:

- Developing breast cancer.
- Having shorter survival time if they do develop breast cancer.
- Relapsing from the disease regardless of the number or lack of lymph nodes involved.
- Dying from breast cancer.[55]

## Signs to Watch For

Life after breast cancer can be likened to a tennis match: You go back and forth in your mind about the meaning of symptoms and new aches and pains. Try not to panic when new conditions arise. Instead, mention them to your doctor for evaluation. Some symptoms to mention (and which can have nothing to do with cancer) are:

- Lump, redness, rash, or pimples on the chest wall or under the arms.
- Dimpling of the skin.
- Thickening in the breast area.
- Swelling.
- Lumps anywhere on body.
- Pain that persists for more than a few days.
- Trouble walking or bone pain, back pain, leg weakness. (Mention it even if you think it may be related to arthritis or stiffness.)
- Dry cough, trouble breathing, shortness of breath.
- Problems with balance, vision, headaches.
- Progressive abdominal discomfort.

### *Metastasis*

Every cancer patient would like to hear the words, "We got it all." Unfortunately, there is no guarantee with treatment for breast cancer. When breast cancer spreads, it usually spreads to the lungs, bone, liver, or brain.

Bone metastasis is the most common in patients with breast cancer. Either the tumor can invade the bone or the cancer can cause hormonal changes that lead to bone loss. The destruction of bone produces a substance that actually aids the growth of the cancer.

The first symptom of bone metastasis is usually bone pain or a fracture. X-rays, bone scans, or PET scans may be done to confirm a diagnosis. A biopsy is usually not done because of the risk of breaking a bone.

Complications with bone metastases may include the release of massive amounts of calcium, which weakens bone further, or the compression of the spinal cord, which is painful and could eventually lead to paralysis.

Bone metastases can be treated with medication, radiation, surgery, or a new type of drug called bisphosphonates. Two leading drugs of this type are Aredia and Zometa, which harden the bones so it is harder for the cancer to penetrate them. They are usually given intravenously, Zometa for 15 minutes once a month and Aredia for two hours once a month. Oral bisphosphonates are Fosamax and Actonel. Common side effects, which usually disappear after a few treatments, are elevated temperature, transient chills, increased bone pain, and renal complications. Your doctor will monitor your kidney function closely while you are on these drugs.

Because most fractures occur with falls, it is important to do exercises for balance such as t'ai chi and strengthening exercises. Repetitive impact exercise can lead to weakening of bone, so don't do any exercise for more than 15 minutes. Avoid heavy weights and power sit-ups that may endanger the spine.[56]

## *Breast Examinations*

One activity you should make a priority whether or not it was part of your previous routine is breast examinations—*even if you had a double mastectomy.*

Because you can know your body better than anyone, it is important to examine your breasts or chest wall monthly for any changes. Be sure to include the axillas (armpits), up to the jawbone, and down to the ribs. Premenopausal women should do the exam about the 10th day of their cycle. Postmenopausal women should pick a day that is easy for them to remember and train themselves to perform the exam each month.

It is also important to have a medical doctor perform an exam at least annually. Ask your gynecologist, oncologist, or family practitioner to do this.

In the breast exam you are on the alert for asymmetry (something on one side and not the other), for changes from the last exam, and for lumps that seem attached to skin or muscle (don't move), seem hard, are or are not painful, and are irregular in shape.

## How to Do a Breast Self-Exam

- Look in a mirror for any changes in your breasts: dimples, shape, color, lumps. Clasp your hands behind your head and look some more.

- Lie down. With the finger pad of the opposite hand, press your breasts around the entire breast area either in a circular pattern or up and down or side to side. Notice any changes, particularly any hard lumps.
- Gently squeeze each nipple to see if there is any discharge.

A breast pad may help your exam. The soft-plastic, fluid-filled square enhances what you are feeling. Baby powder on your skin may help also.

Smooth, round, soft lumps tend not to be cancerous; cancerous lumps tend to be hard, irregular, and firmly attached to breast tissue. If there are any changes from your last exam or you have a nipple discharge, see your doctor. There are many benign reasons for breast changes and lumps, but only a doctor can assess them accurately.

## How Can I Get Involved in the Fight against Breast Cancer?

Many breast cancer survivors and their friends and family exit the treatment phase with a desire to give back, to make a difference in the fight against breast cancer. The ways to do this are as unique as each individual. These ideas might spark your thinking:

- Be a stand-in-the-gap friend to the next person you know who is diagnosed with breast cancer.
- Sign up as a telephone buddy through a cancer organization.
- Consider participating in a clinical trial in the next phase of your treatment.
- Participate in a cancer race or other fund-raising event.
- Volunteer to speak to groups in schools, the community, or workplace about breast cancer.
- Facilitate or participate in a support group, even after your treatment ends. Begin a support group at your church or community center.
- Be an example of a healthy lifestyle and be ready to tell people why you made the changes you did.
- Take advocacy training to influence policy on a state or national level.
- Write to your local politicians about breast cancer-related legislation.
- See Resources for ways to donate free mammograms or purchase products that earn funds for research.
- Support a local organization that provides mammograms and other services for low-income or uninsured women. Donate to organizations that conduct breast cancer research.
- Donate books on breast cancer to a library.

We all wish there were answers about the causes of breast cancer and recurrence. Until those answers are determined, all we can do is educate ourselves about healthy living in general and adopt as many healthy behaviors as possible. Only you can decide which precautions seem worth the effort.

For results of studies about lifestyle and breast cancer specifically, review the Websites listed in Resources.

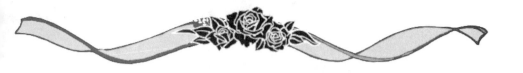

# Conclusion

It happened although you didn't invite it. You dealt with it although you hated some of the process. You are different now. Relish those differences.

Breast cancer will most likely shadow your thoughts for the rest of your life. Acknowledge the fear or anxiety when it comes and determine not to let the disease rob you of your joy. Even in the midst of sickness or weakness from treatment, joy is all around you if you train your eyes, ears, and heart to look and listen.

You've had a wake-up call—to change unhealthy lifestyle factors, to reassess priorities, to mend and deepen relationships. You can turn breast cancer into a bend in your life journey toward a fuller, more meaningful life. It may take courage and fortitude to make changes you decide you want to make. Raymond Lindquist said, "Courage is the power to let go of the familiar." Because breast cancer patients cannot return to exactly the place/attitude/outlook we had before diagnosis, we may as well take advantage of our newfound wisdom and begin living the life we've always wanted. There is freedom in that thought that overshadows the fear of recurrence.

I hope this book has given you many ideas to help you move through treatment easier. I also hope you embrace the rest of your life with renewed optimism, healthier choices, and joys that astound you.

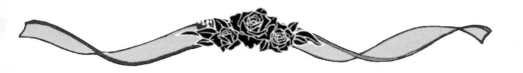

# Notes

## Chapter 1

[1] *The Harvard Report on Cancer Prevention*, cited in AICR, *Stopping Cancer before It Starts*, 1999.

[2] Ibid.

[3] National Cancer Institute (NCI), "Closing in on Cancer," 47.

[4] *Stopping Cancer*, 19; DeGregorio, Michael, *Tamoxifen and Breast Cancer* (Yale University Press, 1999), p. 13.

[5] American Cancer Society (ACS), *Breast Cancer Facts & Figures 2001–2002*, 2.

[6] "Beyond Tomorrow: A New Look at Breast Cancer," *www.healthtalk.com*, Oct. 25, 2000, 14.

[7] Susan Love, *The Breast Cancer Course for Researchers: An In-Depth Interdisciplinary Review of the State of the Science*, *www.susanlovemd.com*, March 21, 2004.

[8] Anne McTiernan, *Breast Fitness: An Optimal Exercise and Health Plan for Reducing Your Risk of Breast Cancer* (St. Martin's Press, 2000), 20.

[9] Ibid., 98.

[10] Ibid., 20.

[11] Ibid.

[12] Love, *Breast Cancer Course*, March 21, 2004.

[13] O'Donnell, Rosie, *Bosom Buddies: Lessons and Laughter On Breast Health and Cancer* (Warner Books, 1999), 95.

[14] "What is Meant by 'Breast Cancer Risk'?" *www.natlbcc.org/bin/index.asp?strid=567&depid=9&btnid=2*, Jan. 29, 2004.

[15] *Stopping Cancer*, 197.

[16] Jane A. Plant, Ph.D., *No-Dairy Breast Cancer Prevention Program* (Thomas Dunne Books, 2001), 16.

[17] Marcus Laux, "Naturally Well Today: Insider's Guide to Cancer-Proofing Your Body," 2.

[18] Susan Lark, "The Women's Pharmacy," 5.

[19] NCI, "Cancer Facts: Lifetime probability of breast cancer in American women," 2002.

[20] Plant, 16.

[21] ACS, *www.cancer.org/docroot/CRI/CRI_2x.asp?sitearea=LRN&dt=5*, April 11, 2004.

[22] ACS, "Surveillance Research, 2001" in *Breast Cancer Facts & Figures 2001–2002*, 9.

[23] National Breast Cancer Coalition, "Facts about Breast Cancer in the United States: Year 2003," *www.nabco.org/index.php/435*, Jan. 28, 2004.

[24] Link, John, *Breast Cancer Survival Manual: A Step-By-Step Guide for the Woman With Newly Diagnosed Cancer* (Owl Books, 2000), p. 163.

[25] *www.natlbcc.org*, Jan. 29, 2004.

[26] Nancy Evans, ed., "State of Evidence: What Is the Connection Between Chemicals and Breast Cancer?", Breast Cancer Fund and Breast Cancer Action, Feb. 2002, 10.

[27] *www.nabco.org/index.php/435*, Jan. 29, 2004.

[28] *Harvard Health Letter*, June 2002, p. 5.

[29] Helen Hill Schnipper, LICSW, *After Breast Cancer: A Common-Sense Guide to Life After Treatment* (Bantam Books, 2003), 236.

[30] Brown et al., Journal of NCI 1993, slide show, "Flaxseed and the Cancer Survivor," Wendy Demark-Wahnefried, Duke University Medical Center.

## Chapter 2

[1] O'Donnell, 58–9.

[2] NCI, "Understanding Breast Changes," 7–8.

[3] ACS, *Cancer Facts & Figures 2003*, 30.

[4] Daniel W. Nixon, M.D., *The Cancer Recovery Eating Plan: The Right Foods to Help Fuel Your Recovery* (Alison Brown Crerier Book Development, Inc./Times Books/Random House, 1996), 87–88.

[5] Ibid., 88–89.

[6] Coalition of National Cancer Cooperative Groups, flier, C3.

[7] DeGregorio, 96.

[8] Stephen Sinatra, "Hidden Dangers of Vitamin Overdosing," Phillips Health LLC, 2003, 2, 4.

[9] Ibid., 4.

[10] *Arthritis Today*, November/December 2002, 69.

[11] American Institute for Cancer Research (AICR), *Dietary Options for Cancer Survivors,* 2002, 3.

[12] *Tufts University Health & Nutrition* ad #35.

[13] O'Donnell, 178.

[14] Center for Science in the Public Interest, *Nutrition Action Healthletter*, October 2001, 12.

[15] *Cancersupportivecare.com/neuropathicpain.html*, "Post Breast Therapy Pain Syndrome," 4–5.

[16] Marisa C. Weiss, M.D., and Ellen Weiss, *Living Beyond Breast Cancer: A Survivor's Guide for When Treatment Ends and the Rest of Your Life Begins* (Three Rivers Press, 1998), 84.

[17] *Nutrition Action*, January/February 2004, 11.

## Chapter 3

[1] "On the Side: Anemia," *LifeLine*, Y-Me newsletter, winter 2004, 18.

[2] Roper Cancer Center handout.

[3] *Natural Health*, April 2003, 77–8.

[4] Roper Cancer Center flier "Elimination Problems."

[5] "Unleash the inner healing power of foods, nausea & vomiting," source not identified.

[6] Stephen Sinatra, *Consumer's Guide to Herbal Remedies* (Phillips Health LLC, 2003), 4.

[7] *Natural Health*, December 2002, 45.

[8] Ibid., May/June 2003, 83.

[9] Ibid., 125.

[10] Ibid., 67.

[11] WHEL (Women's Healthy Eating and Lifestyle) newsletter, University of California, San Diego.

[12] Debbie Deangelo, *Sudden Menopause: Restoring Health and Emotional Well-Being* (Hunter House, 2001), 17.

[13] Abstract 655 at 26th Annual San Antonio Breast Cancer Symposium (2004) showed that black cohosh was safe and effective against hot flashes and did not stimulate growth of cancer cells.

[14] Susan Love, M.D., *Dr. Susan Love's Hormone Book* (Three Rivers Press, 1998), 160.

[15] *Nutrition Action*, January/February 2004, 11.

[16] Ibid., 9.

[17] "Tips to Avoid Infections," *www.cancerlynx.com*, Jan. 28, 2004.

[18] *Natural Health*, March 2003, 70.

[19] Louden, Jennifer, *Woman's Comfort Book, A Self-Nurturing Guide for Restoring Balance in Your Life* (HarperSanFrancisco, 1992), 150.

[20] Love, *Hormone Book*, 182.

[21] *Harvard Health Letter*, May 2002, 2.

[22] Ibid.

[23] Louden, 151.

[24] Amy Halverstadt, and Andrea Leonard, *Essential Exercises for Breast Cancer Survivors: How to Live Stronger and Feel Better* (Harvard Common Press, 2000), 15.

[25] Ibid., 36.

[26] Saskia R.J. Thiadens, R.N., "18 Steps to Prevention of Upper Extremities," National Lymphedema Network, January 2002, 1.

[27] Weiss, 130.

[28] Love, *Hormone Book*, 11.

[29] Deangelo, 15.

[30] Holly Clegg, and Gerald Miletello, M.D., *Eating Well Through Cancer* (Aventis, 2001), p. 134.

[31] "Taking time to dunk that tea bag can be a mini meditation during the day. In fact, I have often wondered if green tea is healthy due solely to its chemical constituents or if health benefits are also conferred due to the relaxation obtained from the preparation process and drinking slowly while chatting with friends or family." C. Astill et al., *Journal of Agricultural Food Chemicals*, November 2001, 49 (11):5340-7, "Factors affecting the caffeine and polyphenol contents of black and green tea infusions."

[32] WHEL (Women's Healthy Eating and Lifestyle) clinical trial, March 2003 cooking class, "Tasty Tummy Tamer," M. D. Anderson Cancer Center, Houston.

[33] Clegg, 133.

[34] *www.cancerlynx.com*, January 28, 2004.

[35] N. Kumar, K.A. Allen, D. Riccardi, et al., "Fatigue, weight gain, lethargy and amenorrhea in breast cancer patients on chemotherapy: is subclinical hypothyroidism the culprit?" *Breast Cancer Research and Treatment*, 83(2):149–59. On PubMed, March 14, 2004.

[36] *Arthritis Today*, July/August 2002, 35.

[37] Nixon, 85.

[38] McTiernan, 123.

[39] *Food & Fitness Advisor*, Weil College of Medicine of Cornell University, January 2003, 4.

## Chapter 4

[1] "NCCAM Five-Year Strategic Plan, 2001–2005," part 1, "Appeal of Nontraditional Approaches," *www.nccam.nih.gov/about/plans/fiveyear/index.htm*, March 15, 2004, 7.

[2] Ibid., part 1, 8.

[3] Link, 144.

[4] "The ABCs of Complementary and Alternative Therapies and Cancer Treatment," *internalmedicine.medscape.com/ACCC/OncIssues/2000/v15.n06/oil506.03.moor/pnt*, January 22, 2001.

[5] *MD News* reprint, Dr. Christina Stemmler's office, Houston, Texas, no date.

[6] Plant, 228.

[7] Lark Letter ad, 14.

[8] Dianna Hale, "Why Prayer Could Be Good Medicine," *Parade*, March 23, 2003, 4.

[9] Father Whitney Miller, Cenacle Silent Retreat, Houston, Texas, June 2001.

[10] *www.cancer.ucsd.edu/outreach/cams/traditionalchinese.asp*, February 8, 2004.
[11] Love, *Hormone Book*, 153.
[12] *Johns Hopkins Medical Letter*, July 2002, 3.

## Chapter 5

[1] Marty Marder, et al., *www.cancersupportivecare.com*, January 29, 2004.
[2] Quoted in *Network*, M. D. Anderson Cancer Center, winter 2002, 2.
[3] McTiernan, 147.
[4] Stephen Sinatra, M.D., *Consumer's Guide to Supplements* (Phillips Health, LLC, 2003), 6.
[5] *Natural Health*, May/June 2003, 63.
[6] "Doctor, doctor," M. D. Anderson Cancer Center newsletter, no date, author's file.
[7] *Food & Fitness*, August 2003, 9.
[8] *Natural Health*, October/November 2002, 104.
[9] Ibid., May/ June 2003, 67.
[10] *Food & Fitness*, August 2003, 9.
[11] *MAMM*, May 2001, 62.
[12] Marcus Laux, "Naturally Well Today: Insider's Guide to Fighting Fatigue," 6.
[13] *Natural Health*, May/June 2003, 64.
[14] David Spiegel, M.D., *New Woman*, October 1994, 136.
[15] Louden, 149.
[16] *Natural Health*, May/June 2003, 63.
[17] Hill Schnipper, p. 76, quoting Ganz, et al., 1998, *Journal of Clinical Oncology*, 16, 501–514.

## Chapter 6

[1] *www.cancerlynx.com/health_insurance.html*, January 28, 2004.
[2] *Arthritis Today*, no date, 77.

## Chapter 7

[1] Pamela Haylock, *Men's Cancers* (Hunter House, 2001), 136.
[2] "Young Women and Breast Cancer," *LifeLine*, Y-Me, winter 2004, 3.
[3] Teleconference, Young Survivors, LBBC (Living Beyond Breast Cancer), March 17, 2004.
[4] "Breast Cancer and Pregnancy," PDQ, National Cancer Institute, January 15, 2004, 6.
[5] John Link, *Take Charge of Your Breast Cancer: A Guide to Getting the Best Possible Treatment* (Owl Books, 2002), 146.
[6] 26th annual San Antonio Breast Cancer Symposium, Abstract 651, author's files.
[7] Weiss, 220.
[8] Ibid., 228.

[9] Transcript, "Fertility and the Safety of Pregnancy after Breast Cancer," *www.lbbc.org*, March 21, 2004.
[10] ACS, *Breast Cancer Fact & Figures 2001–2002,* 5.
[11] Ibid., 4.
[12] O'Donnell, 7.

## Chapter 8
[1] ACS, Look Good…Feel Better instruction book, 4.
[2] *Natural Health*, April 2003, 39.
[3] *www.headwear-etc.com.*

## Chapter 9
[1] McTiernan, 204.
[2] ACS, Breast Cancer printout; McTiernan, 52.
[3] *Stopping Cancer*, 96.
[4] Link, *Breast Cancer Survival Manual*, 147.
[5] AICR newsletter, fall 2003, 8.
[6] AICR newsletter, "Taking a Closer Look at Calories, Exercise, & Cancer."
[7] *Food & Fitness*, January 2003, 4.
[8] *Food & Fitness*, November 2001, 2.
[9] AICR newsletter, spring 2003, 5.
[10] Marcus Laux, "Naturally Well Today: Insider's Guide to Healthy Hormones," 5.
[11] *Natural Health*, September 2003, 41.
[12] Summarized in Rosebuds Support Group newsletter, April 2004. From Daniel Q. Haney, Associated Press.

## Chapter 10
[1] ACS, "Nutrition and Physical Activity During and After Cancer Treatment: An American Cancer Society Guide for Informed Choices," *A Cancer Journal for Clinicians*, September/October 2003, 287.
[2] *Stopping Cancer*, 3.
[3] Association of American Medical Colleges, *www.aamc.org*, January 28, 2004.
[4] *www.cancerrd.com*, November 2003.
[5] "Ask Dr. Etingin," *Women's Health Advisor*, July 2001, 8.
[6] Ibid.
[7] *Health*, May 2001, 137.
[8] Plant, 123.
[9] Ibid.
[10] Ibid., 123–4.
[11] AICR newsletter, spring 2003, p. 9.
[12] *Food & Fitness*, September 2003, 2.
[13] Link, *Breast Cancer Survival Manual*, 130.
[14] Lark, *The Women's Pharmacy*, 7.

[15] Laux, "Cancer-Proofing Your Body," 2.

[16] *www.nal.usda.gov/fsrio/ppd/fda07e.htm*, April 3, 2004.

[17] *Food & Fitness*, February 2003, 7.

[18] Link, *Breast Cancer Survival Manual*, 143.

[19] *Arthritis Today*, January/February 2003, 10.

[20] Clegg, p. 197; UCSD Cancer Center, *www.cancer.ucsd.edu/outreach/cams/greentea.asp*, March 25, 2004.

[21] *www.agmrc.org/vegetables/profiles/carrotprofile.pdf*, April 3, 2004.

[22] Lark Letter, "Fibroids and Endometriosis," 2003, 3.

[23] *Mind/Body Health Newsletter*, Vol. VIII, No. 1, 1999, 2.

[24] *Food & Fitness,* October 2003, 5.

[25] *Stopping Cancer*, 162.

[26] Lark Letter ad, 11.

[27] Laux, "Healthy Hormones," 4.

[28] Nixon, 32–33.

[29] *Food & Fitness*, March 2003, 2.

[30] Plant, 97.

[31] Ibid., 103.

[32] Ibid., 127.

[33] *Stopping Cancer*, 75.

[34] Nixon, 217.

[35] ACS, "Nutrition and Physical Activity," 7.

[36] *Food & Fitness*, October 2003, 9.

[37] *www.agmrc.org/vegetables/profiles/carrotprofile.pdf*, April 3, 2004.

[38] Oils are extracted from foods in three ways. Cold pressing keeps temperatures low so temperature-sensitive vitamins are not disturbed. The technique is more expensive because of copious waste, but it is the most nutritious. Screw or expeller pressed oils have undergone high pressure, which generates high heat that destroys some vitamins. Solvent extraction produces the highest yield, so is the cheapest. The grains or seeds are steamed and mixed with solvents, heated, bleached, and filtered. Then the oil is heated again and chemicals are sometimes added to prevent rancidity. Not many nutrients can withstand the processing.

[39] WHEL News, January/February 2004, 3.

[40] *www.chemocare.com*, May 20, 2003.

[41] Plant, 227.

[42] Evans, 2003.

[43] Ibid., 6.

[44] Link, *Breast Cancer Survival Manual*, 131.

[45] Evans, 6.

[46] "Rethinking Environmental Estrogens," *www.mamm.com*, April 14, 2004.

[47] *www.techcentralstation.com/060302B.html*, "Pesky Pesticide Tests," June 2002.

[48] Stephen Sinatra, "How to Survive—and Thrive—in a World of Hidden Toxins," 10.

[49] Ibid., 7.

[50] *www.natlbcc.org*, "Breast Cancer and the Environment," January 29, 2004, 3.

[51] Ibid., 1.

[52] Robinson, Rebecca, *Step-by-Step Guide to Dealing with Your Breast Cancer* (Citadel Trade, 1997), 126.

[53] Nixon, 91.

[54] Lark, Susan, "How Natural HRT Works," 2.

[55] Nixon, 84.

[56] *www.cancercare.org,* December 18, 2003.

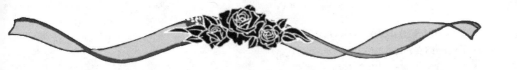

# Resources

A listing here does not imply an endorsement of any organization, philosophy, or product.

## Organizations
### Advocacy
Breast Cancer Action
*www.baction.org*
   Aims to influence policy changes necessary to end the breast cancer epidemic.

Breast Cancer Fund
*www.breastcancerfund.org*, 800–487–0492
   Advocates for elimination of environmental and other preventable causes of breast cancer. Sponsors Expedition Inspiration, a mountain climb by breast cancer survivors.

Breast Cancer Resource Committee
*www.afamerica.com/bcrc*, 202–463–8040
   Educates the African-American community about breast cancer.

Hurricane Voices
*www.hurricanevoices.org*, 866–667–3300
   Raises public consciousness about causes of and cures for breast cancer. See its study on breast cancer and the environment.

National Breast Cancer Coalition
*www.natlbcc.org*, 800–622–2838
   Sponsors a free (except for travel and lodging) training course, called Project LEAD, to provide breast cancer advocates with knowledge to influence research and public policy. Scholarships available.

National Patient Advocate Foundation
*www.npaf.org/index.php*, 202–347–8009
   Creates insurance funding for evolving therapies and therapeutic devices and agents through legislative and policy reform.

## Breast Cancer Information

Breast Cancer Alliance
   *www.breastcanceralliance.org*
      Breast cancer research, education, and outreach.

BreastCancer.Net
   *www.breastcancer.net*
      Daily e-mails on new breast cancer articles on the Web.

Breastcancer.org
   *www.breastcancer.org*
      Treatment, research, recovery, and more. Founded by Dr. Marisa Weiss.
      Monthly online conferences.

Canadian Breast Cancer Foundation
   *www.cbcf.org*, 800–387–9816
      Leading volunteer-based breast cancer organization in Canada. Promotes
      research, awareness, and survivor issues.

Casting for Recovery (CFR)
   *www.castingforrecovery.org*, 888–553–3500
      Provides no-cost fly-fishing retreats for women with breast cancer.

Healthtalk Breast Cancer Education Network
   *www.healthtalk.com*
      Archives discussions with top experts; interviews with breast cancer survivors.

Living Beyond Breast Cancer
   *www.lbbc.org*
      Public forums for young survivors and women with metastatic disease;
      conferences; newsletter.

Living With It
   *www.livingwithit.org*, 877–548–4649
      Also in Spanish. Money matters, medical information, lifestyle tips, and
      recurrence information from Aventis Pharmaceuticals Inc.

Medscape's Breast Cancer Resource Center
   *www.medscape.com/resource/breastcancer*
      Breaking medical news and information on breast cancer prevention,
      diagnosis, and treatment.

Mothers Supporting Daughters with Breast Cancer (MSDBC)
   *www.mothersdaughters.org*, 410–778–1982
      Bulletin board and information for mothers whose daughters have breast
      cancer.

National Breast Cancer Foundation
   *www.nationalbreastcancer.org*
      Educational information and free mammograms for the underserved,
      minorities, and working poor.

Sharsheret
*www.sharsheret.org*
   Connects young Jewish women recently diagnosed with breast cancer with volunteers who can share their experiences.

Sisters Network
*www.sistersnetworkinc.org,* 866–781–1808
   For African-American breast cancer survivors.

Susan G. Komen Breast Cancer Foundation
*www.komen.org,* 972–855–1600, HelpLine: 800–462–9273
   Supports research and outreach programs through U.S. and international affiliates and events such as Race for the Cure.

Susan Love, M.D.
*www.SusanLoveMD.org*
   News and information on breast cancer.

Women's Information Network Against Breast Cancer
*www.winabc.org,* 866–294–6222
   Information and resources on breast cancer.

Y-Me National Breast Cancer Organization
*www.y-me.org,* 800–221–2141, Spanish 800–986–9505
   Translators in 150 languages. Information, monthly teleconferences, and support programs.

Young Survival Coalition
*www.youngsurvival.org,* 212–206–6610
   Advocacy, awareness, and support of young breast cancer patients. Bulletin board.

## Clinical Trials
CenterWatch
*www.centerwatch.com*

Coalition of National Cancer Cooperative Groups Inc.
*www.cancertrialshelp.org*

National Cancer Institute
*cancertrials.nci.nih.gov*

National Institutes of Health
*clinicaltrials.gov*

National Surgical Adjuvant Breast and Bowel Project
*www.nsabp.pitt.edu,* 412–330–4600

OncoLink
*www.oncolink.org/treatment/matching.cfm*

## Complementary/Alternative Medicine (CAM)

Alternative Medicine-On Line
*www.alternativemedicine.com*, 800–515–4325
CAM techniques and practitioners.

American College for the Advancement of Medicine
*www.acam.org*
Latest in alternative medicine; physician referrals.

Federal Trade Commission (FTC)
*www.ftc.gov*
Enforces consumer protection laws.

Food and Drug Administration (FDA)
*www.fda.gov*
Regulates drugs and medical devices to ensure safety and effectiveness.

Laughter Clubs
*www.worldlaughtertour.com*, 800–NOW–LAFF

M. D. Anderson Cancer Center's Complementary/Integrative Medicine Education Resources
*www.mdanderson.org/cimer*
Herbal information, drug interaction advisory, reviews of therapies.

Memorial Sloan-Kettering Cancer Center
*www.mskcc.org*
Look at Site Map/Integrative Medine/About Herbs, Botanicals & Other Products.

National Center for Complementary and Alternative Medicine (NCCAM)
*nccam.nih.gov* or *www.nlm.nih.gov/nccam/camonpubmed.html*
Part of National Institutes of Health. Extensive information on many CAM therapies.

University of California San Diego Cancer Center
*www.cancer.ucsd.edu/outreach/cams/index.asp*
Extensive information on CAM therapies.

USDA Food and Nutrition Information Center
*www.nal.usda.gov/fnic/pubs/bibs/gen/dietsupp.html*
Latest research on supplements.

## General Cancer Information

Abramson Cancer Center of the University of Pennsylvania
*oncolink.upenn.edu*

American Cancer Society
   *www.cancer.org*, 800–ACS–2345
   •Hope Lodges, free temporary housing for cancer patients and families.
   •I Can Cope, educational series about cancer treatment, side effects, nutrition, etc.
   •Kids Count Too, six-session program for children age 3 through teens.
   •Look Good...Feel Better, workshop on beauty techniques to enhance self-image during treatment.
   •Reach to Recovery, one-on-one support for breast cancer patients.

Beth Isreal Deaconess Cancer Center at Harvard University Medical School
   *cancercenter.bidmc.harvard.edu*

CancerCare
   *www.cancercare.org*, 800–813–HOPE
   Counseling, education, information and referral, support groups, and financial assistance.

Cancer Glossary
   *www.meds.com/glossary.html*
   Compiled by the Nursing Advisory Board of Pharmacia and Upjohn.

Cancer Links
   *www.cancerlinks.org*
   Lists many Websites about cancer.

Cancer Prevention Coalition
   *www.preventcancer.com*, 312–996–2297
   Information on avoidable causes, prevention, and politics of cancer.

Health On the Net Foundation (HON)
   *www.hon.ch*
   A not-for-profit Swiss organization to guide nonmedical users to reliable online medical and health information.

Kimmel Cancer Center at Thomas Jefferson University
   *www.kcc.tju.edu*

Mary-Helen Mautner Project for Lesbians with Cancer
   *www.mautnerproject.org*, 503–332–5536
   Education and support.

Mayo Clinic Cancer Center
   *www.mayoclinic.com*

National Cancer Institute
   *www.cancer.gov/cancerinfo*, 800–4–CANCER
   For a content list of its fax service, dial 301–402–5874 from a fax machine. To "chat" with a live person via e-mail, click the "LiveHelp" button on the Website. For a listing of NCI-designated cancer centers, go to *www3.cancer.gov/cancercenters/centerslist.html*.

National Coalition for Cancer Survivorship
*www.canceradvocacy.org*
　　Network of independent groups that deal with advocacy, support, and survivorship. Extensive database. Some publications in Spanish. Sponsors "Cancer: Keys to Survivorship" programs around the country. Listen to its Cancer Survivor Toolbox audio series at *www.cancersurvivaltoolbox.org* (negotiating your rights, communicating, etc.).

National Comprehensive Cancer Network
*www.nccn.org,* 888–909–NCCN
　　Alliance of 19 of the world's leading cancer centers offers clinical practice guidelines.

PDQ
*www.cancer.gov/cancerinfo/pdq*
　　Comprehensive database maintained by the National Cancer Institute. Information, clinical trials, alternative medicine, screening, and supportive care.

People Living With Cancer
*www.plwc.org*
　　Patient portion of American Society of Clinical Oncology Website.

Sidney Kimmel Comprehensive Cancer Center at Johns Hopkins
*www.med.jhu.edu/cancerctr*

## General Medical Information

American Red Cross Family Caregiving Program
*www.redcross.org/services/hss/care/family.html*
　　Series of workshops for caregivers on finances, general caregiving skills, healthy eating, etc.

Drugs.com
*www.drugs.com*
　　Consumer information on thousands of prescription medications.

Hardin Library for the Health Sciences, University of Iowa
*www.lib.uiowa.edu/hardin/md*
　　Exhaustive medical directory.

Harvard Medical School
*www.intelihealth.com*
　　Medical information for the layman.

Medline, National Library of Medicine
*www.nlm.nih.gov*
　　World's largest medical library.

Medscape
*www.medscape.com*
Latest medical news, resources, and links.

Pubmed, National Library of Medicine
*www.pubmed.com*

U.S. Department of Health and Human Services
*www.healthfinder.gov*
Links to more than 1,700 health-related organizations.

WebMD
*www.webmd.com*
General medical information and news.

## Herbs/Supplements

American Botanical Council
*www.herbalgram.org*, 512–926–4900
Science-based and traditional information to promote responsible use of herbal medicine.

American Herbal Products Association
*www.ahpa.org/companies.htm*
Sets standards, and links to those who meet those standards.

Consumer Lab
*www.consumerlab.com*
Independent test results and information to help consumers evaluate health, wellness, and nutrition products.

Herb Research Foundation
*www.herbs.org*
Information on medicinal plants and herbs.

National Institute of Environmental Health Services-Herbal Medicines
*www.niehs.nih.gov/external/resinits/ri-16.htm*
Reviews of literature and consumer information on herbal medicine.

National Institutes of Health Office of Dietary Supplements
*dietary-supplements.info.nih.gov*
Information on dietary supplements, dietary reference intakes (DRIs), and safety notices about supplements.

## Nutrition Information/Recipes

American Institute for Cancer Research
*www.aicr.org*
Information on role of nutrition in cancer; healthy recipes.

Cancer Nutrition Info, LLC
*www.cancernutritioninfo.com*
Complex nutrition-cancer research in layman's language.

Center for Food Safety and Applied Nutrition
*vm.cfsan.fda.gov/list.html*
Information on labeling, nutrition, and dietary supplements; consumer advice; and pesticides and lead in food.

Diana Dyer, MS, RD
*www.cancerrd.com*
Dietician's information on nutrition, eating out, recipes, etc.

Eat Wild
*www.eatwild.com*
Comprehensive information about grass-fed and organic beef, pork, lamb, bison, dairy products, and poultry and list of suppliers.

Food Routes
*www.foodroutes.org*
Find local growers.

International Vegetarian Union
*www.ivu.org/recipes*

National Agricultural Library
*www.nal.usda.gov*
Food and nutrition safety, research, and agricultural policy.

National Center for Nutrition (American Dietetic Association)
*www.eatright.org*, 800–366–1655
Position papers and help finding a dietician.

Nutrition Data
*www.NutritionData.com*
Free online resource of 7,500-plus foods using USDA data and restaurant data.

Nutrition Navigator
*www.navigator.tufts.edu*
Rates nutrition Websites.

Produce for Better Health Foundation
*www.aboutproduce.com*
Recipes and information on fresh fruits and vegetables.

U.S. Department of Agriculture
*www.nal.usda.gov*, 800–535–4555
Food safety hotline. To view listing of more than 6,000 foods, go to *www.nal.usda.gov/fnic/cgi-bin/nut_search.pl*. For a list of cookbooks, magazines, and Websites on nutrition and healthy eating, go to *www.nal.usda.gov/fnic/pubs/bibs/gen/eatsmart.html*.

Vegan Chef
  *www.veganchef.com*
    Recipes.
Vegan Cooking
  *www.vegancooking.com*
    Recipes.
Vegetarian Resource Group
  *www.vrg.org*, 410–366–8343
    Recipes, news, and information on vegetarianism.
VegWeb
  *www.vegweb.com*
    Recipes.

## Reconstruction

U.S. Food and Drug Administration
  *www.fda.gov/cdrh/breastimplants*, 800–532–4440
    About the safety of breast implants.

U.S. Food and Drug Administration's Center for Devices and Radiological Health
  *www.fda.gov/cdrh/breastimplants/indexbip.html*
    See a 2000 report on breast implants.

## Related Sites

American Bar Association
  *www.abanet.org/women/tensteps.html*
    Information on legal topics involving breast cancer.

Association of Cancer Online Resources
  *www.acor.org*
    Cancer-related Internet mailing lists and Web-based resources, including Breast Cancer List (Breast Cancer ListServ), an e-mail forum and discussion group.

Breast-Cancer Mailing List
  *www.bclist.org*
    International list that discusses all aspects of breast cancer.

Cancer Hope Network
  *www.cancerhopenetwork.org*, 877–467–3638
    One-on-one support for patients going through cancer treatment.

Dave Dravecky's Outreach of Hope
  *www.outreachofhope.org*, 719–481–3528
    Christian ministry to cancer patients. Prayer support and nonmedical resources.

FORCE (Facing Our Risk of Cancer Empowered)
*www.facingourrisk.org*, 954–255–8732
Chat room and resources on genetic risk for breast or ovarian cancer.

Kids Konnected
*www.kidskonnected.org*, 800–462–9273
Support groups through Susan B. Komen Foundation for kids whose mothers have breast cancer.

Team Survivor
*www.teamsurvivor.org*
Program of weekly exercise sessions, walking and biking programs, educational forums, instructional clinics, and special events for women with breast cancer.

YWCA Encore Plus
*www.ywca.org*, 800–95–EPLUS
Referrals for breast cancer screening and support and exercise programs for breast cancer patients.

# Books

## Complementary/Alternative Medicine (CAM)

Borysenko, Joan, *Minding the Body, Mending the Mind* (Bantam Books, 1988).
Personal stories teach the reader how to use mental and physical exercises to transform one's life.

Dossey, Larry, M.D., *Reinventing Medicine: Beyond Mind-Body to a New Era of Healing* (HarperSanFrancisco, 1999).
Scientific and medical proof that the spiritual dimension works in healing.

Hobbs, Christopher, L.Ac., *Herbal Remedies for Dummies* (IDG Books Worldwide, Inc., 1998).
Benefits of using herbal remedies, their selection and safe use, and growing and making herbals at home.

Kabat-Zinn, Jon, *Full Catastrophe Living* (Dell Publishing, 1990).
Practical guide to mindfulness, meditation, and healing.

Koenig, Harold, M.D., and Harvey Jay Cohen, *The Link Between Religion and Health: Psychoneuroimmunology and the Faith Factor* (Oxford Press, 2002).
How faith can affect health outcomes.

Moss, Ralph W., Ph.D., *Herbs Against Cancer. History and Controversy.* (Equinox Press, Inc., 1998).
History and controversies around using herbs to treat cancer.

O'Toole, Carole, and Carolyn B. Hendricks, *Healing Outside the Margins: The Survivor's Guide to Integrative Cancer Care* (Lifeline Press, 2003).
Review of complementary and alternative medicine approaches to cancer.

Weiss, Marisa C., M.D., and Ellen Weiss, *Living Beyond Breast Cancer: A Survivor's Guide for When Treatment Ends and the Rest of Your Life Begins* (Three Rivers Press, 1998).
Fear of recurrence, lingering side effects, etc.

## Cookbooks and Nutrition

American Institute for Cancer Research, *Dietary Options for Cancer Survivors* (AICR, 2002).
Research on foods, herbs, and dietary regimes and their effects on cancer.

Barnard, Neal, M.D., *Eat Right, Live Longer* (Harmony Books, 1995).
How foods affect our bodies, well documented by studies in medical journals. Vegetarian recipes.

Clegg, Holly, and Gerald Miletello, M.D., *Eating Well Through Cancer: Easy Recipes & Recommendations During and After Treatment* (Wimmer Cookbooks, 2001).
Recipes for day of chemotherapy, loss of appetite, etc. Free to cancer survivors from *www.livingwithit.org*.

Davis, Gail, *So Now What Do I Eat? The Complete Guide to Vegetarian Convenience Foods* (Blue Coyote Press, 1998).
Directory of vegetarian convenience foods. Not a cookbook.

Feldt, Linda Diane, *Spinach and Beyond: Loving Life and Dark Green Leafy Vegetables* (Moon Field Press, 2003).
One hundred recipes for greens of all types.

Keane, Maureen, MS, and Daniella Chace, MS, *What to Eat if You Have Cancer* (McGraw-Hill/Contemporary Books, 1996).
More than 100 easy-to-prepare recipes that meet the unique dietary needs of cancer patients.

Madison, Deborah, *Vegetarian Cooking for Everyone* (Broadway, 1997).
Basic vegetarian cooking techniques and 1,400 recipes.

Magee, Elaine, MPH, RD, *Tell Me What to Eat to Help Prevent Breast Cancer* (Career Press, 2000).
Dozens of recipes, plus supermarket and restaurant advice.

Nixon, Daniel W., M.D., *The Cancer Recovery Eating Plan: The Right Foods to Help Fuel Your Recovery* (Alison Brown Crerier Book Development, Inc./ Times Books/Random House, 1996).
Role of nutrition in cancer recovery and great low-fat recipes, including many desserts.

Pennington, Jean, et al., *Bowe's and Church's Food Values of Portion's Commonly Used* (Lippincott, Williams, and Wilkins, 2004).
More than 8,000 foods analyzed by brand name.

Pensiero, Laura, RD, and Susan Oliveria, ScD, MPH, with Michael Osborne, M.D., *Strang Cancer Prevention Center Cookbook* (McGraw-Hill, 2004).
Cutting-edge nutritional and scientific data on cancer; 100 recipes.

Polunin, Miriam, *Healing Foods: A Practical Guide to Key Foods for Good Health* (DK Publishing Inc., 1999).
Foods that have health-enhancing powers and healthy recipes.

Quillin, Patrick, Ph.D., *Beating Cancer with Nutrition* (Bookworld Services, 2001).
Recipes and menu plans for cancer patients.

Schlosser, Eric, *Fast Food Nation: The Dark Side of the All-American Meal* (HarperCollins, 2002).
An exposé of the fast food industry.

Weihofen, Donna, *The Cancer Survival Cookbook* (John Wiley & Sons, 1998).
Two hundred quick and easy recipes.

Wilson, Randy, and Mark Piper, *The I-Can't-Chew Cookbook: Delicious Soft Diet Recipes for People with Chewing, Swallowing, and Dry Mouth Disorders* (Hunter House, 2003).
Appealing recipes for patients unable to chew.

## Emotional Aspects

Callanan, Maggie, and Patricia Kelley, *Final Gifts, Understanding the Special Awareness, Needs, and Communications of the Dying* (Bantam, 1997).
Explains "nearing death awareness" and helps patients and family understand the difficult process of dying.

Delinsky, Barbara, *Uplift: Secrets from the Sisterhood of Breast Cancer Survivors* (Washington Square Press, 2003).
Practical and inspirational advice from survivors.

Fintel, William A., M.D., and Gerald R. McDermott, Ph.D., *Dear God, It's Cancer: A Medical and Spiritual Guide for Patients and Their Families* (Word Publishing, 1997).
Weaves medical information with spiritual questions that arise during crises such as cancer.

Kaye, Ronnie, *Spinning Straw into Gold: Your Emotional Recovery from Breast Cancer* (Lamppost Press, 1991).
Sensitive treatment of breast cancer emotions.

Siegal, Bernie, *Love, Medicine & Miracles* (HarperPerennial, 1998).
The primer on patient empowerment.

## Exercise

Halverstadt, Amy, and Andrea Leonard, *Essential Exercises for Breast Cancer Survivors: How to Live Stronger and Feel Better* (Harvard Common Press, 2000).
Role of exercise in breast cancer treatment.

McTiernan, Anne, M.D., Ph.D., Julie Gralow, M.D., and Lisa Talbott, MPH,
*Breast Fitness: An Optimal Exercise and Health Plan for Reducing Your Risk of
Breast Cancer* (St. Martin's Press, 2000).
Scientific evidence for role of exercise in breast cancer.

Stumm, Diana, PT, *Recovering from Breast Surgery...Exercises to Strengthen Your
Body and Relieve Pain* (Hunter House, 1995).
How to enhance recovery from breast cancer surgeries and complications.

## General Breast Cancer

*Art.Rage.Us.: The Art and Outrage of Breast Cancer,*
*www.breastcancerfund.org.*
Powerful juried collection of art, photos, essays, and more by women with
breast cancer.

DeAngelo, Debbie, RNC, BSN, *Sudden Menopause: Restoring Health &
Emotional Well-Being* (Hunter House, 2000).
How being catapulted into menopause produces different and more intense
symptoms than natural menopause and how to cope.

Link, John, M.D., *The Breast Cancer Survival Manual: A Step-by-Step Guide for the
Woman with Newly Diagnosed Breast Cancer* (Henry Holt and Company, 2000).
Clear medical information on treatment, etc.

Love, Susan, M.D., *Dr. Susan Love's Breast Book* (Perseus Publishing, 2000).
The bible of breast care. Updated information on breast cancer.

———. *Dr. Susan Love's Menopause and Hormone Book: Making Informed Choices*
(Three Rivers Press, 2003).
Explores options for handling menopause, including HRT and alternative
methods.

Mayer, Musa, *Advanced Breast Cancer: A Guide to Living with Metastatic
Disease* (Patient-Centered Guides, 2003).
Information is presented in a sensitive and factual manner.

Schnipper, Hester Hill, LICSW, and Joan Feinberg Berns, Ph.D., *Woman to
Woman: A Handbook for Women Newly Diagnosed with Breast Cancer* (Avon
Books, 1999).
Two breast cancer survivors, one an oncology social worker, give "friendly
advice" on treatment, side effects, etc.

*Surviving the Legal Challenges: A Resource Guide for Women with Breast Cancer,*
available in English, Samoan, and Spanish. Download text at *www.cwlc.org* or
call 213–637–9900.

Zuckweiler, Rebecca, MS, RN, *Living in the Postmastectomy Body: Learning to
Live in and Love Your Body Again* (Andrews McMeel Publishing, 1998).
Issues related to selecting prostheses, sexuality and intimacy, and
professional counseling.

## General Healing

American Institute for Cancer Research's Program for Cancer Prevention,
   *Stopping Cancer Before It Starts* (Golden Books, 1999).
      Separates new research from old myths about cancer; menus and recipes.

Lerner, Michael, *Choices in Healing: Integrating the Best of Conventional and
   Complementary Approaches to Cancer* (MIT Press, 1994).
      Overview of conventional and alternative medicine cancer treatments.

Louden, Jennifer, *Woman's Comfort Book, A Self-Nurturing Guide for Restoring
   Balance in Your Life* (HarperSanFrancisco, 1992).
      Timeless ideas for pampering yourself.

## Survivor Stories

Bischke, Scott, *Crossing Divides: A Couple's Story of Cancer, Hope, and Hiking
   Montana's Continental Divide* (American Cancer Society, 2002).
      After Scott's wife is treated for breast cancer, they embark on a three-
      month hike along the Continental Divide, a metaphor for the cancer
      experience.

Plant, Jane A., Ph.D., *The No-Dairy Breast Cancer Prevention Program: How
   One Scientist's Discovery Helped Her Defeat Her Cancer* (Thomas Dunne
   Books, 2001).
      Scientist provides controversial evidence of possible links between dairy
      products and breast cancer.

# Periodicals

*A Friend Indeed*
   *www.afriendindeed.ca*
      Newsletter on menopause with emphasis on alternative therapies.

*Alternative Therapies in Health and Medicine*
   *www.alternative-therapies.com*
      Physician-reviewed journal of CAM clinical studies.

*American Journal of Clinical Nutrition*, American Society for Clinical Nutrition
   *www.faseb.org/ascn*
      Online; latest diet and nutrition research.

*Breast Cancer Week*
   *www.breastcancerweek.org*
      Online; latest news on prevention, diagnosis, and treatment of breast
      cancer.

*lynx.com*
   'r cancer patients and professionals.

*CancerWise Consumer*
  *www.cancerwise.org*
    Monthly, online cancer news from M. D. Anderson Cancer Center.

*Coping*
  *www.copingmagazine.com*, 615–791–3859
    Magazine for cancer survivors, caregivers, and healthcare workers.

*Cure*
  *www.curetoday.com*, 800–210–CURE
    Free quarterly magazine on general cancer treatment, news, education, etc.

*Food and Fitness Advisor: Helping Women Live Healthier, More Active Lives*,
  Weil Medical College of Cornell University
  *www.foodandfitnessadvisor.com*, 800–829–2505
    Practical tips on supplements, exercise, nutrition.

*Harvard Women's Health Watch*
  *www.health.harvard.edu*
    Breast cancer, nutrition, hormone therapy, vitamins, etc.

*Heal*
  *www.curetoday.com*, 800–210–CURE
    Free quarterly magazine for cancer survivors.

*HerbalGram*, American Botanical Council
  *www.herbalgram.com*, 512–926–4900
    Educates on safe and effective use of medicinal plants.

Laux, Marcus, M.D., *Naturally Well Today: Healing with Nature's Medicine*
  *www.drmarcuslaux.com/c/contact_us.asp*
    A naturopathic physician reports on clinical studies, new natural
    remedies, etc.

*MAMM*
  *www.mamm.com*, 212–243–2916
    Magazine for women with breast and reproductive cancers.

*Medical Herbalism: A Journal for the Clinical Practitioner*
  *www.medherb.com*
    General information on herbs.

*Our Call*, by Lluminari
  *www.lluminari.com/products_newsletter.asp*
    A group of breast cancer researchers/doctors evaluates research studies
    in the media in free monthly online newsletter.

Sinatra, Stephen, *Sinatra Health Report: An Insider's Guide to Smart Medicine
  and Longevity*
  *www.drsinatra.com*
    A medical doctor takes you into the world of alternative and herbal
    medicine and nutritional supplements.

Tufts University Health & Nutrition
  *healthletter.tufts.edu/*
    About half devoted to nutrition.

## Videos/Tapes

American Cancer Society, *A Significant Journey: Breast Cancer Survivors and the Men Who Love Them*
    800–850–9445 (Item #7686)

*Between Us and Beyond Flowers: What to Say and Do When Someone You Know Has Breast Cancer*
  *www.betweenus.org/video_synopsis.html*
    Videos of real women with breast cancer.

Exercise, National Institute of Aging
    800–222–2225
    Low-impact stretching, balance, and strength-building exercises for beginners.

Kabat-Zinn, Jon, *Mindfulness Meditation Practice Tapes*
  *www.mindfulnesstapes.com*

Kidscope, *My Mom Has Breast Cancer*
    Video for parents and young children. Available at libraries, Blockbuster Video, or community organizations or 404–892–1437, *www.kidscope.org*.

*Rachel's Daughters: Searching for the Causes of Breast Cancer*
  *www.wmm.com*
    Looks at environmental possibilities.

Stanford University
  *healthlibrary.stanford.edu/resources/videos.html*
    A few online videos on breast cancer.

## Financial/Insurance Help

  *Check for patient assistance program on the Website of the manufacturer of the drug you need.*

Air travel, free and discounted, to medical treatment
    Cancer Links, *www.cancerlinks.com/air.html*; Corporate Angel Network, *www.corpangelnetwork.org*; National Patient Travel Helpline, *www.patienttravel.org*, 800–296–1217.

Alliance of Claims Assistance Professionals
              *rg*
                in getting insurers to pay for experimental treatments and
                rsement and billing problems.

Benefits Checkup
*www.benefitscheckup.org*
Finds programs for people 55 and older that may pay for some prescription drugs, healthcare, utilities, and other services.

CancerCare
*www.cancercare.org,* 800–813–4673
May be able to assist with financial concerns for disease-related costs such as medication, transportation, homecare, and childcare. Extensive list of resources by state.

Cancer Supportive Care Programs
*www.cancersupportivecare.com/drug_assistance.html*
Lists many drug manufacturers' patient assistance programs.

Medicare
*www.medicare.gov*
Information on public and private programs that offer discounted or free medication.

Medicare Rights Center
*www.medicarerights.org*
Information on state and private-assistance programs, mail-order discount pharmacies, Internet-based discount programs, and prescription discount cards.

Medicine Program
*www.themedicineprogram.com*, 573–996–7300
For $5 per prescription drug request, this group will wade through the paperwork and coordinate free drug distribution to eligible applicants.

National Association of Hospital Hospitality Houses Inc.
*www.nahhh.org*, 800–542–9730
A network of houses providing lodging for people out of town for medical treatment.

Needymeds.com
*www.needymeds.com*
Information about patient assistance programs.

Patient Advocate Foundation
*www.patientadvocate.org*, 800–532–5274
Active liaison between patient and insurer, employer, and/or creditors to resolve insurance, job retention, and/or debt crisis matters relative to diagnosis.

Pharmaceutical Research and Manufacturers of America (PhRMA)
*www.helpingpatients.org*
Search for patient assistance program by drug manufacturer.

Taking Care of Money Matters, American Cancer Society
   *www.cancer.org/docroot/SHR/SHR_2.asp*
      Workshop on money issues that arise around cancer treatment.

# Helping Out
Breast Cancer Site
   *www.thebreastcancersite.com*
      Click on the pink ribbon once a day to generate free mammograms, paid
   by sponsors. Also sells gifts and clothing with pink ribbons.
Breast cancer stamp
      A 45-cent breast cancer research stamp (postage value: 37 cents) is on
   sale through the end of 2005. Through October 2003, its sale had earned
   more than $34.5 million for research. Available through most post offices or
   by calling 800–782–6724.
Living Beyond Breast Cancer
   *www.lbbc.org*
      Sells a scarf, shirts, cards, and a poster.
M&Ms
      Each purchase of an 8-oz. package of pink and white M&Ms earns 50
   cents for the Susan G. Komen Breast Cancer Foundation.
Making Memories Breast Cancer Foundation
   *www.w-h-b.com/helping*, 800–236–1942
      Donate a wedding gown or jewelry to fund wishes for breast cancer
   patients. Damaged gowns are donated to quilting groups that make them
   into quilts to be sold for $2,000 or more for the foundation. Take gowns to
   Women's Health Boutique near you.
Susan G. Komen Breast Cancer Foundation
   *www.efastcom.com/Marketplace/control/giftshopmain*
      Apparel, jewelry, stationery, etc.
Y-Me
   *www.y-me.org*
      Fifteen percent of every purchase from its Holiday Card Store supports
   programs and services. There are cards for Thanksgiving, Christmas,
   Hanukkah, and Kwanzaa.

# Headwear/Postsurgical Clothing
Chemo Savvy
   *www.chemosavvy.com*, 888–599–3560
      Hats, wigs, turbans, wraps, caps, berets.

Headwear Etc.
*www.headwearetc.com*
   Chic hats, headwear, scarves.

Ladies First, Inc.
*www.ladiesfirst.com*
   Breast forms, lingerie.

Lands' End
*www.landsend.com*
   Mastectomy swimsuits.

National Wholesale Co., Inc.
*www.shopnational.com*
   Mastectomy bras, lingerie, nightclothes, loungewear.

Paula Young
*www.paulayoung.com,* 800–343–9695
   Wigs.

Thämert (UK) Ltd.
*www.conturabelle.co.uk/*
   Mastectomy bras with matching panties.

TLC, catalog of the American Cancer Society
*www.tlccatalog.org,* 800–850–9445
   Wigs, hairpieces, breast forms, prostheses, bras, hats, turbans, swimwear, accessories.

TWC (The Wig Company)
*www.twcwigs.com,* 800–444–1788
   Wigs, accessories.

Women's Health Boutique
*www.w-h-b.com*
   Headwear, breast forms, swimsuits, accessories, compression garments, mastectomy garments.

Y-Me Prosthesis and Wig Bank
*www.y-me.org,* 800–221–2141
   They loan wigs and breast prostheses.

# Going Natural

Bardey, Catherine, *Secrets of the Spas* (Black Dog & Leventhal, 1999).
   Easy recipes for soaps, creams, lotions, and salves from natural ingredients.

Chemical-free furniture: Organic Cotton Alternatives, *www.niccottonalts.com,* 888–645–4452. Sofa U Love, *www.sofaulove.com,* 323–464–3397. Shaker Workshops, *www.shakerworkshops.com,* 800–840–9121.

Herb Products Co.
   *www.herbproducts.com*, 800–877–3104
      Herbs, fragrances, oils, botanicals, tinctures, extracts, personal care products, potpourris. Books on herbs, botanicals, aromatherapy, and making soap; some in Spanish.

*SaffronRouge.com*
      Skincare products that meet strict ecological and all-natural standards.

Siegel-Maier, Karyn, *The Naturally Clean Home: 101 Safe and Easy Herbal Formulas for Non-Toxic Cleansers* (Workman Publishing, 1999)
      Laundry detergents, insect repellants, bathroom cleaners, etc.

True Food Shopping List
   *www.truefoodnow.org*
      More than 2,000 foods with genetically engineered ingredients to avoid. A project of Genetic Engineering Action Network (GEAN).

Weleda natural toothpaste and cosmetics
   *usa.weleda.com,* 800–241–1030

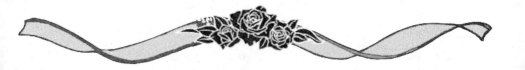

# Index

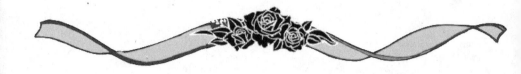

# About the Author

*By training, a journalist.*

*By chance, a breast cancer patient.*

*By grace, a survivor.*

That's the way Judy King summarizes her path that led to this book.

After earning a journalism degree with honors from the University of Texas at Austin, Judy worked as a book editor, public relations professional, newspaper reporter, and freelance writer. *Breast Cancer Answers* is her fifth book. She owns Judy King Editorial Services in Houston, Texas.

When she was diagnosed with breast cancer in 1999, she quickly had to become educated about the disease because her insurance company refused to send her to an oncologist and insisted she have an immediate mastectomy. Always one to get second opinions on major medical decisions, Judy sought the opinion of three breast cancer specialists and learned that, for her particular circumstances, chemotherapy was the place to begin. After chemo she had surgery, radiation, and hormonal therapy. Then two years later metastasis to the bone was discovered.

All through treatment Judy researched issues, attended support group meetings and conferences to hear the concerns and experiences of other survivors, and was an active participant in her treatment decisions. As she visited with other patients, she discovered that the same questions were asked and she realized she could apply her training in writing to share information she had gathered and benefited from. After more research and consultations with experts in many fields, she compiled the book she wishes she had had when she was going through treatment.

Besides sharing her hard-won knowledge about breast cancer and helping other authors polish their work, Judy enjoys spending time with her husband, two children, and seven grandchildren.